Praise for *Making a Baby*

"Finally! A user-friendly, easy-to-understand guide to help you navigate through the basics of infertility!"

—STEPHEN G. SOMKUTI, M.D., PH.D.
Abington Reproductive Medicine
Medical Director, IVF Program
Toll Center for Reproductive Sciences
Abington, Pennsylvania

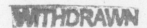

Making a Baby

Everything You Need to Know to Get Pregnant

Debra Fulghum Bruce

and

Samuel Thatcher, M.D., Ph.D.

Ballantine Books ⚞ New York

A Ballantine Book
Published by The Ballantine Publishing Group
Copyright © 2000 by Debra Fulghum Bruce
Introduction copyright © 2000 by Dr. Bernard Cantor

www.randomhouse.com/BB/

LIBRARY OF CONGRESS CATALOG CARD NUMBER: 00-190529

ISBN 0-345-43543-5

Text design by Holly Johnson

Cover photo © Kazu Studio Ltd./FPG International

Manufactured in the United States of America

First Edition: July 2000

10 9 8 7 6 5 4 3 2 1

To my husband, Bob,
whose infinite love and encouragement
provided the motivation and persistence needed
to write this book and all the rest

—*Debra Fulghum Bruce*

Contents

Acknowledgments

In my quest to provide accurate and up-to-date information on infertility and its treatment, I have sought and received generous assistance from a gifted and select group of health care professionals. I express my gratitude to them all.

Samuel Seldon Thatcher, M.D., Ph.D.: reproductive endocrinologist, Center for Applied Reproductive Science, Johnson City, Tennessee (medical editor).

Bernard Cantor, M.D., FACOG: obstetrician and gynecologist and reproductive endocrinologist; chairman, Department of Obstetrics and Gynecology, Mount Sinai Medical Center, Miami, Florida (introduction).

David Bruce Sable, M.D.: obstetrician and gynecologist and reproductive endocrinologist, Saint Barnabas Medical Center, New Jersey (assisted reproduction and in vitro fertilization).

Randy S. Morris, M.D.: obstetrician and gynecologist and reproductive endocrinologist, The Center for Human Reproduction, Chicago, Illinois (assisted reproduction therapies and complications).

W. F. Howard, M.D.: obstetrician and gynecologist and reproductive endocrinologist, private practice, Carrollton, Texas (fertility testing and endometriosis).

Phillip G. Wise, M.D., FACS: urologist with a fellowship in male reproductive medicine and surgery, La Jolla, California (tests for male infertility).

Marc Goldstein, M.D., FACS: urologic surgeon, professor of urology, Cornell University Medical College; director, Center for Male Reproductive Medicine and Microsurgery, The New York Hospital–Cornell Medical Center, New York, New York (causes of male infertility).

Haval Ravin, Ph.D., HCLD: scientific director, Fertility Center of California, Orange, California (sperm washing techniques).

D. Lawrence Mohyi, M.D. (REI): obstetrician and gynecologist and reproductive endocrinologist, Fertility Center of California, Orange, California (sperm washing techniques).

Carolyn Coulam, M.D.: obstetrician and gynecologist and reproductive endocrinologist, medical director, Sher Institute for Reproductive Medicine, Chicago, Illinois (recurrent pregnancy loss).

Louis Weckstein, M.D.: obstetrician and gynecologist and reproductive endocrinologist, Reproductive Science Center of the San Francisco Bay Area, San Francisco, California (treating women over 40).

Harris McIlwain, M.D.: rheumatologist and geriatric medicine specialist, Tampa Medical Group, Tampa, Florida (osteoporosis).

Stephen G. Somkuti, M.D., Ph.D.: obstetrician and gynecologist and reproductive endocrinologist, medical director, IVF Program, Toll Center for Reproductive Sciences; assistant professor, Ob/Gyn, Jefferson Medical College, Abingdon, Pennsylvania (environmental factors and infertility).

Pamela J. Prager: attorney, Finley, Alt, Smith, Scharnberg, Craig, Hilmes & Gaffney, P.C., Des Moines, Iowa (insurance coverage for infertility).

Jennifer Sippel Springer, R.Ph.: pharmacist, Orlando, Florida (infertility medications).

Mike Berkley, L.Ac: New York State licensed and board certified in acupuncture, diplomate National Commission for the Certification of Acupuncturists, New York Center for Acupuncture and Alternative Medicine, LLP, New York, New York (acupuncture).

RESOLVE, a national nonprofit consumer organization that exists to provide timely, compassionate support and information to individuals experiencing infertility and to increase awareness of infertility issues through advocacy and public education (choosing a reproductive endocrinologist and fertility clinic).

Jeff and Rachel Hoyer for sharing the miraculous story of the birth of Calista Catherine Hoyer.

Melissa Himelein, Ph.D., and Dale Wachowiak, Ph.D., for personal and professional insight on stress and infertility and for sharing the birthing story of Emma Irene and McKenzie Lee Himelein-Wachowiak.

Robert G. Bruce, III, Claire Van Leuven Bruce, Brittnye H. Bruce,

M.S., Ashley Elizabeth Bruce, Laura E. McIlwain, M.D., Kimberly L. McIlwain, Michael F. McIlwain, Ginah McIlwain, Hugh H. Cruse, M.P.H., and Jessica Taub for research and editing skills.

My agent, Denise Marcil, for moral support during the researching and writing phase.

My editors, Elisa Wares and Elizabeth Zack, for innovation, excellent editing skills, and personal enthusiasm for this project.

Foreword

Recently my wife's family visited, and we took a trip to a nearby outlet mall. On this day, people-watching was more interesting to me than shopping. Although I deal with infertility each day, this day I attempted to see the world with a different perspective, through "infertile eyes." Everywhere I looked, it seemed as if the entire world was either pregnant or had children in tow. I thought about my patients, many of whom had enough money to buy anything they wanted at this mall—and how they would exchange all that money for just one healthy pregnancy.

As an infertility specialist, I feel that I have the most fulfilling career in the world. I usually deal with healthy, intelligent individuals who are totally committed to their medical care. These men and woman want and deserve to know the reasoning behind their fertility problem, along with the options for their therapy. Their commitment to knowledge and understanding is consistent with the field of reproductive endocrinology, which is also on the cutting edge of human understanding, where medical practice differs little from medical research. Highly sophisticated techniques are used for gathering the best of both surgical and medical subspecialties. Still, it's sobering to think of the self-doubt and emotional hardship that passes through an infertility clinic each day.

My own career in reproductive medicine started several years before the 1978 birth of Louise Brown, the first test-tube baby. How well I can remember the public outcry against this "unnatural" process. I also remember a discussion in which it was agreed that assisted reproduction was an interesting experiment that would have little clinical utility. I hypothesized that the success rate would not reach much over 5 percent and that few could ever afford the technology. There was also the added fear of creating birth defects. I was so wrong in my predictions that I now refuse to reject any new technology without sufficient grounds!

Just recently Natalie Brown, the sister of Louise Brown and the fortieth in vitro fertilization (IVF) pregnancy in the world, successfully delivered her own healthy baby. Today, there are several hundred thousand IVF babies worldwide, and almost everyone knows of a woman who has utilized IVF technology. Success rates continue to climb, although the basic procedure is very much unaltered. In fact, the chance of starting an IVF cycle and carrying home a baby from that attempt is now at least 25 percent in most centers.

Not only has IVF become a mainstream procedure, male infertility is almost a disease of the past. Perhaps the largest advance in therapy since IVF began has been the development of the technique called intracytoplasmic sperm injection (ICSI), in which a single sperm is directly injected into the egg and pregnancy occurs. In the past, the only option for male infertility had been adoption or donor insemination using donor sperm.

On the female side, our biggest barrier today is advanced age. Women have postponed childbearing to realize other life objectives, while others are at the end of a trip through infertility therapy. Because of the effect of aging on fertility, egg donation has started to rival sperm donation as a means of third-party reproduction.

Despite all the breakthroughs in the field of reproductive endocrinology, there is so much more to come. We still have areas for significant improvement, including reducing the chances of multiple pregnancy and increasing the accessibility of the therapy to all. Yet whether you are considering baby-boosting medications, IVF, sperm injection, egg donation, or any other high-tech procedure, the ride through infertility covers unknown terrain and is a bit frightening. Moments of anticipation and hope are quickly changed to despair and isolation when a period starts, and, once again, there is the realization that a pregnancy did not occur. Nonetheless, for most couples, the story will have a happy ending. While all will not be successful in the establishment of a pregnancy, with breakthrough technologies and greater understanding of the human body, most couples will meet their goal of a healthy baby.

How do you survive infertility? Strength comes through understanding and knowledge. You must realize the size of your universe, have a great awareness of normal processes of fertility for both men and women, and know the abnormal processes that lead to infertility. And let's not forget to mention that you must have hope and confidence that you can be successful.

The days of a physician's assuming unilateral responsibility for diagnosis, with a patient's input and understanding extremely limited, are over. Both men and women must be aware of the basic physiologic processes and their options for treatment. It is through this understanding that comfort and perseverance arise. Your goal? To move from infertility to a successful pregnancy as quickly, safely, and efficiently as possible.

The goals of this book are to offer suggestions on how to fight infertility without resorting to advanced therapies, and to allow you to become an informed consumer in the complex medical market. For some, this may mean going back to the basics of lifestyle alteration. For others, it may provide a better understanding of ovulation and intercourse, while still others may need to progress directly to the most advanced assisted reproductive technologies. Seek answers, and let your doctor help guide you.

I was pleased and honored when Debra Fulghum Bruce asked me to participate in her project of creating a consumer-friendly book on infertility. Debra is a respected published author with many books to her credit. She is also a skilled medical journalist with an uncanny ability to make complicated medical procedures and terminology readily understandable and accessible. With *Making a Baby*, she has emphasized the value of creating an environment that is conducive to maximizing fertility potential. Knowing the risks and benefits of various tests, techniques, and therapies will allow you to make the safest decision possible.

No matter what your age or situation is, it is now my sincere hope that this book will aid in your ultimate objective of "making a baby."

—*Sam Thatcher, M.D., Ph.D.*
Johnson City, Tennessee

Introduction

It is estimated that there are 5 to 8 million couples in the United States who are having difficulties conceiving. The sexual revolution of the 1960s and 1970s resulted in an epidemic of sexually transmitted diseases and the resulting damage to fallopian tube function. Then during the 1980s and 1990s more couples delayed childbearing, thus making the biological clock play a key role in blocking conception. My current infertility patients are on average ten years older than those I treated when I first began my practice in the seventies! These and other factors have created challenges to the modern reproductive endocrinologist, which we continually strive to overcome.

As a reproductive endocrinologist dealing with infertile couples for the past thirty years, I have been privileged to participate in the growth of our specialty. I have observed an astounding array of technological breakthroughs that make reality of what was considered science fiction less than a generation ago. For example, the development in the sixties of a technique to measure minute quantities of hormones circulating in the bloodstream led to major breakthroughs in our understanding of how ovulation is controlled. Now we routinely use this information to control and manipulate ovulation. Experiments to understand the physiology of the fallopian tube and its unique environment and function resulted in the development of microsurgical techniques to correct dysfunction and damage. Ultimately, this information led to the development of tissue culture media that can sustain the fertilization and growth of an embryo in the laboratory for up to five days, providing an artificial tubal environment.

Imaging Gives New Insight into Infertility

I have seen the development of ultrasound imaging from its beginnings to techniques so sophisticated that we can see blood vessels around a maturing egg in the ovary and accurately measure structures as small as a tenth of a millimeter. This imaging has opened a world of knowledge about normal and abnormal functioning in the ovary, fallopian tube, and uterus.

From the discovery of the double helix of DNA in 1953, we have now come to understand how cells function. With that information we can use sophisticated diagnostic testing to determine genetic abnormalities from a single cell of an embryo growing in the laboratory. The technology that allows us to sample a single cell has also brought us the ability to fertilize eggs in the laboratory with a single sperm of a man who ten short years ago would have been considered sterile.

The amazing growth of technology in this generation has brought joy to many infertile couples. Frequent advances in the knowledge and understanding of infertility continually expand our capabilities to achieve success.

The Causes Have Not Changed

Yet, despite the amazing growth in our knowledge and ability to treat infertility, the underlying causes remain the same. Problems with egg production (ovulation), anatomic problems such as fallopian tube blockage, endometriosis, cervical mucus problems, and male factors such as low sperm counts or poor motility have continued to create problems for couples wanting a child.

Seeking Help

If you believe you are experiencing infertility problems, find someone well qualified, with a subspecialty in reproductive endocrinology, with whom you feel a rapport. Many general gynecologists have little formal training in the nuances of infertility diagnosis and treatment. Once the basic evaluation is completed or simple techniques are unsuccessful after a few attempts, you should seek out a reproductive endocrinologist in your area who can efficiently guide you to more effective approaches. Hope is available for everyone!

Experts Across the Nation Collaborate in *Making a Baby*

Unlike some books on the market today, *Making a Baby* is not filled with old wives' tales on how to get pregnant. Instead, it provides you with solid medical information and the latest scientific studies, along with high-tech, low-tech, natural, and even complementary methods for making a healthy baby.

Along with the pros and cons of current tests and treatments, the available options for reversing infertility are clearly explained in this book, so you, the reader, can make an informed decision in partnership with your physician. My thirty years of experience tells me that you will find hope and joy in these pages.

—*Bernard Cantor, M.D., FACOG*
Chairman, Department of Obstetrics and Gynecology
Mount Sinai Medical Center, Miami, Florida

Part One

The Causes of Infertility

Chapter 1

What You Must Know About Infertility

"This was the first time in my life that I was faced with failure," 31-year-old Megan said about her inability to get pregnant. "Since I was a child, I always set lofty goals and worked hard to meet these. When my doctor said we had 'unexplained infertility,' it was as if my life was in chaos and out of my control."

Lorri had a successful dental practice and finally married her college boyfriend at age 34. "I could not believe that I was a successful pedio-dontist, dedicating my life to helping young children, yet I could not have my own baby. After three years of trying to conceive, we finally turned to in vitro fertilization and now are the parents of twins. But I will never forget the emotional upheavals and feelings of grief and anxiety we went through."

When 36-year-old Rob played college basketball, he suffered a groin injury that resulted in a ruptured testicle. "It doesn't take a rocket scientist to know that this problem slashes the chances of making a baby. After undergoing a battery of tests, my urologist said I have a low sperm count. Yet medical technology is amazing. Our team of doctors used some high-tech methods to retrieve sperm to fertilize my wife's eggs so we could make a healthy baby. The result? Two active boys, now ages two and four. They are my life!"

Remember how, when you were eight, you dreamed of having a family someday? For 32-year-old Jennifer, being a mother was her ultimate childhood wish.

My good friends talked about having children but also about being teachers or doctors. Not me. I just wanted to stay at home and take care of babies, and I wanted a houseful! Mark and I waited until our late twenties to start a family, then tried for over a year to get pregnant with no luck. You probably know how I felt when my doctor said I was infertile due to ovulation problems. I wanted to run, to cover my head, so I didn't have to hear the words. But I couldn't escape this reality.

That was two years ago. Tonight Mark is struggling with a colicky baby who refuses to honor one o'clock in the morning as quiet time. I am rocking her twin sister, who is lying in my arms wide-eyed and grinning. I'm reminded of the old saw "Be careful what you wish for, you just might get it." Of course, we did more than just wish for a baby, we engineered it. At times, it has felt like we were birthing a Martian rover rather than a storybook bundle of joy.

Many people dream of having a family someday, even before they meet Mr. or Ms. Right. In fact, most of us assume that making a baby the old-fashioned way is a natural birthright. After all, we are made to be sexual beings, so anyone can get pregnant, right? Wrong. For an estimated 5 to 8 million infertile couples in the United States, making a baby is difficult, if not seemingly impossible. Whether from your irregular menstrual cycles, from his reduced sperm count, or for unknown reasons, infertility is a fact of life and a vastly growing concern.

"My friends tell me it's all in my head," 37-year-old Allison said. "We've tried to get pregnant for three years now, and all my friends are either expecting or pushing strollers. If it is in my head, I need to know what therapist can help me reverse it—now." Infertility is not in your head. It is not the result of something you did as a child or rebellious acts as a teenager. Nonetheless, a chief barrier to overcoming infertility occurs when well-meaning friends and family members suggest that infertility is "imagined." You have probably heard the following statements:

- Maybe if you weren't so obsessed with getting pregnant, it would just happen.
- Since the medicine the doctor gave you didn't work, maybe it's a mental thing.

- Just relax! You're so uptight, no wonder you can't get pregnant.
- Isn't it about time you had one of your own?
- Your sisters and cousins had no problem conceiving. I just can't imagine why you can't have a child.
- You can always adopt. Then you will surely get pregnant.

Who's in the Driver's Seat Now?

After trying for months to conceive—with no results—you may start to think that perhaps the high anxiety you feel is keeping you from getting pregnant. The first insidious feeling of infertility is the sense of a loss of control. Up until this point in your life, you have been in the driver's seat, controlling most of your major life decisions—whether or not to attend college, whom to marry, when to marry, what to do as your life's work, and where to live. Now, no matter what you do or how hard you try, you cannot conceive a child. This may be the first major decision in your life over which you have no control.

You must know that infertility—no matter which type you encounter (see Table 1.1)—is *not* in your head; it is a very real disease of the reproductive system that impairs one of your body's most basic functions: the conception or making of a baby.

Table 1.1 Types of Infertility

Infertile   When a successful pregnancy has not occurred after more than one year of unprotected sex

Primary infertility   Infertility without a previous pregnancy

Secondary infertility   Infertility with a previous pregnancy

Sterility   No chance of conceiving

You Have Great Company

Studies show that 15 to 20 percent of reproductive-age couples in the United States have difficulty becoming pregnant, and the causes are multifaceted. Some cases are due to easily identified medical problems or diseases, and success depends on conventional medical treatment, including drugs and surgery. Other causes include lifestyle problems such as diet, overuse of alcohol, or the use of recreational drugs. These problems require a natural, drug-free, mind/body approach.

Fertility Treatments Have Come a Long Way

Although twenty years ago the diagnosis of infertility was etched in stone, times have dramatically changed since then. Comprehensive research indicates about 90 percent of all diagnosed infertility cases can be linked to definite reasons, and two out of every three infertile couples who seek medical answers are able to have children. Seeking medical answers is the first step to increasing your odds of getting pregnant. Once you understand the causes of infertility—know which treatments are likely to be effective, and which probably will not work well—you can begin to manage infertility just as you do other areas of your life.

Treatment may be as simple as proper timing of intercourse with ovulation. Other, more aggressive therapies might include ovulation drugs (see Chapter 13) to assisted reproduction, or donation of eggs and/or sperm, as discussed in Chapter 14. Knowing that the statistics of making a baby may be changed in your favor can motivate you to dig in and understand what causes infertility, get to know your own body, make important lifestyle changes you can control, and experiment until you find the best treatment available.

Truth or Myth?

If you or someone you love has been diagnosed as infertile, much of the anxiety and distress may result from a lack of knowledge about this disease. Not only are there fears about upcoming medical tests or invasive procedures, but the uncertainty about your future family can be overwhelming. While a quick fix for infertility may not be possible, by using the large amount of information in this book you can learn how the reproductive system functions, along with low- and high-tech solutions to making a baby.

Before you begin reading the ins and outs of infertility and treatment, check the following beliefs to determine your Baby-Making IQ (Infertility Quotient).

BABY-MAKING IQ (INFERTILITY QUOTIENT)

TRUE FALSE

___ ___ 1. Infertility is a woman's problem.

___ ___ 2. Everyone else gets pregnant when they choose.

___ ___ 3. If I could just relax or quit my job, I know I'd get pregnant.

___ ___ 4. I think infertility is all in my head.

___ ___ 5. If we try long enough, we're bound to get pregnant someday.

___ ___ 6. Maybe we're not meant to be parents.

___ ___ 7. If we adopt a newborn, it's easier to get pregnant.

___ ___ 8. Infertility is a sign that we're not sexually compatible.

___ ___ 9. My doctor tells me that I'm too thin, but I think if I could lose a bit more weight, it might be easier to get pregnant.

___ ___ 10. Because my doctor said I'm infertile, that means I'm sterile.

___ ___ 11. We're in our late thirties, so it's too late to even consider making a baby.

___ ___ 12. If we delay having children while we develop our careers, the chances of having a baby grow dim.

___ ___ 13. I'm not only infertile, but I'm single, and there's no hope for me to have a baby.

___ ___ 14. We cannot afford infertility treatments, and health insurance companies don't touch this.

___ ___ 15. We need to have sexual intercourse at least once a day to overcome infertility.

Ignore the Myths

So how did you answer? If your answers were *true* to any of these statements, you are not alone—but you are wrong! Although these common beliefs have the sound of authority, the answer to each is *false*. They are just myths and are based on *misinformation, old wives' tales,* or *folk wisdom* without any scientific substantiation. Yet despite the scientific research on infertility and its effects on millions of couples, confusion still prevails among most people. The following pages will discredit each of these myths (and many more!), and allow you to explore all the available options—medical and complementary—to solve your infertility problem.

Getting Prepared for Pregnancy—Know the Rules

RULE 1: NO ONE IS TO BLAME FOR YOUR INFERTILITY. Would you blame someone for having diabetes or cancer? Of course not! Infertility happens. Whether for specific medical reasons or for no reason at all, some couples are infertile. Research shows that infertility is a female problem in about 35 percent of the cases; a male problem in 35 percent of the cases; a combined problem in 20 percent of the cases; and unexplained in 10 percent of the cases.

RULE 2: REMEMBER THE MULTIPLICATION PRINCIPLE. For many couples it is a variety of factors distributed between both partners that contribute to infertility. However, before you misinterpret the statistics and how they affect you, it's important to understand the multiplication principle. If you are 60 percent fertile, perhaps due to irregular ovulation, and your partner is 60 percent fertile due to lower sperm motility, it does not mean as a couple that you are 60 percent fertile. Rather, it means you are only 36 percent fertile. With each additional infertility factor, the percentage lessens. If you take away another 10 percent for frequency or timing of intercourse, soon a couple may be infertile without one clear cause.

RULE 3: RECOGNIZE THE DIFFERENT FACTORS THAT CONTRIBUTE TO INFERTILITY. Some of these are listed in Table 1.2, including the overall health of both male and female, lifestyle factors (smoking, drug use, alcohol), age, diet, and obesity, among many.

Making a Baby

In order for you to understand why you may be infertile, you must first look at how this process works. Actually, conception is an extremely complicated process that requires the joining of two special cells—sperm

Table 1.2 Common Causes of Infertility

Women	Men
ENDOCRINE	**ENDOCRINE**
Ovulation problems	Sperm production
ANATOMIC	**ANATOMIC**
Ovarian cysts	Testicular cancer
Prior abortion	Testicular injury
Cervical stenosis	Undescended testicle
Endometriosis	Prior vasectomy/reversal
Fibroids or polyps	Varicocele
Scar tissue or adhesions	Mumps
Blocked fallopian tubes	
Birth defects of the uterus	

Shared

Chronic illness
Hyper- and hypoactive thyroid disease
Stress
Smoking, alcohol, and recreational drugs
Sexually transmitted diseases
Weight and exercise
Sperm allergies
DES exposure in the womb
Sexual dysfunction
Prior surgeries

from the male and an egg (oocyte) from the female. Each sex cell contains half the normal amount of DNA. These sex cells fuse (fertilization) to restore the normal amount of DNA, and this blueprint creates a unique individual.

Keep in mind that human reproduction is an incredibly inefficient and complex process. Even something as benign as an infection or a slight hormone imbalance can throw off this process, resulting in infertility. Women are born with hundreds of thousands of eggs, more than they will ever ovulate, and no new eggs are ever made. Women may ovulate only as many as 400 times between puberty and menopause. Most ovulated eggs do not become pregnancies, even if there is adequate sperm for their fertilization at the time they are released. Conversely, men continually produce millions of sperm throughout their reproductive life, and reduction of sperm count is not seen until a relatively old age. It is not known why it takes millions of sperm in each ejaculation to successfully fertilize a single egg. Some have hypothesized that it would take fewer if sperm would just stop to ask for directions! Still, deficiencies in the production and release of his sperm and ovulation of her eggs are the basis of most cases of human infertility.

While the man can readily release sperm just about anytime, the woman releases only a single mature egg every four weeks or so through a carefully coordinated and timed process called ovulation. Yet for conception to occur, the reproductive systems must function without a hitch. Studies show that even the most fertile couple having intercourse at the exact right moment in the woman's cycle will still fail to conceive *three times out of four*. If there are any internal abnormalities or conditions that are less than perfect, the odds of conception are dramatically reduced. It's not as simple as you once thought, is it?

Examining the Female Reproductive System

To better understand the process of conception, let's examine your reproductive organs and see how they work in union with your menstrual cycle and reproductive hormones to make a healthy baby. (You can keep your clothes on for this exam!)

The Rites of Passage

From the bottom up, the female reproductive tract (see Figure 1.1) starts with the vagina, a tubular, muscular structure sometimes called the birth canal. This passage leads from the outside of your body to the cervix. Sperm are deposited at the top of the vagina and behind the cervix during intercourse. This is called the seminal pool.

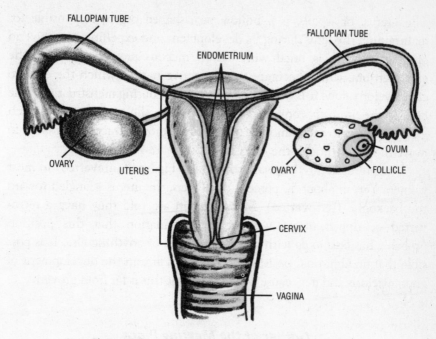

Figure 1.1   The Female Reproductive System

Enter Through the Official Gate

The cervix is the lowest part of the uterus, the organ in which the pregnancy develops. It is the official "gate" into the uterus that controls sperm entry into your reproductive tract. The cervix produces different types of mucus, depending on the time of the month—a thick and impenetrable mucus during most of the cycle and a thin, clear, elastic, nutrient-rich mucus near ovulation.

The sperm swim through the cervical opening (os) into the body of the uterus. The preovulatory mucus produced by the cervix is very receptive to sperm, and the inside folds of the cervix act as a reservoir to allow the slow release of sperm into the uterus over several days. The sperm travel through the uterus and into the fallopian tube. Fertilization, if it occurs, takes place in the outer third of the tube.

Protected in the Nest

The uterus, or womb, is a hollow pear-shaped organ, responsible for maintaining the fetus during its development and expelling it at the end of pregnancy. It is lined with a rich mucous membrane called the endometrium, which becomes the protective nest in which the embryo can develop safely. It is this lining which is lost during menstruation. The bulk of the uterus is composed of muscle cells, the myometrium, which greatly expand to accommodate a pregnancy and contract during labor to move the baby through the birth canal.

The uterus is tilted forward toward the bladder (anteverted) in most women. Yet, in about 30 percent of women, the uterus is angled toward the backbone (retroverted). Many women are told they have a retroverted or tipped uterus without an explanation that this position probably has *little to do* with getting pregnant or anything else. It is possible that an abnormal position of the uterus aids in the development of endometriosis and may cause pelvic pain, but this is far from proven.

Gather at the Meeting Place

The fallopian tubes are attached to the uterus and open near the ovaries. They are about 4 inches long and about as big around as a ballpoint pen refill. At the ovarian end of each tube are small finger-like projections, fimbriae, that help to capture the egg as it is released from the ovary at ovulation. Fertilization takes place in the outer third of the tube. During the next three to four days, the tube serves as temporary lodging for the fertilized egg and, later, for the embryo.

The inner lining of the tube has cells that produce a nutritive fluid that nudges the sperm and egg toward each other and the embryo into the uterus. Infections can damage these cells and increase the risk of a tubal pregnancy. The cellular layer is surrounded by a layer of muscle cells that rhythmically work together to contract and further aid in transport. This contraction increases significantly during intercourse, and it takes only several minutes for the sperm deposited in the vagina to reach the site of fertilization. Although sperm travel quickly, it can be several hours before the capacity to fertilize an egg is gained.

Baby Buster

In a birth-control procedure known as tubal ligation, the fallopian tubes are cut and tied to block the release of eggs.

The fallopian tubes have four crucial functions:

1. To transport sperm to the site of fertilization
2. To pick up the egg at ovulation
3. To provide a proper environment for fertilization to take place
4. To nourish and transport the resulting embryo into the uterus

Waiting in Your Storehouse

Adjacent to the fallopian tubes are your ovaries, one on either side of the uterus. The ovaries, like your partner's testes, serve as the storehouse of sex cells. Normally, once a month at midcycle, a preovulatory follicle ruptures in a process called ovulation. This rupture may be a source of pain known as mittelschmerz. If you've felt this pain, chances are that's a good sign that ovulation has occurred. (Still, many women have pain and do not ovulate.) After ovulation, the ruptured follicle fills in with cells and is called the corpus luteum. If there is no pregnancy, the corpus luteum shrinks and the cycle of follicle growth restarts. If the ovum is not fertilized by sperm before it reaches the uterus, it dissolves and is flushed away during menstruation along with blood and other fluids.

The size of your ovary depends on the stage of menstrual cycle. Early in the cycle it may be about the size of an almond, but it enlarges by two or three times as the follicle grows. (A follicle is a small, transparent, fluid-filled sac that contains the egg.) At the beginning of the cycle, the follicle is microscopic, but it grows to about the size of a half dollar (20 to 25 mm) just before ovulation. The egg is smaller than a pinhead and changes little during the follicle growth.

Harmonious Hormones or Raging Hormones?

Hormones are minute chemical messengers that are carried by the bloodstream to relay information from one part of your body to another. Secreted into the bloodstream, then circulated throughout your body, reproductive hormones rise and fall throughout your monthly menstrual cycle. The two major female sex hormones are estrogen and progesterone, both produced by the ovaries.

Virtually all hormones are released in short bursts (pulses) every 1 to 3 hours. Because of this, your hormone levels in the bloodstream fluctuate. (Of course, you and your partner probably already knew that one!)

Many hormones influence your ability to conceive, including two hormones produced in the pituitary gland. Follicle-stimulating hormone (FSH) and luteinizing hormone (LH), called gonadotropins, stimulate the growth of ovarian follicles. FSH stimulates your ovaries to produce follicles which primarily produce estrogen. Natural cycles usually result in the release of a single egg. Overriding the body's normal levels of FSH results in the release of extra eggs and higher hormone levels. This is a process that is the basis for the gonadotropin medications (Pergonal, Metrodin, Fertinex, and Humagon), as described in Chapter 13. A rise in FSH levels early in the menstrual cycle can suggest a problem with egg quality, making FSH testing an important diagnostic procedure (see Chapter 11).

While FSH stimulates the follicle to enlarge and mature, another gonadotropin, LH, helps in the production of estrogen and is critical for ovulation and formation of the corpus luteum. Ovulation is usually preceded by a sudden rush of LH called the LH surge. The detection of this surge is the basis for home ovulation kits. High LH levels are also common in polycystic ovarian syndrome, or PCOS (discussed in Chapter 4), which is an increasingly common hormonal imbalance that leads to infertility in women.

The third key hormone is the gonadotropin-releasing hormone (GnRH). Sometimes called the conductor of the reproductive hormones, GnRH is released in very precise fashion by the hypothalamus (the part of the brain concerned with regulating your survival functions—temperature control, appetite, growth, metabolism, and salt and water regulation). Pulses of GnRH are sent to the pituitary, a pea-sized gland found directly below the hypothalamus, where it stimulates the release of the gonado-tropins FSH and LH. These two gonadotropins stimulate the production of sex hormones in the gonads (testes for men; ovaries for women).

Your Hormones Influence the Menstrual Cycle

Your menstrual cycle is the part of your reproductive system that you are most aware of and is the result of hormonal influence. Starting shortly after the onset of puberty, it can be as long as five years from the beginning of your period before ovulation occurs regularly. At menopause, or approximately thirty-five years later, about 400 cycles (400 ovulations) are possible before your egg pool is exhausted.

Contrary to popular opinion, your menstrual cycle does not coincide with the lunar cycle, nor does it necessarily repeat itself like clockwork. Your cycle can vary, and only about 10 to 15 percent of cycles are exactly 28 days. So, don't feel like you're the *only* one who's not on the textbook 28-day chart. The problem arises with cycles under 26 days or over 32 days, as they are clearly associated with increased chances of infertility.

The Ovarian Cycle

Virtually all discussion of female endocrinology revolves around the menstrual cycle. One *cycle* is defined as being from Day 1 of bleeding to the next Day 1 of bleeding. If medications are used during this time, this is called *one treatment cycle*. Hormones change on a daily basis (from harmonious to raging!). These hormones are secreted in short bursts, or pulses, which vary from hour to hour and even minute to minute. Hormone release varies between night and day and from one stage of the menstrual cycle to another. Usually when we speak of the menstrual cycle we are talking about the combined ovarian and uterine cycles. However, even though the uterus is important, it is really quite submissive and does exactly what the ovary tells it. It is the ovarian cycle that commands the pelvic operations.

There are four major hormones involved in the ovarian cycle. Follicle-stimulating hormone (FSH) and luteinizing hormone (LH) are called gonadotropins (*gonad* = ovary; *trop* = make grow) and are made and secreted from the pituitary gland. Estradiol (E2) and progesterone (P4) are steroid hormones, which are made and secreted by the ovary. How do they work harmoniously? Follow the arrows.

> → FSH stimulates the growth of follicles.
>> → Growing follicles make E2.
>>> → Rising E2 levels trigger LH release.
>>>> → LH results in ovulation and P4 production.
>>>>> → If no pregnancy occurs, P4 levels drop and there is a period.
>>>>>> → As P4 levels fall, FSH starts to rise, and the cycle begins again.

Glitches in Your Cycle—and What They Mean

The follicle is a structure comprised of the egg and its surrounding supporting cells. Scientists do not know the exact signal that causes the follicle growth, but a small group of follicles, collectively known as a cohort, begins the path toward ovulation two to three cycles before the chosen follicle will ovulate.

In the first stages, follicle growth is slow. Most of the follicle growth occurs after the follicle gains the capacity to respond to FSH, or in the last three weeks before it is ovulated. Under the stimulus of FSH, the follicle cells start to multiply, and the follicle develops into a small cyst, called the *graafian follicle*. All fertility drugs aim to increase FSH, which in turn causes more follicles to develop (see Chapter 13). But here's the catch: If your FSH is too high at the start of your cycle, it may signal a problem with the follicle (egg) number or quality. As follicles are depleted from the ovary, the pituitary tries to compensate by releasing more FSH. One way to think of this is that your ovary is hard of hearing and your pituitary gland starts to shout louder, "Make more! Make more!"

As the follicles grow, they make estradiol (E2), the principal estrogen before menopause. It is estradiol, not testosterone, that separates men from women. Not only is estradiol responsible for your female characteristics, but it probably is the source of most gynecologic problems such as endometriosis, fibroids, and even cancer. All estradiol is produced from testosterone, the principle male hormone (ah, the Adam's rib theory!). If there is a block in the conversion of testosterone to estradiol, your follicle health suffers. Polycystic ovarian syndrome (PCOS) is one example of this disordered conversion process (see Chapter 4).

Scientists just don't know what causes the sudden release of LH (the LH surge). The LH surge is what you will look for with the ovulation predictor kit. Except at the time of the LH surge, your LH levels are low. Again, an exception is sometimes with PCOS, which may be characterized by high "basal" LH levels, resulting in false positive ovulation predictor kits. The LH surge seems to be related to follicle growth and E2 secretion, but scientists are unsure as to how all of this works.

It is known that the LH surge is involved in three critical processes:

1. The resumption of meiosis
2. Ovulation
3. Luteinization

RESUMPTION OF MEIOSIS. Until the LH surge, the egg (oocyte) has been arrested in its development since before you were born. This means that there have been at least fifteen years—maybe up to forty years—that the egg has been sitting there waiting for some signal to start rearranging its chromosomes for that hopeful meeting with your partner's sperm. During this time, changes might occur in the DNA of the oocyte which might make this seemingly exhilarating meeting less than blissful. This form of aging is one major cause of decreased fertility, increased risk of miscarriage, and birth defects seen in the later reproductive years (see Chapter 6).

OVULATION. The LH surge is a critical part of the precisely orchestrated process of ovulation. Given the rupture of the preovulatory follicle and release of an egg, you may think that ovulation is also explosive. Not so. It is a meticulous and orderly process in which the follicle wall dissolves, with the oocyte flowing out for pickup by the tube, which is hopefully nearby. Ovulation is thought to occur about 24 hours after the LH surge peak, or 36 to 48 hours after the surge onset.

LUTEINIZATION. The third function of the LH surge is to perform luteinization. Under the influence of luteinizing hormone the preovulatory follicle, which has produced only estradiol, ovulates and changes into the corpus luteum, which makes both estradiol and progesterone. (Just think of it as the same structure, with a different appearance and a different name.) In the human female, the corpus luteum is bright yellow, which is why it's called "yellow body." As the corpus luteum forms, the follicle cells become a ball about an inch in diameter. When the follicle has been ill prepared to respond to the LH surge, it will turn into a cyst.

Now, an LH surge does not equal ovulation. There may be an inadequate amount of LH or an altered capacity of the follicle to respond to LH such that these events do not happen.

The corpus luteum has a finite life span of 10 to 14 days. The luteal phase or luteal function is considered inadequate if the luteal phase is less than 10 days, or if the progesterone level is low. The most common cause of an inadequate luteal phase is lack of ovulation. There may be a follicle that forms but does not ovulate. While a small amount of progesterone may be produced, it is not enough to support the uterus for the full 12 to 14 days. Maximum progesterone production occurs at about 7 days after ovulation, or 7 days before menstruation. The life of the corpus luteum is more predictable than the process of follicle growth. If implantation, which is usually about 6 to 7 days after ovulation, does not occur, progesterone levels will fall and menstruation occurs.

The ovarian cycle is divided into two major sections:

1. The *follicular phase* lasts from the onset of bleeding until ovulation. Two hormones of the follicular phase are sex steroid estrogen and gonadotropin FSH.
2. The *luteal phase* is from ovulation until bleeding begins. It is characterized by gonadotropin LH and steroid hormone progesterone.

STAGES OF OVARIAN AND UTERINE CYCLES

OVARY	UTERUS	HORMONE
Follicular	Menstrual proliferative	FSH
		Estradiol
Luteal	Secretory	LH
		Progesterone

The Uterine Cycle

The uterine cycle has three phases and mirrors the ovary's endocrine activity.

MENSTRUAL PHASE. The menstrual cycle starts on the first day of bleeding, even spotting. Usually there are 2 to 3 days of relatively heavy bleeding with 2 to 4 days of lighter flow. Sometimes more painful periods (dysmenorrhea) are associated with a greater chance of ovulation. The less pain and the shorter the cycles, the greater the chance of ovulation failure. On the other hand, painful periods may also be a sign of endometriosis (see Chapter 3). The menstrual fluid is a mixture of uterine lining, tissue fluid, and blood, and normally lasts from 3 to 7 days. The blood loss varies in amount from half an ounce to 10 ounces (averaging 4 to 5 ounces). To give you an idea of how much this entails, a sanitary pad or tampon holds about an ounce.

It probably feels like the menstrual phase is the prime time when there is a lot happening in your pelvis, but this is not true. On cycle day 2 to 3, both hormonally and anatomically, your reproductive system has reached the baseline. This is the time when the most accurate hormone testing and ultrasound scan (baseline scan) can be performed. The endometrium is thin, and the ovaries are quiet without the evidence of cysts.

PROLIFERATIVE PHASE. With estrogen production from the follicle, the endometrial cells start to multiply. This is called the proliferative phase, which lasts until progesterone from the ovary, or a synthetic progestin, is given. As the wall of the uterus thickens, bleeding stops. If there is no progesterone, such as with failure of ovulation, there is continued estrogen production and proliferation. This unopposed estrogen is thought to be the source of many female problems such as hyperplasia (overgrowth) of the endometrium, and maybe even cancer. Virtually all cases of uterine cancer before age 35 are associated with polycystic ovarian syndrome.

SECRETORY PHASE. With the production of progesterone from the corpus luteum, the endometrium is converted from the growing proliferative phase to a very lush nutritional environment in preparation for implantation, called the secretory phase. If a pregnancy occurs, a signal is sent (human chorionic gonadotropin, or hCG) to the ovary to continue progesterone production and maintain the favorable lining. If there is no pregnancy, progesterone falls. The endometrial cells start to break down, menstruation occurs, and the cycle begins again.

The Hypothalamic-Pituitary-Ovarian (HPO) Axis

There is still one more system to consider: how the reproductive system relates to your brain and to the outside world. This happens through the hypothalamic-pituitary-ovarian axis. At the base of your brain is the hypothalamus. The hypothalamus is a great switching station for endocrine activity as well as that part of the brain concerned with regulating your survival functions—temperature control, appetite, growth, metabolism, and salt and water regulation. It receives signals from throughout the nervous system, which in turn has received them from the entire world outside. Numerous neurotransmitters produced by the brain (dopamine, adrenaline, and serotonin) all interact at the level of the hypothalamus. Transmissions from every direction are converted into a single signal stimulating the gonadotropin-releasing hormone (GnRH). GnRH release occurs in pulses that vary in amplitude and frequency, depending on the stage of the menstrual cycle.

Hormone Testing

As you begin investigating infertility causes, tests, and treatments, you need to understand the significant hormones that play key roles in keeping your reproductive tract optimally balanced and functioning in top order. Your doctor may test the following:

ANDROGENS. Androgens are produced by the ovary and the adrenal gland (a hormone-producing organ next to the kidney). While all women produce androgens, elevations in androgens can interfere with normal egg development and release. In severe cases, excessive androgen production can cause unwanted facial or body hair (see Chapter 4).

ESTRADIOL (E2). E2 levels are used as a measure of ovarian follicle health and growth. Monitoring of estradiol levels is an important aspect of cycle monitoring, especially if you are using injectable fertility drugs such as gonadotropins. When estradiol levels fail to rise appropriately in response to stimulation, there may be possible egg problems.

CORTISOL. Cortisol is a major and important adrenal hormone. Excess amounts can cause Cushing's disease, with symptoms of weight gain, irregular periods, and hypertension. These symptoms are often shared by women with polycystic ovarian syndrome.

DHEAS (DEHYDROEPIANDROSTERONE SULFATE). DHEAS is a weak androgen that's produced in large quantities almost exclusively by the adrenal gland. In cases of androgen excess (with usual symptoms of irregular menstrual function and excess facial or body hair), a DHEAS level is usually drawn. Using the results, your doctor will decide if the extra hormone is coming only from the adrenal gland and whether you may respond to adrenal suppressive therapy, either by itself or in conjunction with fertility medications.

HUMAN CHORIONIC GONADOTROPIN (hCG). hCG is a gonadotropin, like FSH and LH, but it has a different origin. This gonadotropin is from the cells that will become the placenta (afterbirth) rather than being produced from the pituitary gland. hCG is the hormone that is measured with a pregnancy test. Home pregnancy tests (HPT) usually turn positive at the time of a missed period, and the hCG level at that time may be from 25 to 200 IU/l, depending on the day of ovulation. The hCG level then doubles about every 48 hours. When the level reaches about 1,500 (750 to 2,500), a pregnancy should be able to be identified in your uterus. Dropping hCG levels are a bad sign. One possibility for abnormal hCG is an ectopic pregnancy (see Chapter 8).

17-HYDROXYPROGESTERONE. The combination of an irregular menstrual pattern and excessive facial or body hair growth can indicate a disorder of adrenal androgen release. One such disorder is called congenital adrenal hyperplasia, or CAH. In some cases, your doctor may screen for this rare disorder by testing for the hormone 17-hydroxyprogesterone soon after your period starts. A more sensitive test using synthetic pituitary hormone adrenocorticotropic hormone (ACTH) to simulate production is sometimes used. 17-hydroxyprogesterone is also produced normally from the corpus luteum, and some doctors have used it as a marker of fetal health.

INSULIN. It is becoming more common to test women with polycystic ovarian syndrome (PCOS) for insulin resistance and glucose tolerance.

Basic testing involves fasting glucose and insulin levels. Even more diagnostic is the glucose tolerance test, where fasting insulin and glucose levels are compared to those after a challenge with glucose. The higher the insulin level, the more likely you will respond to the new insulin-lowering agents. Also, the higher the insulin level, the greater the risk of developing Type 2 diabetes later in life.

PROGESTERONE (P4). After ovulation, the cells that surrounded the just-released egg switch much of their hormone production from estradiol to progesterone. Progesterone levels rise markedly in the second half of the cycle and probably contribute greatly to nurturing the very early pregnancy. Continued release of progesterone requires the presence of the pregnancy hormone (hCG). In the absence of hCG, progesterone levels fall, menstrual bleeding begins, and the period comes. With hCG present, further release of progesterone by the ovaries continues to support the lining. Progesterone supplementation is a common and logical treatment both in the treatment of infertility and protection against miscarriage, although its benefits are uncertain.

PROLACTIN (PRL). Prolactin is released by the pituitary gland. High prolactin levels (hyperprolactinemia) can interfere with ovulation, or interfere with the efficiency by which the eggs are matured. Breast secretion (galactorrhea) is a common and important sign of elevated prolactin. Prolactin levels should be measured if your periods are irregular or absent.

Even if you do not have hyperprolactinemia, your lab may indicate signs of this as a result of the blood-drawing procedure itself or if you:

- Have the lab test done at the wrong time in your cycle
- Have taken certain medications or have used recreational drugs
- Have had recent breast stimulation
- Are under stress

To make sure the test results are accurate, prolactin levels should be drawn early in the menstrual cycle, then redrawn if they are elevated. Hyperprolactinemia can be a sign of a prolactin-producing pituitary gland tumor (prolactinoma). These tumors, which are usually benign, are diagnosed by magnetic resonance imaging (MRI) and are easily treated with oral medications. Less often, hyperprolactinemia may be an indication of other structural abnormalities of the brain. Hyperprolactinemia is often found in patients with hypothyroidism. A prolactin level is a common early test in an infertility workup.

SEX HORMONE BINDING GLOBULIN (SHBG). Testosterone and estradiol are transported in the blood. They are mostly bound to the protein SHBG. Androgens decrease the level of SHBG, while estrogens increase the level. Low levels are associated with hyperandrogen states such as polycystic ovarian syndrome. SHBG is a useful but not commonly used marker of PCOS. Elevated insulin, age, weight, diet, and steroid and thyroid hormone levels all affect the concentration of SHBG. Low levels of SHBG are associated with increased androgen levels and serve as an indirect indicator of insulin resistance. Individuals with insulin resistance have a greater lifetime risk of Type 2 diabetes.

TESTOSTERONE (T). While many people associate testosterone with men, it is released into the bloodstream by your ovaries in relatively small quantities. Most testosterone binds to sex hormone binding globulin and remains inactive. High levels of testosterone are common with polycystic ovarian syndrome (PCOS), as explained in Chapter 4.

THYROID-STIMULATING HORMONE (TSH). The thyroid is a crucial hormone-releasing organ that is located on the front of the neck just below the Adam's apple. Under- or overrelease of thyroid hormones (also called thyroxine) can interfere with the menstrual cycle and contribute to infertility. The most accurate measurement of thyroid activity is checking TSH, a hormone from the pituitary that controls the activity of the thyroid. Many women with thyroid problems see their doctor because of irregular bleeding.

Thyroid disease is common and is easily treated with proper medication.

There *Are* Answers

"I can understand how reproduction works, but how is this information going to help me to make a baby?" We know that the main reason you opened this book is not to read about the reproductive system. However, it has long been recognized that when many couples are given the diagnosis of infertility, much of their anxiety and distress results from a lack of knowledge about the illness. Not only are they frightened about the inability to conceive, but they are also uneasy about the future of their family.

No matter what is causing infertility, there are answers. Using the information given in this book, along with an acute awareness of how your body functions and your specific infertility problem, you will be equipped to take control of your illness. And the general rule of thumb is that if you've been trying to conceive without birth control for more than 12 months, it's time to see what is causing the problem. If you are over thirty, have a history of pelvic inflammatory disease, painful menstrual periods, irregular menstrual cycles, or miscarriage, or if your partner has a known low sperm count, you may want to seek help now. Your doctor will run tests described in Chapters 11 and 12 to look at specific causes of infertility, then find the best treatment for your situation.

Relax! The Statistics Are in Your Favor

Studies show that most infertile couples will conceive children with medical treatment. Even more will conceive if they remain open to all the available options. A woman who does not ovulate regularly may become pregnant after treatment with an ovulation-inducing medication. A man may have an infection that when treated allows conception to take place. Couples may conceive with the assistance of donor sperm or donor eggs. New techniques and technologies are enabling doctors to treat a greater variety of conditions associated with infertility.

Understanding infertility and how it manifests itself in men and women to block conception is crucial. Still, what can you do now to get pregnant and stay pregnant? You can keep reading! Learn about the current methods of diagnosis, weigh the advantages of the latest medications and low- or high-tech conception methods, and make the necessary lifestyle changes today to ensure making a healthy baby.

Chapter 2

Checking Out Your Personal History— *Before* You Get Pregnant

"Although Mike and I dreamed of the day we would have our first baby, I wasn't quite sure I was ready for this big step and was still taking birth control pills to prevent any accidents," 29-year-old Ellen said. "It was by mere chance (or good luck!) that I checked in with my ob-gyn to get my pills refilled and to talk more about getting pregnant. During the visit, he asked me about any past illnesses and my immunizations—whether I had received the hepatitis B series and if I'd ever had the German measles. I honestly did not know the answers. Later I called my pediatrician from childhood and learned I still needed to get the hepatitis series and a tetanus shot. According to my charts, I'd never had the German measles, so my ob-gyn immunized me against that, too—while I stayed on the pill for three more months to make sure I didn't get pregnant. I also got a TB test during this visit. I never realized how much preparation is needed to ensure a healthy pregnancy, but I'm glad I found out ahead of time."

Knowledge is power, especially when you need extra help in getting pregnant. There are simple steps you can take today to convert your body into a baby-friendly environment, making it easier to get and stay pregnant.

Some causes of infertility are entirely preventable, such as sexually transmitted diseases, which cause pelvic scarring. Other causes such as endometriosis, fibroids, or hormonal imbalances may not be foreseen or prevented. Nonetheless, in many cases, we can have enough control of our health to make a major difference, and prepregnancy planning can prepare the groundwork for successful conception.

Schedule a Preconception Checkup

"But I haven't had a comprehensive physical in a long time." Then you owe it to yourself to schedule an appointment for a thorough preconception checkup. Give yourself six months before a pregnancy is planned to allow time for any health modifications. This will help ensure that you have a healthy body to sustain your future baby. After all, your body will provide that perfect nurturing environment for more than nine months.

The preconception exam will let your doctor evaluate your overall health, pinpoint potential or even serious problems, and provide necessary treatment before you get pregnant. It is a chance to talk and to learn. Your doctor may find specific medical problems such as uterine malformations, autoimmune diseases, genital infections, or endocrine abnormalities and be able to treat these early on. Working together, you and your doctor can also pinpoint important lifestyle measures that may benefit your making a baby. Your doctor will obtain a detailed medical history, including any information on symptoms, feelings, your activity level and diet, your home and work environment, and your family history, and then do a thorough physical examination.

Depending on your age and health history, tests may include any or all of the following:

- Blood pressure
- Complete blood count (CBC)
- Blood chemistries, including lipid profile and glucose
- Urine testing
- Pelvic exam with Pap smear
- Colon cancer screening (if family history indicates)
- Chest x-ray (if a nonpregnant smoker over age 35)
- Baseline mammogram at age 35 to 39 (or earlier if family history of breast cancer)
- Bone density test to check for osteoporosis (in selected individuals)

- For those over age 35, a baseline electrocardiogram, a rectal exam, and colon cancer screening

Your doctor will also review your personal risk factors for coronary heart disease, cancer, diabetes, and osteoporosis, and discuss removal or control of these risk factors. Hearing, eye, or dental examinations, a skin test for tuberculosis, and other tests may be planned.

During the exam, your doctor will check your breasts for abnormal lumps or changes. If you don't already practice breast self-examination (BSE), this is a good time to learn this important preventive measure. Your doctor will make sure your reproductive organs are of normal size and shape and do a Pap smear—a test for distinguishing normal from abnormal cells of the cervix. If cervical abnormalities or cancer is detected early, it is usually treatable.

Be prepared to address the following questions:

- When did you start menstruating (menarche)? (*Getting your period late could signal a hormone problem.*)
- Are your periods regular? (*An irregular cycle can mean anything from ovulation disorders to a thyroid problem, polycystic ovaries, endometriosis, or even an early menopause for those women over age forty.*)
- Can you describe the frequency, regularity, duration, and amount of flow of your menstrual period? (*An inconsistent flow could signal an ovulation disorder, while a heavy flow could mean a fibroid tumor on your uterus.*)
- What are the dates of your last two menstrual periods? (*Irregular menstrual periods could signal a problem with ovulation.*)
- Do you have bleeding or spotting between periods? (*Unexplained bleeding could signal hormone problems, fibroids, polyps, or problems with your uterus or cervix.*)
- Do you have pain during periods, during intercourse, or under other circumstances? (*Pain during intercourse could signal pelvic inflammatory disease or endometriosis.*)
- Have you had any gynecologic infections, injuries, or pregnancies?
- Have you been diagnosed with any reproductive disorder?
- Have you had surgery for any problem of the reproductive system?
- Have you ever had an abnormal Pap smear?

- Have you ever had breast problems—pain, redness, discharge from the nipples, growths, or specific areas of tenderness?
- Do you have PMS? What are your symptoms?
- Have you ever been diagnosed with a fibroid tumor? Was this surgically removed?
- Have you had pain and mucus changes at midcycle?
- What type of birth control have you used?
- Is there a family history of infertility, hormonal problems, long spacing between children, or female cancer?

Openly Discuss Your History and Concerns

"But I hate talking about gynecological concerns with a stranger, even if it is my doctor." Talking about personal issues so embarrassed Kerri that she waited until every test was done to quietly mention that she hadn't had a period for almost a year. Elizabeth was no different. She reluctantly told her doctor about her heavy, lengthy periods only after her lab work came back showing she was anemic.

During the consultation and examination, be frank and accurately describe your concerns. Honest communication will save you time, money, and your reproductive health, as any diagnosis will be easier to make. To help with this evaluation, take a copy of your previous medical records with you to your initial appointment. Be sure to keep a copy for yourself. You may also list questions on a piece of paper and bring this with you to the appointment. Be open with any unusual symptoms and feelings so your doctor can best interpret the overall results of the discussion, including the physical examination and laboratory testing. You have the right to know the findings of your evaluation.

Blood Tests Can Assess Your Health

During the office visit your doctor may get a sample of your blood for a complete blood count (CBC) and chemical profile. The CBC measures the amount of red and white blood cells and shows how your vital organs such as the kidney and liver are functioning. From the CBC, your doctor can tell whether you are anemic or have an infection. These results will also help assess your general health and eliminate any disease that you may have. Tests for AIDS and hepatitis B and C are routinely done. A rubella titer should be obtained to check for immunity if status is unknown.

Why Your Sexual History Is Important

Sexual history is an extremely important factor to discuss as you prepare your body for pregnancy. If you have been sexually active with more than one partner, discuss this openly with your doctor and consider testing for STDs (sexually transmitted diseases) such as chlamydia, gonorrhea, syphilis, herpes, and the human papilloma virus. Pelvic inflammatory disease (PID), resulting from chlamydial or gonococcal infection, is a *preventable* cause of infertility. But STDs transmitted during pregnancy or birth result in the deaths or birth defects of 100,000 infants annually.

Each year, more than 12 million people become infected with a sexually transmitted disease (STD), and millions have *no symptoms* at all. For example, chlamydia is the most common sexually transmitted disease in the United States and infects more than 4 million Americans annually. However, up to 70 percent of women and 30 percent of men have no symptoms of chlamydia. The bad news is that past chlamydial infection is a major cause of permanent pelvic scarring.

Herpes is a lifelong sexually transmitted disease affecting roughly one in five Americans over age twelve. Herpes is caused by a virus called *Herpes simplex* and is spread by skin-to-skin contact during genital, oral, or anal sex, not from toilet seats.

The symptoms of genital herpes include many painful sores on the genital area, fever, enlarged lymph nodes in the groin area, burning on urination, headache, and flulike symptoms. A first outbreak can last several weeks. Subsequent outbreaks occur as frequently as several times a year. About 70 percent of the 40 million Americans with genital herpes have no symptoms at all. Herpes does not cause infertility and an infection is no more shameful than a cold sore on your lip. However, an active outbreak during the rupture of membranes or at the time of delivery can be a life-threatening condition for your newborn. It is important that your doctor know of any herpes infections you may have had.

Doctor's Rx

There are two blood tests for HIV that signal the presence of antibodies to the virus. One test is called the enzyme-linked immunosorbent assay (ELISA). If the ELISA result is positive, your doctor may use the Western blot test to be sure the first result was correct. Saliva tests are also available.

Cures are available for gonorrhea, syphilis, chlamydial infection, and chancroid. HIV infection, genital herpes, and human papilloma virus *are not curable*, but helpful treatments are available. See your doctor regularly if you are diagnosed with any of these conditions.

Questions to consider:

- Have you been sexually active with more than one person?
- Have you had blood transfusions in the past? When was this?
- Have you had sex with multiple partners within the past five years?
- Have you tested HIV positive? Has your partner?
- Are you or have you been an intravenous drug user? Is your partner?
- Is your partner a hemophiliac who has not been tested for HIV?
- Have you ever had an STD? How was it treated? Are you being treated?

Chronic Illness Can Affect Fertility

For women like Liz, who has asthma, it's important to have your medical condition controlled before you get pregnant. Liz worked with an allergist to get off oral medications and began using inhaled medications to control her asthma. Her allergist and obstetrician consult periodically now that she is pregnant to make sure she has a safe and healthy delivery.

If you have any type of ongoing or chronic medical condition, such as diabetes, allergies and asthma, high blood pressure, or serious forms of arthritis (rheumatoid arthritis or lupus), be sure to make your doctor aware of the problem, especially if another specialist is treating the condition. Make sure the illness is well controlled before you get pregnant to ensure safety for you and your future baby.

Get All Medications and
Herbal Supplements
Approved

Studies show that 40 percent of women take prescription or over-the-counter drugs during the first few weeks of pregnancy—before they realize they are pregnant. Yet some medications may greatly increase your chance of infertility (see Table 2.1). For example, in scientific studies, antidepressants have resulted in abnormally high prolactin levels. Some women have a loss of libido (interest in sex), and intercourse may become painful because of vaginal dryness.

Who would have thought that something as seemingly benign as Motrin could keep you from making a baby? While medications are necessary to relieve symptoms or clear up an infection, they may hinder conception. It makes sense that all substances ingested by the body can affect your biochemistry. These responses may contribute to infertility.

Researchers have found cases where the use of nonsteroidal anti-inflammatory drugs (NSAIDs, pronounced en-*sayd*), including Advil, Aleve, and aspirin, may cause problems with ovulation. In studies, scientists found that these medications can cause a failure of the follicles to burst and release eggs—called luteinizing unruptured follicle syndrome (LUF or LUFS). Studies reported in *The British Journal of Rheumatology* (January and May 1996) reported cases of three young women with ankylosing spondylitis, rheumatoid arthritis, and seronegative inflammatory polyarthritis. These women took NSAIDs for arthritic conditions and suffered infertility. On the other hand, there are some reports that small doses of aspirin improve fertility.

Other newer drugs such as Acutane, used to treat severe cases of acne, and Propecia, for male baldness, should never be used until you have completed your family. Both medications, while beneficial for the specific condition, may be associated with miscarriage or an increased risk of birth defects.

Place all medications, vitamins, and supplements in a brown paper bag, and cart these to your preconception checkup. Because some medications can add to the chance of infertility, your doctor will help you make adjustments ahead of time and then alert you to the medications that can and cannot be taken after conception.

Questions to consider:

- Do you have any previous or present health problems?
- Were these problems cured?
- Was surgery required?
- What medications did you take?
- What medications are you taking now?

Table 2.1 Commonly Used Prescription Medications That May Zap Fertility

GENERIC NAME	BRAND NAME
Spironolactone	Aldactone
Thioridazine	Mellaril
Cyclophosphamide	Cytoxan
Naproxen	Anaprox, Naprosyn
Indomethacin	Indocin
Metoclopramide	Reglan
Amitriptyline	Elavil
Desipramine	Norpramin
Nortriptyline	Pamelor

Update Your Immunizations

During the preconception evaluation, ask your doctor about any necessary immunizations. Most women in the United States should be immune to measles, rubella, tetanus, mumps, diphtheria, and polio. If you have not been infected with or vaccinated against these diseases, your doctor may recommend immunization at least three months before you become pregnant. (Make sure you are not pregnant before receiving the vaccine.) There are also other diseases—hepatitis B, pneumonococcal pneumonia, influenza, and chicken pox (varicella)—which vaccines can prevent. Not only will the vaccination protect you from potentially serious illnesses, it will protect your future child as well. Also, ask about the Mantoux test for tuberculosis. This painless skin test is an excellent primary screening method to determine if you have been exposed to tuberculosis.

Make sure you are current on your tetanus booster. Adults need a tetanus booster every ten years.

Because the possible effects of some vaccines on fetal development may not be known, trust your doctor to advise you about the amount of time necessary to wait before trying to conceive.

Family History Gives Clues

Both you and your husband should tell the doctor about your family health history. Some medical problems such as birth defects, mental retardation, cystic fibrosis, Tay-Sachs disease, sickle cell anemia, muscular dystrophy, and Huntington's disease may be genetic or inherited in nature. Your doctor may advise you to undergo genetic counseling and discuss any possible risks for your future child.

Finding Your Ideal Weight for Conception

Your weight—whether you are significantly overweight or underweight— is an important factor that influences fertility and can affect ovulation. If you are underweight, you may not have an adequate fat-to-body-mass ratio. Some athletes, especially women who vigorously exercise, may have a change in menstrual periods or may stop menstruating altogether (amenorrhea). This is especially common in long-distance runners (more than four to five miles daily), gymnasts, and other athletes who exercise vigorously for long periods. Being underweight, especially with a low amount of body fat (less than 10 percent), may alter the ovarian function necessary to get pregnant. Treatment would be to stop losing weight, to gain weight, if necessary, or to take medications to correct the hormonal imbalance.

Conversely, women who are significantly overweight may have disruptions in their menstrual cycles due to an excess of androgens. There is also a correlation between being overweight and the production of insulin, which can occupy the hormone receptor sites necessary for ovulation. Treatment would begin with a sensible weight loss program that includes regular exercise. Sometimes medication is prescribed to help lower androgen levels.

What Is Normal for You?

Just how much should you weigh? Your weight can depend on many variables, including your height, age, bone structure, and weight-cycling history. The best weight for you is the one that is closest to the recommended normal level and at which you can conceive a baby. Traditionally, height/weight charts gave an accurate portrayal of overweight. Yet now experts believe that your body mass index (BMI) may give a more accurate picture of health. BMI is defined as body weight (in kilograms) divided by height (in square meters). The BMI number or value correlates to your risk of adverse effects on health, with higher numbers showing an increased risk. According to the American Dietetic Association, people with a higher percentage of body fat tend to have a higher BMI than those who have a greater percentage of muscle. It is this extra body fat, not muscle, that may be altering your hormones, leading to infertility. Both the National Heart, Lung, and Blood Institute and the World Health Organization have defined *overweight* as a BMI of 25.0 to 29.9, while *obesity* is a BMI of 30 or greater.

Using the body mass index (see Table 2.3), locate the weight closest to your weight in the left-hand column. Then locate the height closest to your height along the top. For your convenience, these are figured in pounds and inches. Where these two numbers meet on the chart is your BMI. For example, if you weigh 180 pounds and are 5 feet 4 inches tall, your BMI is 31. A BMI of 31 or greater puts you at greater risk for health problems related to body weight (see Table 2.2).

Table 2.2   BMI Index

BMI	RISK FOR CHRONIC HEALTH PROBLEMS RELATED TO BODY WEIGHT
20–25	Very low risk
26–30	Low risk
31–35	Moderate risk
36–40	High risk
40+	Very high risk

Table 2.3 Body Mass Index (BMI)

HEIGHT (INCHES)	19	20	21	22	23	24	25	26	27	28	29	30	31	32	33	34	35
58	91	96	100	105	110	115	119	124	129	134	138	143	148	153	158	162	167
59	94	99	104	109	114	119	124	128	133	138	143	148	153	158	163	168	173
60	97	102	107	112	118	123	128	133	138	143	148	153	158	163	168	174	179
61	100	106	111	116	122	127	132	137	143	148	153	158	164	169	174	180	185
62	104	109	115	120	126	131	136	142	147	153	158	164	169	175	180	186	191
63	107	113	118	124	130	135	141	146	152	158	163	169	175	180	186	191	197
64	110	116	122	128	134	140	145	151	157	163	169	174	180	186	192	197	204
65	114	120	126	132	138	144	150	156	162	168	174	180	186	192	198	204	210
66	118	124	130	136	142	148	155	161	167	173	179	186	192	198	204	210	216
67	121	127	134	140	146	153	159	166	172	178	185	191	198	204	211	217	223
68	125	131	138	144	151	158	164	171	177	184	190	197	203	209	216	223	230
69	128	135	142	149	155	162	169	176	182	190	196	203	209	216	223	230	236
70	132	139	146	153	160	167	174	181	188	195	202	209	216	222	229	236	243
71	136	143	150	157	165	172	179	186	193	200	208	215	222	229	236	243	250
72	140	147	154	162	169	177	184	191	199	206	213	221	228	235	242	250	258
73	144	151	159	166	174	182	189	197	204	212	219	227	235	242	250	257	265
74	148	155	163	171	179	186	194	202	210	218	225	233	241	249	256	264	272
75	152	160	168	176	184	192	200	208	216	224	232	240	248	256	264	272	279
76	156	164	172	180	189	197	205	213	221	230	238	246	254	263	271	279	287

BODY WEIGHT (POUNDS)

Talk About Your Nutritional History

Whatever your dieting history, nutritious healing food is vital fuel for both you and your future child. When you eat a nutritional, well-balanced diet, many other factors fall in place. For example, foods that are nutrient-dense help fight infections and may help to prevent illness. Ironically, in some cases of infertility, it is the extremely low-fat diet that may hinder making a baby.

Understanding Eating Disorders

Eating disorders and exercise obsession are increasingly common problems that result in dramatic changes in weight. For many women, these changes may decrease their chance of getting pregnant. Bulimia nervosa is an increasingly common problem among teens and young adults and affects as many as 5 *percent* of American women. This emotional disorder usually starts in late adolescence and early adulthood and manifests itself in cycles of binging or rapid consumption of foods followed by purging (vomiting, laxative use, diuretics, or hours of aerobic exercise). Warning signs include extreme preoccupation with weight, strict dieting followed by high-calorie eating binges, overeating when distressed, feeling out of control, disappearing after a meal, depressive moods, alcohol or drug abuse, frequent use of laxatives or diuretics, excessive exercising, and irregularities in menstrual cycle.

Anorexia Can Be Fatal

Bulimia is not the only serious eating disorder that may hinder conception. Remember how anorexia (self-starvation) took the life of gifted singer Karen Carpenter? While eating disorders are escalating, especially among young adult women, studies underscore the importance of getting a nutritional and eating disorder history from women who are diagnosed as infertile. In a study of sixty-six infertile women, eating disorders were reported in 16.7 percent. Anorexia nervosa or bulimia nervosa was found in 7.6 percent. For those women who had amenorrhea or oligomenorrhea, the association with eating disorders was significantly higher (58 percent) in this study population.

Females with anorexia nervosa have low serum levels of LH and E2, blunted responses to GnRH, high levels of cortisol, and a failure to ovulate in response to clomiphene citrate. Thyroid function tests are also frequently abnormal, and basal TSH levels may be low or normal. Similar findings were observed in simple weight-loss amenorrheics—women who had abnormal menstrual cycles from weight loss, yet who were not suffering from anorexia nervosa. Women with anorexia nervosa are also at higher risk for osteoporosis, or porous bones.

Dying to Be Thin?

It makes sense that if your body is starving for nutrition, it's not the best time to conceive a healthy baby. If you have an eating disorder, talk with your doctor. Treatment is effective if started early and usually consists of outpatient behavior therapy, group support, nutrition education, and sometimes antidepressant medication. Because eating disorders appear to run in families in which there is also substance abuse or higher than average incidences of depression, researchers are now focusing on serotonin and other brain neurochemicals, hoping to find a biological clue to the problem. For fertility, it is probably better to maintain a heavier weight than to yo-yo up and down in weight.

Table 2.4   Signs and Symptoms of Anorexia Nervosa

- A distorted body image
- Skipping meals
- Unusual eating patterns
- Oversensitivity to criticism
- Perfectionistic behavior (excellent grades or performance)
- Absence of menstrual cycle (amenorrhea)
- Withdrawal from friends or unusual immersion in activities
- Inflexibility
- Frequent weighing

Lifestyle Choices Can Hinder Fertility

Of all the risk factors for infertility, making healthy lifestyle choices is something you can control. Study after study (as outlined in Chapter 7) reports that drinking alcohol, smoking cigarettes, or using recreational drugs (marijuana or cocaine) even in moderation can have a detrimental effect on your fertility. Talk with your doctor about any past or present lifestyle habits that may interfere with getting pregnant. Then ask for a plan that can help you detoxify your body while eliminating these unhealthful habits.

Questions to consider:

- Do you drink regularly? How much?
- Do you smoke cigarettes? How many?
- Have you ever taken recreational drugs? What type? How often?
- Do you use recreational drugs now?

Chapter 3

Top Threats to Making a Baby—and How to Manage Them

"The world of infertility treatment is a gamble," Pete, a 43-year-old, said. "All along the way, you are quoted in 'odds,' and most of the time, Erin and I were bucking them. The chances of a successful reversal of my vasectomy were somewhere below fifteen out of a hundred. There is about a 20 percent chance of a successful IVF cycle. The chances of miscarrying at Erin's age (37) were probably greater than 20 percent. There is one in sixty chances of Down's syndrome in twins of parents our age.

"We knew that people don't always win at the craps table. We realized that the same goes for the world of infertility."

You're infertile. The diagnosis is always unexpected and painful. After you get over the shock, then you begin with questions: "Why am I infertile? What can be done to help me get pregnant?" In many cases, certain risk factors are excellent markers to alert you to the underlying problem of infertility. Some common threats are:

- Extremes of thinness or obesity
- Substance abuse such as nicotine, caffeine, alcohol, and recreational drug use
- Advanced maternal age
- Recurrent pregnancy loss
- Male factors

There are other medical conditions that threaten your ability to conceive. Some of these conditions are out of your control, such as having ovarian dysfunction, endometriosis, or a fibroid tumor. However, some of these conditions can also be managed and treated, giving you a greater chance to make a baby. For example, a lingering infection might easily be treated with antibiotic therapy. A surgical procedure to clear up endometriosis can also help you to get pregnant. Early diagnosis and treatment of a pelvic infection will let you avoid the serious scarring that can lead to infertility. Practicing safe sex and having a monogamous sexual relationship can help you to avoid sexually transmitted diseases, a common cause of pelvic inflammatory disease.

Let's look at the top threats to making a baby and how you can regain control.

Ovulatory Defects

Ovulatory disorders are the most common cause of female infertility, and may account for more than 50 percent of cases. The wide array of problems include:

- A complete lack of ovulation (anovulation)
- Infrequent and/or irregular ovulation
- Luteinized unruptured follicle (LUF) syndrome (development of a follicle but a lack of ovulation)
- Luteal phase defects (ovulation but poor hormone production/ endometrial development)
- Delayed ovulation—ovulation after day 16 (increases risk of infertility and miscarriage)
- Spontaneous abortion (follicle development, ovulation, implantation, but pregnancy loss)

If you have no menstrual periods (amenorrhea), or intervals between your menstrual periods of more than 35 days (oligomenorrhea) or less than 25 days, look no further: you have an ovulatory disturbance. Even if you have normal periods, you could still have problems with ovulation. If the menstrual cycles are irregular, there is not much need to go through the motions of ovulation detection such as temperature charts and ovulation prediction kits. See your doctor. It's time for an evaluation and appropriate medical therapy to get ovulation in sync.

Who's at Risk?

Age plays a key role in ovarian disorders, and women over age 35 are prime targets. Other signals for ovarian disorders include:

- Irregular menstrual cycles
- Midcycle spotting or bleeding
- History of skipping periods any time during your life
- Onset of menstrual period after age 16
- Failure to have pain and/or mucus changes at midcycle
- History of increased hair growth, breast secretion, thyroid disease, or diabetes
- Eating or weight disorder
- History of early pregnancy loss
- Aggressive exercises
- Use of cardiac drugs or antidepressants
- Infertility when male and anatomic factors have been excluded

What Causes It?

Ovulation is a very exacting process that is easily altered by a number of factors. Most ovulatory disturbances, however, are the result of hormonal imbalances that affect follicle development. A precise balance of the reproductive system is vital for ovulation. In some women, there is an inherent defect in the quality of eggs. Other women have a significant reduction in the number of follicles or eggs in the ovary. There is no way to halt this decline. Genetic predisposition, prior ovarian surgery, smoking, and endometriosis can accelerate the rate of egg loss or cause a decrease in egg quality. Aging also causes a progressive decline in the number and quality of a woman's eggs.

What You May Feel

You may have no symptoms of ovulatory dysfunction other than infertility. In fact, you might think you are perfectly ovulatory even though something can be seriously wrong. A big clue is change in the characteristics of your cycle, including:

- Shortened or lengthened cycles
- Lighter or heavier bleeding
- Loss of "feeling" of ovulation
- Hot flashes, especially during your menstrual period
- Lack of cervical mucus changes

Making the Diagnosis

- **Chart your basal body temperature (BBT).** The easiest way to find out if you have an ovulatory defect is to track your menstrual cycle characteristics. This can be done at home by charting your basal body temperature (BBT), as described in detail on page 145. While this method does not tell you that you are going to ovulate, it can tell you that you have ovulated. Take the temperature using the instructions included with the special BBT thermometer (available at pharmacies). Typically in ovulatory cycles, there is a temperature drop on the day of ovulation followed by a rise of 0.5 to 1.0 degrees F., which is called the shift. A biphasic chart suggests ovulation, and a temperature rise lasting 10 or more days suggests normal luteal function. This is when ovulation has occurred and the ovaries start producing progesterone. Progesterone is thermogenic—that is, it causes your temperature to rise. After charting your BBT for several months, it's helpful to look back to this information to figure out a pattern in your menstrual cycles.
- **Use an ovulation predictor kit (OPK).** You can also use an ovulation predictor kit (OPK), which is available at most drugstores, to determine if your cycle is ovulatory. This can also help you determine the best time for intercourse.
- **Measure progesterone.** An additional blood test 6 to 8 days after the BBT rises and the OPK turns positive can measure progesterone, which is of even greater benefit in determining ovulation.

- **Check midcycle symptoms.** Look for midcycle symptoms such as pain (mittelschmerz) or mucus changes.

You can almost guarantee that ovulation is occurring if you have:

- Midcycle pain
- Mucus changes
- Biphasic BBT with a shift on days 12 to 16
- An OPK that turns positive
- A serum progesterone level above 20 PG/ml

If all this occurs, then it's time to start looking for another cause of your infertility. The only absolute test for ovulation is a positive pregnancy test. Sometimes ovulation defects may be subtle and require more serious detection, including tests of endocrine function (LH, FSH, prolactin, thyroid-stimulating hormone).

A properly timed ultrasound scan can give information on the development of follicles and the endometrium. One or two ultrasound evaluations may be used to track the natural cycle to see if a follicle develops and the uterus responds. Ultrasound is usually limited to monitoring follicle growth when infertility medications are used. The endometrial biopsy, long considered the gold standard, is expensive, painful, somewhat unreliable, and usually does not change the course of therapy.

Saving Your Fertility

Treatment of ovulation disorders may vary from ovulation induction, as described in Chapter 13, to birth control pills to keep hormone levels balanced or to allow a cyst to dissolve. Treatment of PCOS is explained in Chapter 4. Ovarian cysts are often "watched" for several menstrual cycles to see if they disappear.

A Word About Ovarian Cancer

Ovarian cancer is the sixth most common cancer in females and is a leading cause of death from gynecological cancer in the United States. Despite advancement in many fields, there has not been improvement in

Table 3.1   Common Ovarian Disorders

Polycystic Ovarian Syndrome (PCOS)

Description	A form of hypergonadism with hyperandrogenism. The follicle development is arrested in the stage of follicle growth, during which the follicles produce relatively large amounts of androgens.
Signs and symptoms	Women with PCOS often have cycles over 35 days in length, obesity, excessive hair growth, or acne.
Making the diagnosis	The diagnosis is made by a high LH/FSH ratio, increased DHEAS and testosterone levels, and multiple small cysts on ultrasound scan. Consideration should be given to the evaluation of insulin resistance by fasting insulin level and glucose tolerance test.

Hypothalamic Hypogonadism

Description	The brain/pituitary axis is suppressed; often referred to as stress amenorrhea. The ovary is "shut down" when a variety of different stressors are perceived to protect the body from pregnancy. Often seen in women of very high or low body weight, Type A personalities, and athletes.
Signs and symptoms	Often irregular period with absent or light bleeding.
Making the diagnosis	Diagnosis is made by excluding other problems.

Premature Ovarian Failure (POF)

Description	Occurs when menopause is before age 40 and is the second most common cause of lack of periods (amenorrhea) after polycystic ovarian syndrome (PCOS). Can be caused by family history, infection, chemotherapy, or pelvic surgery. Also thought to result from smaller stock of eggs (follicles) in the ovary present from birth, an accelerated loss of eggs, or a specific disease entity that destroys the egg store. Many cases are thought to be autoimmune, related to the body's own self-directed destruction of eggs or follicles by unknown triggers.
Signs and symptoms	Erratic or absence of bleeding before age 40, unless the ovaries have been removed.

| Making the diagnosis | Test levels of FSH; search for other autoimmune endocrine diseases, specifically adrenal and thyroid disease. |

Ovarian Cysts

Description	Soft, fluid-filled sacs that appear on the ovaries and can be functional cysts, originating from either a follicle or a corpus luteum and disappearing on their own after a few months. Less frequently they can be long-lasting (benign) cysts (adenomas, teratomas) that must be removed. Very rarely are they cancerous cysts (carcinomas) that must be aggressively treated. Any cyst can disrupt ovulation and normal ovarian function.
Signs and symptoms	Some cysts may be asymptomatic and found on a routine pelvic examination or ultrasound. There could be discomfort on one side, generalized pelvic pain, or pain with intercourse. Cyst rupture is extremely painful, but the discomfort is usually temporary. (Any persistent pain should be reported to your physician.)
Making the diagnosis	Diagnosis is made by taking clinical history and ultrasound scan. Sometimes more extensive tests are performed to help determine the type of cyst. Most benign cycts can be removed through laparoscopy.

survival rates of ovarian cancer largely because of its silent progression and discovery at late stages. Luckily the occurrence rate appears stable.

A decrease in the incidence of ovarian cancer is seen in women who have been pregnant, used oral contraception, or have an early menopause. Each of these groups have had a protective time-out from ovulation in one way or another. This time-out results in a reduced number of instances in which the ovarian surface is distorted during the usual monthly ovulation process. Also, these women are less exposed to the high levels of estradiol seen in the preovulatory period. A possible connection has been the presence of relatively large amounts of follicular fluid that spread over the surface of the ovary at ovulation and into the pelvis. This fluid may contain growth-promoting factors that increase the risk of cancer by their stimulatory effects on cells.

Conception 101

From 5 to 10 percent of breast and ovarian cancer can be attributed to an inherited mutation in the BRCA1 genes. Women who inherit a BRCA1 mutated gene have a greater than 80 percent lifetime risk of breast cancer and a 45 percent chance of ovarian cancer by age 70. DNA testing has been recommended only for women judged to be at high risk. The CA125 blood test has been used to follow response of cancer to therapy. Some have suggested that it be used for screening purposes, but this has not been approved.

There are few symptoms of ovarian cancer until it is found in its later stages—and even then, the symptoms are vague. The diagnosis is usually made by an ultrasound scan. Despite aggressive attempts, there are no approved screening tests for ovarian cancer at this time.

Recognizing the Most Underdiagnosed Disease

Sometimes tagged as the most underdiagnosed disease of women, endometriosis can prevent conception and has been linked to early pregnancy loss. The endometrium is the inner lining of the uterus that is shed each month during menstruation. Endometriosis is a condition where small patches of endometrium are found outside the uterus. These patches first appear as small abnormalities around blood vessels associated with clear and red blisters. With further progression and deeper invasion of the endometriotic implants, the lesions start to chronically bleed, especially at the time of menstruation. In the body's attempt to heal itself, these small sores are walled off and take on the appearance of powder burns. Eventually these sores heal as deep scars, but in the meantime, they may disrupt normal reproductive function and lead to infertility. Certainly, moderate and severe cases of endometriosis "cause" infertility, and fertility is improved by treatment. The effect of treatment for minimal and mild endometriosis is much less clear. The ovary is the most common site for endometriosis, where it may become walled off in a cyst called an endometrioma. It forms a blood-filled or "chocolate" cyst—called thus because the endometrial fluid has the consistency of chocolate syrup—which restricts egg development and release.

Endometriosis may cause infertility in multiple ways:

- Scarring that blocks the tubes or tube movement
- Compromise of ovarian function by endometriomas
- Destruction of the egg store of the ovary
- Chronic inflammation, causing a heightened immune response
- Pelvic pain, reducing intercourse frequency
- Possible reduction in sperm and egg quality
- Possible reduction in uterine receptivity

Who's at Risk?

Although the exact percentage of women who have endometriosis is unknown, the estimates vary widely from 2 percent to more than 50 percent. It is estimated that 30 percent of infertile women have endometriosis. Previously it was believed that endometriosis most often occurred in thin, Type A professional women who had regular menstrual periods and postponed childbearing. Now researchers know that endometriosis affects all ages and races. While endometriosis is not directly inherited, it is more common in some families. Risk factors for endometriosis include:

- Menstrual cycle less than 28 days
- Bleeding more than 5 days
- Painful periods
- Infertility
- Congenital abnormality of the uterus
- Abnormally tight cervical opening
- Family history of endometriosis

What Causes It?

Most experts agree that endometriosis is associated with the backflow of menstrual fluid and tissue through the tubes and out into the pelvic cavity (retrograde menstruation). These implantation locations are mostly in the pelvis, but in some cases endometriosis can be found outside the pelvis. The effect on infertility by endometriosis depends upon how widespread the disease is, where the tissue is located, and how deeply it has invaded. These factors then influence how much damage is done to the pelvis.

If you have endometriosis, then your body produces more prostaglandins, chemicals in the body that cause inflammation and pain. Nonsteroidal anti-inflammatory drugs (NSAIDs) such as ibuprofen block prostaglandins and are effective in relieving menstrual pain in some women. The new cyclooxygenase-2 (COX-2) inhibitors (Celebrex, Vioxx) also block prostaglandin production and may help end pain without stomach upset.

What You May Feel

With endometriosis you feel a triad of symptoms, including painful menstruation (dysmenorrhea), painful intercourse (dyspareunia), and painful bowel movements (dyskysia). Some women are misdiagnosed with irritable bowel syndrome when diarrhea and constipation along with intestinal pain are related to menstruation. Because hormones control endometriosis, you may have pelvic pain during certain times of the month, such as during ovulation and menstruation.

Making the Diagnosis

If you have symptoms of spastic colon (irritable bowel syndrome), painful periods, chronic urinary bladder pain, painful intercourse, an abnormal bleeding pattern, or no identifiable cause for your infertility, you may suspect endometriosis. During an exam, your doctor may feel nodules along the uterosacral ligaments that attach your cervix to the backbone. Sometimes an ultrasound scan increases the suspicion of endometriosis when a cyst is found that has a "ground glass" appearance of an endometrioma. There are several immunologic tests for endometriosis including CA125, anti-endometrial antibodies, and the Etegrity Test (beta-3 integrin protein), but none have shown to be that helpful in making the diagnosis.

While your doctor may determine that you have endometriosis from evaluating your medical history, the only sure way to diagnose this condition is by surgery, specifically laparoscopy. However, if your condition is minimal or mild, it may just require a very careful inspection of the pelvis by an experienced laparoscopic surgeon. Keep in mind that just because it is mild does not mean that endometriosis is not a cause for your infertility or for pain. Even mild endometriosis can cause severe pain and severe endometriosis may cause little pain at all.

Right now, treatment of endometriosis is controversial, with the choices being surgery, medical therapy, or a combination of the two. Surgery of the endometriosis lesions can be done by laser (evaporation), harmonic scalpel (cutting), and electrocautery (burning). The important goal is to eliminate as much of the tissue as possible without causing harm to pelvic organs, which is probably best done by a surgeon experienced in endometrial surgery.

Medical therapy is very effective in relieving pain and possibly improving fertility, if used aggressively, and current medical treatment includes hormone suppression. The two medications commonly used are GnRH analogs or GnRH-A (Lupron, Synarel, and Zoladex) and Danazol. GnRH-A works by turning off the ovaries, which generate most of the hormone estrogen. Estrogen is "fertilizer" for endometriosis, so reducing its production reduces the stimulation for endometriosis to grow.

While the GnRH analogs treat endometriosis, their side effects are similar to those of menopause—hot flashes, vaginal dryness, insomnia, and bone loss. A newer long-term treatment program involves adding back small amounts of estrogen and progestins to reduce the symptoms and at the same time to keep the endometriosis in check. Danazol has been shown to have a lethal effect on endometriosis cells. Again, the side effects are not pleasant, including weight gain, acne, abnormal hair growth, and occasionally mood changes. An experimental class of hormonal therapy agents called aromatase inhibitors act in a manner similar to Danazol and are now being studied for treating endometriosis.

Other medical therapies, including continuous oral contraceptives and progestin, may retard the development of endometriosis, but are usually second-line therapy.

PID—The Most Preventable Cause of Infertility

Pelvic inflammatory disease (PID) is an infection or inflammation with great potential for permanently scarring the reproductive tract—the uterus, ovaries, or fallopian tubes—leading to infertility. While PID causes scar tissue that can damage or block organs, it is also the most preventable cause of infertility.

Who's at Risk?

PID is one of the most common illnesses affecting women today, with a reported 1 million new cases diagnosed in the United States annually. The disease is most prevalent among young women, those under age 25, who have more than one sex partner, as well as those who have had STDs or a prior case of PID. If your partner has had more than one sexual partner, your risk for PID increases.

What Causes It?

The vast majority of PID stems from sexually transmitted diseases (STDs). In the United States, there are about 1 million cases of gonorrhea and 4 million cases of chlamydia infections annually. The only method of transmission of gonorrhea or chlamydia is by recent sexual contact with an infected person. The organisms do not live outside the body, and an infection from casual contact, sharing towels, or using public toilet seats is highly unlikely. Another common cause of PID is a mixed infection, usually arising from contamination by microorganisms from the intestine or vagina. This form of PID may have no relation to multiple partners.

There are less common causes of PID. For example, a ruptured cyst or appendix, pelvic surgery, or a bowel injury can also cause PID. Infectious PID may also result from unintentional contamination of the pelvic cavity by uterine manipulation such as a hysterosalpingogram (HSG). The most common cause of tubal factor infertility is previous pelvic inflammatory disease (PID).

What You May Feel

Symptoms of PID may be mild and easily dismissed as an intestinal bug, or the symptoms may be severe enough to require hospitalization. Symptoms are usually more pronounced in males. The most common signs and symptoms include:

- Abdominal/pelvic discomfort
- Abnormal bleeding
- Vaginal discharge with an unpleasant odor
- Painful urination
- Fever and chills
- Mild odorous discharge

Making the Diagnosis

If you have symptoms of PID, see your doctor; there is treatment available. It's important to start treatment even if the diagnosis is less than 100 percent. However, this quick-to-treat philosophy has also left some women with a diagnosis of PID when in fact there was an ovarian cyst rupture and no infection. The organisms that cause chlamydia and gonorrhea infection are easily identified on tests of cervical cells, and other blood tests are done to check the severity of infection.

If left untreated, pelvic infections may leave residual scarring that will hamper fertility (see Table 3.2). The fallopian tubes are usually affected. Even if the tubes remain open, they may scar into the pelvic side wall. Or the end of the tube, which is necessary for oocyte collection, may become completely scarred and closed. The tube may later fill with fluid, a hydrosalpinx, and this causes chronic pain. The good news is pelvic infection and its scarring can be reduced by early and aggressive antibiotic therapy.

Table 3.2 PID and Infertility

NUMBER OF PELVIC INFECTIONS	CHANCE OF INFERTILITY
1	30%
2	60%
3	90%

How You Can Avoid PID

- Have a monogamous sexual relationship.
- Use vaginal spermicides (agents that kill sperm).
- Also use barrier methods (condom, diaphragm, cervical cap, sponge).

Is There Hidden Damage in Your Fallopian Tubes?

In vitro fertilization was initially developed as a means of allowing women with blocked or absent fallopian tubes to conceive. Removing the eggs directly from the ovaries, fertilizing them outside the body, and returning the resulting embryos to the uterus completely bypasses the fallopian tubes. Women with fallopian tubes damaged by prior infection or scarring from surgery or endometriosis were considered perfect candidates for the new procedure. Unfortunately, many of these high prognosis young women had an awfully difficult time conceiving through IVF. Cycle after cycle would go by in which the ovaries would respond appropriately to medication, making lots of mature eggs; fertilization would occur and normal-looking embryos would develop. Cycle after cycle, however, resulted in negative pregnancy tests.

Some reproductive endocrinologists have found a high correlation between the presence of a *hydrosalpinx* and very poor pregnancy rates. The cells that line the normally functioning fallopian tube both secrete fluid into the tube and later reabsorb it. As tubes become damaged, they retain the ability to secrete fluid but lose their ability to reabsorb it. Often these tubes are blocked at the end and the accumulated fluid further distends the tube. This fluid, backflowing into the uterine cavity from the tubes, washes away, poisons, or in some other way hinders the growth of the embryos that are implanted. When these damaged tubes are removed prior to IVF cycles, the pregnancy rates in these women rise. While many REs consider this a controversial topic and defer removing the fallopian tubes until after a failed cycle, other experts look for and remove the tubes aggressively.

If you have tubal factor and good embryos yet fail to conceive in an IVF cycle, ask your doctor about having a repeat hysterosalpingogram to determine whether a hydrosalpinx may be hiding behind the uterus or in a difficult-to-detect place.

Be Aware of Uterine Fibroids

Uterine fibroids (myomas or leiomyomas) are the most common tumors in the female reproductive system. Unfortunately, there have been only a few studies that have specifically addressed the role of fibroids in fertility.

Although fibroids may vary greatly size, most experts in the field of reproductive endocrinology believe that the fibroid must be about the size of a golf ball (or above 3 centimeters) for it to have an adverse effect on fertility or pregnancy. Obviously, the position of the fibroid in the uterus may be more important than its size. If the fibroid is not intruding on the uterine cavity and distorting the endometrium, treatment may not be necessary. Your doctor can evaluate this by using hysteroscopy, hysterosalpingography, or sonohysterosalpingography (see Chapter 11). Most physicians agree that even smaller fibroids should be removed if they are distorting the endometrial cavity, and that all fibroids the size of a baseball (greater than 6 centimeters) should be removed regardless of their position. The reason for this is that the hormones produced during pregnancy can stimulate fibroid growth. What was once an asymptomatic and relatively unimportant structure may cause significant pain and even jeopardize the pregnancy. The fibroid in the wall of the uterus may prevent the uterus from properly expanding in pregnancy, or stimulate premature contractions.

Who's at Risk?

If you are female, you are at risk for this common tumor. However, the incidence of fibroids increases with age and by age 50, as many as 50 percent of women have one or more. Fibroids are common in all races, although some studies show that they are more common in African Americans. If you use birth control pills, you may have a lower incidence of fibroid changes than those who do not use the pill.

What Causes It?

Each fibroid begins its development as a single muscle cell, which for unknown reasons begins to duplicate. While it is not known what causes fibroids to grow, these tumors are under the control of estrogen and pro-gesterone, the principal ovarian hormones. After menopause, when the estrogen levels fall, fibroids decrease in size.

What You May Feel

Many fibroids cause nothing more than mild pelvic pressure. However, other common symptoms include:

- Pelvic pain
- Heavy periods
- Painful periods
- Pelvic pressure or fullness
- Frequent urination
- Chronic back pain

Making the Diagnosis

Your doctor may suspect a fibroid tumor during a pelvic examination. Ultrasound scan is an excellent diagnostic tool for fibroids. In select cases, more extensive imaging with an MRI may be necessary.

Stopping the Interference of Fibroids

Treatment may vary from medication to surgery to simply observing the tumor. Nonsteroidal anti-inflammatory drugs (NSAIDs) such as ibuprofen can help to stop cramping and may also decrease blood loss. Since fibroids are under the control of ovarian hormones, treatment may include gonadotropin (GnRH) agonists, which cause a temporary chemical menopause. The reduction in hormonal stimulation may stop fibroid growth and often results in their shrinkage. Unfortunately, although the chemicals may reduce the fibroid size by 50 percent, the fibroid will quickly return to its pretreatment size when the suppressive therapy is stopped.

Submucosal fibroids, those adjacent to the endometrium, may be surgically removed by hysteroscopy. Other times, a procedure called a myomectomy may be used, which helps to preserve fertility. This procedure is performed through an abdomen incision, a laparotomy, or laparoscopy. Some experts believe that a fibroid that is sufficiently easy to remove with laparoscopy may be insignificant in its capacity to affect fertility, but removal may prevent later growth. Once the fibroid is removed, the surrounding muscle is usually closed with sutures, and the area forms a scar. This scar may not expand as well as the muscle during pregnancy and could result in a uterine rupture. If you've had a fibroid removed, ask your doctor about the possibilities of doing a cesarean section.

When You're Faced with Unexplained Infertility

After doing a host of medical tests, your doctor may throw her or his hands up in the air and conclude that you have unexplained infertility. Often this diagnosis is given too freely when there has been only minimal evaluation. Other times doctors are sure that there is a serious problem, but it is beyond our present scope of understanding. Maybe in the future the disorder will not only have someone's name on it but a successful therapy as well. For now, the causes of some infertilities remain elusive.

Although a diagnosis of unexplained infertility seems threatening with no identifiable source, most experts agree that ovarian dysfunction is a primary contributor. Successful treatment of unexplained infertility runs the gamut from intrauterine insemination and ovarian stimulation with medical therapy to in vitro fertilization and even egg donation. Still many couples, especially younger couples, with unexplained infertility will achieve a pregnancy even if therapy is not used.

Now Go Plan Your Family

Using the information in this chapter, work with your doctor to get an accurate diagnosis, then control the factors you can to increase your chances of conceiving. By taking care of these potential threats ahead of time, you can continue your family planning—on schedule.

Chapter 4

The Unrecognized Epidemic of PCOS

"I honestly thought it was normal to have a slight mustache and long hair on my arms," Annie, age 32, said. "But when I could no longer wear a bathing suit because I was just plain too hairy, I knew there was a problem. Little did I know that I had a hormonal imbalance that could affect my ability to have children.

"My ob-gyn diagnosed me with polycystic ovarian syndrome (PCOS) after doing an ultrasound scan and running other laboratory tests. He then suggested that I lose weight, exercise regularly, and take birth control pills to help balance my hormones. I know there's no cure, but I can live with the symptoms now that they are managed, and I work hard to keep my body healthy.

"The best news is that ... it's a girl! Once we stabilized the condition, my husband and I were able to get pregnant and have our first child."

Polycystic ovarian syndrome (PCOS) is a common threat to women's fertility, yet it is vastly unrecognized by doctors and women alike. PCOS is the most common hormonal problem of the reproductive-age woman, affecting up to 30 percent of all premenopausal women.

In 1935 two gynecologists, Irving F. Stein and Michael L. Leventhal, found a definite link between women with enlarged ovaries containing many small cysts and three common clinical characteristics, including:

1. Excessive male-pattern hair growth or hirsutism (the overabundance of body hair, such as a mustache or pubic hair growing upward toward the navel, found in women with excess androgens)

2. Obesity
3. Menstrual cycle disturbances leading to infertility

Stein and Leventhal labeled this condition polycystic ovarian disease. Since then, doctors have realized that because no two women are affected the same way with PCOS, it is not a disease, but rather a syndrome with a broad spectrum of symptoms. For example, although many women with PCOS are obese, there is a distinct group of thin women who may have even more firmly entrenched hormonal and fertility problems. Some women with abnormal hair growth have been given the diagnosis of idiopathic (no known cause) hirsutism. Yet on close examination most of these women will have subtle abnormalities of their hormones or polycystic ovaries on an ultrasound scan. While researchers make the distinction between "PCO-appearing" ovaries on ultrasound and PCOS, not all women with PCOS are infertile or have menstrual cycle abnormalities. Using pelvic ultrasound for screening, researchers estimate that approximately 20 to 30 percent of women of reproductive age have polycystic-appearing ovaries, including some who are fertile and have no other symptoms of PCOS.

How all this fits together is really unknown. Some experts believe that there may be a central problem at the root of PCOS, yet this is inconclusive. Others believe that PCOS is a symptom of a variety of problems, much like a fever is a sign of an infection.

What You May See—Signs and Symptoms of PCOS

While women with PCOS have normal reproductive organs (uterus and fallopian tubes), the following abnormal signs and symptoms are common:

Menstrual Disturbances

Many women with PCOS get their first period at the usual age of twelve to thirteen years, while some may start menstruating earlier or later. Some women never start menstruating. Typically, teenagers are seen by a physician because they have not yet had a period. (If a young woman has not started her period by age sixteen, a physician should evaluate her.)

IRREGULAR OR ABSENT PERIODS. The menstrual cycle of a girl with PCOS may at first be regular, but by the time she is in high school, her cycles start to lengthen and her period may be skipped. Usually during her teenage years, the other symptoms of skin and weight problems also start to be seen. Often during this time, oral contraceptives are started. Although the birth control pill usually regulates the menstrual cycle, it may give a false impression that all is well.

NO BLEEDING TO EXCESSIVE SPOTTING. Some women with PCOS easily get pregnant in these early years. Occasionally, birth control pills may even increase the chance of pregnancy by suppressing abnormal hormonal production. Often the woman is seen by a gynecologist when she is in her twenties after she stops taking the pill and her menstrual periods cease. In fact, some women with PCOS have no menstrual bleeding unless some form of medication, usually a progestin, is given. In others, there is excessive bleeding, or long periods of spotting. Although some women with PCOS have regular 28-day cycles, PCOS should be suspected in women who have cycle lengths of more than 35 days. Menopause in women with PCOS is around age 50, as with other women.

PMS AND PELVIC PAIN. Although not commonly reported, many women with PCOS have chronic pelvic pain and premenstrual (PMS) symptoms. This is the result of chronically abnormal hormonal patterns, the capacity of hormones to alter body fluid, and even the enlarged cystic ovaries.

INFERTILITY AND MISCARRIAGE. FSH (follicle-stimulating hormone) and LH (luteinizing hormone), two hormones secreted by the pituitary gland in the brain, are imbalanced in women with PCOS. Elevated LH levels may also affect the egg quality and lead to an increased risk of miscarriage. The ovary becomes filled with small follicles (cysts) that further disrupt normal follicle development. The ovary's surface is also thickened (sclerocystic), which may impede ovulation. Some women with PCOS, especially those who are markedly obese, may have gonadotropin levels that are suppressed rather than elevated.

Menstrual History Gives Clues to PCOS

Some factors involved in making the diagnosis of PCOS include:

- The time your period started (menarche)
- The pattern of your periods presently and in the past
- The number of days between periods exceeding 35

Hair and Skin Problems

The skin problems associated with PCOS are possibly more common than either menstrual cycle irregularity or obesity. These skin disorders are related to an increase in the level of male hormones (hyperandrogenism). This abnormality may be due to an absolute increase in androgen level or to an alteration in the ratio of hormone levels. A third possibility is an exaggerated response of the skin to relatively normal androgen levels. The end result of all three of these possibilities is the same and includes such conditions as:

- Acne
- Seborrhea
- Hidradenitis suppurativa (inflammation of the specialized sweat glands in the armpit and groin)
- Balding
- Acanthosis nigricans (brown hyperpigmentation of the skin)
- Hirsutism

ACNE AND SEBORRHEA. Many women complain of skin problems to some degree during the menstrual cycle. In women with regular menstrual cycles, the second half of the menstrual cycle is characterized by increased progesterone levels. Progesterone is a weak androgen and may create a situation of relative hyperandrogenism. Around the time of menstruation, estradiol (the principal estrogen released by the ovary) is decreased. Low levels of estrogen (hypoestrogenism) also result in an increase in androgens that causes the increased oiliness, inflammation of the skin, and acne.

Androgens increase sebum (a combination of skin oils and old skin tissue). Increased male hormone levels also cause seborrhea. A particularly common type of seborrhea that one would not associate with hormonal alterations is dandruff. Contrary to what you may have thought, dandruff is caused by oily, not dry, skin.

ALOPECIA (BALDING). A rise in androgens may also result in alopecia (balding). The most androgen-sensitive area of your scalp is the vertex, or the highest point of your head. Women who have severe cases of excessive androgen are prone to frontal balding and anterior hairline recession.

ACANTHOSIS NIGRICANS (AN). AN consists of velvety raised pigmented skin changes, usually seen on the back of the neck, the underarm area, and beneath the breasts. These skin changes are usually found along with skin tags (acrochordons). Possibly the best description of AN is that it looks like the affected skin is dirty and would benefit from scrubbing. Obviously, this is not true! While AN is associated with such conditions as obesity and other endocrine disorders, it should always alert your doctor to a risk of diabetes mellitus, major lipid abnormalities, and hypertension. Although less common, it may be a warning signal of cancer.

HIRSUTISM. Hirsutism is an increase in amount and/or coarseness of hair distributed in the male pattern, such as a mustache or pubic hair growing upward toward the navel (see Table 4.1 for the Ferriman-Gallwey Scoring System for Hirsutism). Other areas of male pattern hair growth include sideburns, lower neck, lower back, and inner thighs. A faint mustache or an occasional stray hair around the breasts is quite common and may be related to your family or an ethnic group rather than to a hormonal imbalance. A good screening test is the amount of hair between your navel and bikini line.

Obesity

About 50 percent of women with PCOS are clinically obese, a condition where you are 20 percent or more over a normal weight. Scientists are unsure whether obesity is a cause or a result of PCOS. The typical obesity of PCOS is described as an apple shape because the fat is located

Table 4.1   The Ferriman-Gallwey Scoring System for Hirsutism

SCORING
scant or mild coverage = 1
marked/complete coverage = 4

____ upper lip
____ face
____ chin
____ jaw and neck
____ upper back
____ lower back
____ arm
____ chest
____ upper abdomen
____ lower abdomen
____ thigh
____ perineum

TOTAL SCORE
>8 = hirsutism

in the center of the body instead of in the thighs and hips. This apple (as opposed to a pear) type of fat distribution is associated with greater risk of hypertension, diabetes, and lipid abnormalities.

While many health concerns may improve with weight loss, weight reduction does not cure PCOS. Almost always, women with PCOS gain weight very easily and lose it only with great effort.

Insulin Resistance Is Prevalent

PCOS increasingly has been linked to abnormalities of insulin and glucose metabolism. Insulin is a hormone released by the pancreas that promotes the storage of calories, increases fat stores, and regulates glucose levels in the blood. Insulin resistance (IR) happens when your body steadily becomes less responsive to the actions of insulin. In IR, blood sugar levels rise despite high levels of insulin, and eventually Type 2 diabetes results. Type 2 diabetes is much more likely to be inherited and passed down through families than Type 1 (see Table 4.2). (This is different from Type 1 diabetes, where the pancreas does not make enough insulin.)

Although the relationship of diabetes to endocrine problems is not new, researchers have found that as many as 50 percent of women with PCOS also have IR. It appears that hyperinsulinemia (excessively high blood insulin levels) actually causes hyperandrogenism. The obese woman with PCOS may have both IR and glucose intolerance, while the thinner woman does not show glucose intolerance as often. IR and hyperinsulinemia are considered significant risk factors in the development of atherosclerosis (hardening of the arteries). This predisposes women with PCOS to increased risk of high blood pressure and stroke. PCOS and obesity are both strongly associated with abnormality in lipid levels in blood (dyslipidemia). This is seen by elevated total cholesterol, high bad cholesterol (LDL), and low good cholesterol (HDL), together with high levels of triglycerides. All women with PCOS should have their lipids checked. Hyperinsulinemia and IR also may be the root of such disorders as:

- Chronic fatigue syndrome
- Immune system abnormalities
- Eating disorders
- Hypoglycemia
- Gastrointestinal disorders
- Depression
- Anxiety

Table 4.2   Type 2 Diabetes Mellitus

WHO IS AT RISK?
More than 20 percent over desirable body weight
First-degree relative with Type 2 DM
High risk ethnic group
Hypercholesterolemia/hyperlipidemia
Delivered a baby weighing more than 9 pounds
Previous gestational diabetes

HOW IS IT DIAGNOSED?
Fasting plasma glucose (>100mg/dl)

The Causes of PCOS

While the cause of PCOS is virtually unknown, heredity does play a role. PCOS may run in your mother's or your father's families, or both, although the characteristic traits may be passed down with varying degrees of severity. When the inherited tendency interacts with dietary and environmental factors, the problems with PCOS may worsen or improve. While PCOS is inherited, the more serious diseases (tumors of the pituitary, adrenal, and ovary) that may masquerade as PCOS are not.

There is evidence that women with PCOS weighed more than average at birth and their mothers may have had gestational diabetes. Likewise, the risk of gestational diabetes and pregnancy-induced hypertension (PIH, toxemia, preeclampsia) may be increased in pregnant women with PCOS. Some of this risk may be independently related to increased prepregnancy weight. Some research suggests that PCOS may be associated with a low birth weight.

Making the Diagnosis

Your medical history is vital in making the diagnosis of PCOS. After doing a physical examination and taking your personal medical history, your doctor will check for symptoms and physical findings, test your hormone levels, and use ultrasound. While most women with PCOS will have abnormalities in all three areas, you may have abnormalities in only one or two.

Laboratory Testing

There are many laboratory tests your doctor may use to diagnose PCOS. Not only will various hormone assays be taken, but the following tests may be useful in making the diagnosis:

COMPREHENSIVE BIOCHEMICAL PROFILE. These blood tests evaluate your body's overall metabolism, salt, and fluid balance as various electrolytes (salts), fats, glucose, and liver enzymes are measured. Overall, these tests are used to evaluate the function of your liver and kidney.

GLUCOSE AND GLUCOSE TOLERANCE TEST (GTT). A GTT may be done, especially if you are more than 120 percent of your ideal weight, have first-degree relatives with diabetes, have elevated serum lipid levels, or have delivered a baby weighing more than 9 pounds. This test can show whether you are diabetic or have impaired insulin resistance (a hallmark of PCOS) that has resulted in elevated glucose levels.

LIPID PANEL. This test measures cholesterol and triglyceride levels—two markers that can determine risk of heart attack and stroke.

Ultrasound

Ultrasound can determine ovarian and endometrial function. The finding of greater than ten cystic structures less than 10 millimeters in either ovary meets the generally established ultrasound criteria of PCOS. Sometimes the ovary is virtually filled with small cysts. Other times the ovary is enlarged with few cysts.

Treating the Symptoms of PCOS

Again, there is no cure for PCOS. However, using a multifaceted treatment program, you can gain control of the symptoms and increase your chances of making a baby.

WEIGHT LOSS. Several studies show that losing weight may correct hyperinsulinemia, reverse other symptoms, and even restore fertility in overweight women with PCOS. With weight loss there is always an improvement in hormone balance and sometimes a return of menstrual periods. Low-carbohydrate/high-protein diets have been used to both lower weight and reduce the amount of circulating insulin. However, weight loss may not affect hirsutism.

Diet plans approved by the American Diabetes Association (ADA) are excellent for PCOS. They are well balanced, and many plans are available. Along with dietary changes to control weight, regular exercise is encouraged and can help you maintain the loss.

PROGESTINS. This medication mimics the action of progesterone and is used to regulate the menstrual cycle and reduce the blood levels of

LH. For women with PCOS who do not ovulate, very little progesterone is produced from the ovary and the interval between menstrual periods is longer (oligomenorrhea). If a progestin alone does not induce menstrual bleeding, treatment may include first using estrogen, then progestin.

ORAL CONTRACEPTIVES. Oral contraceptives (OCs) are a mainstay of treatment of PCOS in women who do not want to become pregnant. They suppress the level of LH and reduce androgen levels by elevating SHBG, which trap active androgens.

There is some evidence that OCs may worsen glucose tolerance.

CORTICOSTEROIDS. Steroids can suppress adrenal androgen production and may be useful in treatment of PCOS with an adrenal component. Overall, their use is better in theory than in practice, for women often stop them because of unwanted side effects.

ANTIANDROGENS. This group of medications, which include spironolactone (Aldactone), Finasteride, and Flutamide, can be used only when not attempting a pregnancy or without some form of adequate birth control. Antiandrogens are used to help improve the skin problems that occur with PCOS.

GnRH ANALOGS. There are two types of analogs, agonists and antagonists. Antagonists directly block the action of GnRH. While there are several antagonists under development, none are currently marketed in the United States because of side effects. Agonists stimulate the release of GnRH, then block it. When GnRH and subsequent LH release are blocked, follicle growth is inhibited, and estrogen and androgen production is markedly reduced. The side effects, which can usually be controlled with estrogen and progestins, are similar to those of menopause, including hot flashes and reversible reduction in bone density.

Protecting Your Fertility

Normally, a single egg ovulates from a single follicle midway through a cycle that is 26 to 32 days long. The processes of follicle growth, ovulation, and production of progesterone from the corpus luteum are controlled by hormones.

In PCOS, these normal mechanisms are disturbed. Your doctor may use fertility drugs, including clomiphene citrate (Clomid, Serophene) and various preparations of injectable gonadotropins, in an attempt to temporarily override this problem and bring about ovulation. One drawback of all fertility drugs is that they tend to work in only one cycle (month). The developing follicle may take as long as three months (cycles) to go through the entire process of growth and maturation. For women with PCOS, this means that the follicle and its egg have progressed through the early stages of growth in an abnormal hormonal environment that may contribute to poorer egg quality despite aggressive stimulation. Use of injectable fertility drugs in PCOS carries a high risk of ovarian hyperstimulation and multiple pregnancy.

In Vitro Fertilization (IVF) Increases Chance of Conception

IVF is increasingly being used for treatment of PCOS as it allows you and your doctor to judge the ability of the egg to be fertilized. Although the chance of IVF failure is higher in women with PCOS, lack of fertilization in one cycle does not necessarily mean that fertilization will fail in subsequent cycles. It may be more the environment in which the oocyte develops than the oocyte itself. An additional advantage is that a more aggressive approach can be taken toward ovarian stimulation. With PCOS, hyperstimulation is somewhat less of an issue because the preovulatory-size follicles are aspirated and a limited number of embryos are replaced. Not only does this decrease the chance of multiple pregnancies, it reduces the risk of more pronounced cystic change. Many women with PCOS either overstimulate or understimulate with gonadotropin therapy. The use of GnRH analogs and gonadotropins in conjunction with IVF may help your doctor to maximize control and ensure the greatest chance of pregnancy in any one cycle.

Procedures That May Help

In the past, ovarian wedge resection, a surgical procedure by which part of the ovary is removed and the ovary sewn back together, was widely used to treat PCOS. This procedure resulted in a significant reduction in LH and androgen production and helped reestablish regular menstrual periods in more than 75 percent of women, with a pregnancy rate of about 60 percent. However, pelvic adhesive disease, which was often severe, occurred in about 30 percent of women. Although wedge resection by laparotomy is rarely used, electrosurgical incisions, or ovarian drilling during laparoscopy has become relatively commonplace. Success rates depend on your surgeon, and while the formation of adhesions may be reduced, it still may occur.

New Hope for Appearance

New lasers especially designed for dermatologic use can accomplish permanent hair removal, which destroys the hair's regeneration mechanism. Contrary to popular belief, shaving and plucking does not induce faster or coarser hair growth. However, electrolysis can be painful and can sometimes cause significant inflammation, infection, and scarring; it should be largely avoided in lieu of medical therapy.

Treating Insulin Resistance with Antidiabetic Medications

By treating the insulin resistance with antidiabetic medications such as metformin (Glucophage) and troglitazone (Rezulin), discussed in Chapter 13, PCOS may also be treated and possibly reversed. A major benefit of these medications is that the entire spectrum of signs and symptoms of PCOS may be improved. Some women with PCOS have successfully restored normal menstruation and fertility. These antidiabetic medications may provide a useful alternative when other therapies have failed.

Doctor's Rx

There are risks with the antidiabetic medications. These should be discussed in detail with a specialist familiar with insulin resistance and the specific medications before therapy is started.

Future Thoughts on PCOS

Hopefully, with new tools made available by molecular biology, there may be significant advances in the next several years, so PCOS may become a problem of the past. In the meantime, if you have any of the signs of PCOS, talk with your doctor about a thorough evaluation and start treatment to save your fertility.

Chapter 5

Not for Women Only: Identifying Male Factor Infertility

"My expectations were influenced by that Billy Crystal movie Forget Paris, *in which he plays an NBA referee," said 44-year-old Pete. "When he has to produce a sperm sample, they usher him into a room fully equipped with a library of pornography and a VCR with tapes addressing every sexual predilection.*

"Unfortunately, my fantasies were quickly dashed. We were ushered into a small examination room with nary a People *magazine in sight."*

While many hold to the myth that infertility is a woman's problem, you know that this is not true. Nonetheless, it often surprises people to learn that while factors to do with the mother are primary in approximately 40 percent of couples, in another 30 to 40 percent factors to do with the father predominate. A combination of male and female factors account for the remaining 20 to 30 percent of cases. New statistics reveal that in more than 50 percent of couples seeking infertility evaluation, a male factor is contributory. This statistic may seem difficult to believe, especially when healthy men release between 120 million and 600 million sperm during one ejaculation (400,000,000,000 sperm in one lifetime!).

All It Takes Is One Sperm

Still, that one sperm has to perform at its best! If your body is not functioning the way it's supposed to, it is time to find out why. A host of anatomical reasons can cause you to have a low sperm count, poor motility or movement of the sperm, poor sperm quality, or sperm that lack the ability to penetrate your partner's egg. Occasionally, the presence of other diseases, such as diabetes mellitus, central nervous system problems, and pituitary tumors, can affect fertility. With all the groundbreaking medical discoveries in the field of reproductive endocrinology, most of these problems can now be solved to allow conception to take place.

We know there are certain measures men and women can take to safeguard their reproductive health . . . and the health of their future children. If you are contemplating making a baby, the smartest thing you can do is to start making the necessary lifestyle changes, as well as protecting yourself from toxins, medications, and other hazards that could injure your sperm.

Reproductive specialists maintain that couples should enter into their fertility evaluation with equal expectations and equal responsibility. Getting your reproductive system checked out by your doctor is part of this responsibility—just to make sure all the parts are working as they should. Before we discuss common barriers to your fertility and how these are treated, let's take a quick course in male anatomy and outline the problems that may increase your chances of infertility.

Male Anatomy 101

The reproductive anatomy of the male is mostly outside the body except for the seminal vesicle.

THE PENIS. This is the erectile organ responsible for the release of urine and for the transfer of sperm to the female's vagina. The penis varies more in size in the flaccid state than when it is erect. (If it is any consolation, size does *not* matter when it comes to making a baby, and circumcision does not affect fertility either!)

The penis is divided into two external parts (the body and glans). Within the body of the penis are three sections:

- The corpus spongiosum, which contains the urethra, the tube that carries either urine or semen.
- Two corpora cavernosa, sometimes called erection chambers, are

responsible for causing an erection. Within each corpus cavernosum is an actual artery supplying blood for erections. An additional dorsal artery travels along the upper surface of the penis to supply the glans, located at the top of the penis.

- The glans penis is the end portion of the penis and is made up of the expansion of the corpus spongiosum. The glans is covered with a thin, sensitive skin. During circumcision, part of the foreskin that covers the glans is removed.

The veins that drain the blood away from the penis combine to join larger veins in the pelvis and carry the blood back toward the heart. Nerve impulses to the penis that cause erections originate from the lower portion of the spinal cord. The testes are outside the body to provide a lower temperature, which is important for normal sperm production.

THE SEMINAL VESICLES. The seminal vesicle is inside the body adjacent to the prostate. Working with the prostate gland, the seminal vesicles provide a fluid environment for sperm. In fact, 95 percent of ejaculate is made up of a fluid from these glands, while less than 5 percent is made up of sperm cells.

The seminiferous tubules are tightly coiled tubules within the testes. Sprinkled around the seminiferous tubules are the Leydig cells, which make testosterone. Also within these tubules, more than thirty million sperm are produced daily and are stored in the epididymis, a tightly coiled thin-walled tube in which they mature. The sperm travel through the vas deferens, a thick, muscular tube, and mix with other secretions to form the semen. Then they enter the urethra at the base of the penis. It takes about 75 days in the testis and another several days to weeks in transit after leaving the testis to develop a mature sperm. Interestingly, this is about the same amount of time for the development of a mature preovulatory follicle in the female. If the sperm are not ejaculated in about one month, they will die, but the supply is constantly being replenished. The male DNA is contained in the chromosomes in the head of the sperm, and the tail helps to get the sperm to the egg.

The urethra, the duct that can carry either urine or semen, begins at the bladder, meets the vas deferens at the base of the penis, runs through the penis, and opens to the outside at the end of the penis.

During ejaculation, the muscles of the epididymis and the vas def-

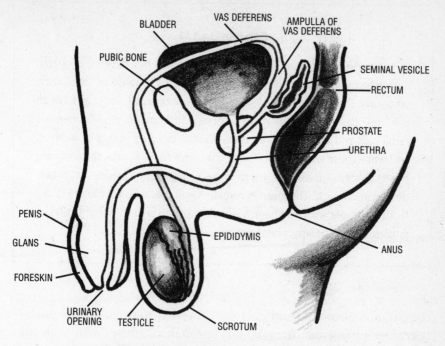

Figure 5.1   The Male Reproductive System

erens work together to force the sperm into the ejaculatory duct. The sperm is then joined with secretions of the seminal vesicles and prostate gland to form semen. At the time of orgasm, the muscles surrounding the base of your urethra make the semen ejaculate out of the penis.

Sperm Development

Pituitary hormones are responsible for maintaining the sperm production process, just as in the case of your partner's eggs. (The pituitary gland is the main endocrine gland producing hormones that control other glands and many body functions, especially growth.) Your hypothalamus, the area of the brain that controls body temperature, hunger, and thirst, emits gonadotropin-releasing hormone (GnRH). GnRH is released in a short pulse about every 90 minutes and causes the release of luteinizing hormone (LH) and follicle-stimulating hormone (FSH) from

---

Conception 101

In Kallmann's syndrome, the hypothalamus does not develop properly. Since the hypothalamus is also responsible for the sense of smell, men who have this syndrome do not have a sense of smell, yet they have all the male parts. With Kallmann's, there is little or no development of facial hair and the testes stay small. Kallmann's also occurs in women, and while those with the syndrome may have female parts, the parts are not activated. In women, there is no estrogen production or breast development, and the ovaries remain small. Because FSH and LH are lacking, people with Kallmann's usually respond well to either GnRH or gonadotropin therapy, and pregnancy is possible.

---

the pituitary gland. LH and FSH work together to stimulate the production of sperm (spermatogenesis) and testosterone (the primary male hormone) in the testes.

Puberty is the awakening of the hypothalamic-pituitary-testicular axis with the resulting first production of mature sperm and testosterone. Testosterone is responsible for the development of the secondary sexual characteristics, such as a beard and growth of the penis.

When you are sexually aroused, your brain sends signals to the nerves in the penis. Touch or direct sensory contact can also simulate these penile nerves. The nerve impulses travel to the two corpora cavernosa, causing the expansion of the penile arteries and an increase in blood flow to the penis. As the two erection chambers fill with blood, this causes pressure on the smaller veins that take blood away from the penis. These spaces change from the low volume of blood normally present to a high volume of blood, making the penis hard and erect. More blood flows in from the arteries and less blood flows out through the smaller veins, leading to an erection.

Researchers have found that the penile nerves produce nitric oxide, the chemical messenger that allows an erection. Nitric oxide causes the blood vessels to relax in the corpora cavernosa. When the spaces containing blood relax, they become filled with blood and the erection occurs.

Baby Booster

Take aim! When giving a sperm sample, you may be asked for a split ejaculate, in which the first, sperm-rich portion is deposited in one cup and the remainder in a second cup. The best sperm are usually present in the first part of the ejaculate. Your sample may be reported as low if that first squirt of sperm is lost.

Only about 5 percent of semen is sperm and epididymal fluid, which is why men with vasectomies do not have a change in semen volume. This seminal fluid (or ejaculate) is deposited into your partner's vagina. After ejaculation, erection diminishes because the spaces that contain blood in the corpora cavernosa become smaller, as the muscles and arteries contract. Likewise, the veins that carry blood out of the penis become less compressed, allowing more blood to flow away from the penis.

Good Sperm, Bad Sperm . . . No Sperm

"Whoa! Several hundred million sperm? Who would have ever thought it took that many to make a baby." Nick's response to this fact was nothing short of disbelief. Most men, like Nick, don't realize that during intercourse several hundred million sperm are released inside their partner's vagina. The sperm travel rapidly to the tubes through the cervix and uterus. This motion is mostly caused by the rhythmic contraction of the female organs and less by the sperm's capacity to swim. Only a few hundred of the original sperm will travel up to the upper third of the fallopian tubes, where fertilization most often takes place. After being ejaculated into the vagina, sperm live and can fertilize an egg for about 2 to 5 days. If during these three days ovulation occurs, one of those sperm could penetrate the egg and start a pregnancy. For the record, Nick, it only takes one sperm to make a baby.

Having insufficient numbers of healthy sperm is perhaps the most frequent diagnosis for male infertility. Only a small percent of infertile men have *zero* sperm counts. To make a baby, your sperm must meet the following criteria:

- **Be present in sufficient volume.** If the amount is less than 20 million sperm per milliliter, the chances for conception decrease.
- **Be active and not clumped together.** Weak, lethargic sperm have a difficult time penetrating the barrier of your partner's cervical mucus, much less fertilizing the egg.
- **Be relatively normal in shape and size.** The head of the sperm should be oval-shaped. Sperm with round heads may lack the packet of enzymes at the tip of the sperm head that allow it to penetrate the egg's outer shell.
- **Not be adversely affected by your or your partner's antibodies.**

Sometimes a low sperm count is temporary and can be brought on by a fever, a virus, or the common cold. An infection that causes your white blood cell count to increase is likely to cause a decrease in sperm. High levels of stress or inadequate sleep may also temporarily cause abnormal sperm shapes or declining numbers.

About 1 out of 20 men with completely absent sperm on ejaculation have retrograde ejaculation (RE). This condition occurs when ejaculate is pushed back into the bladder; it may be treated with decongestants, such as pseudoephedrine, which cause a tightening of the bladder neck and prevent reflux. Retrograde flow of sperm may be caused by medications for high blood pressure or surgery on the bladder. Nevertheless, the bottom line is that if your sperm cannot get to where the egg is, then fertilization cannot take place! Infertility usually results when the testes fail to drop or descend into the scrotum. Also, a fever, chronic disease, or severe physical injuries can harm your ability to produce sperm, or block their delivery.

Varicocele Is Common and Easy to Treat

A varicocele is present in 15 to 25 percent of men with male-factor infertility and is the most common and readily treatable problem. This condition is usually caused by failure of the testicular valves, which results in pooling of blood in the scrotum and an elevated temperature. A varico-cele affects fertility due to the decrease in circulation of blood in the tes-ticular area. While you may experience an aching discomfort in the scrotum, the condition is relatively harmless—unless you are trying to make a baby. In fact, studies show that up to 15 percent of all men have varicocele, and many do not experience any complications with fertility.

Nonetheless, if you are diagnosed with varicocele and have large varicosities and pain, your doctor may recommend a surgical procedure to repair this abnormal collection of veins around the testes. Semen quality is often improved, but it is controversial whether this procedure improves fertility. In rare cases, varicocele could cause permanent damage to the testicles, or cause pain leading to testicular failure. In some cases, the surgery has been known to cause rather than cure infertility, so make sure this is necessary.

Injury or Illness

Sometimes during sports or an accident, an injury can occur to your testi-cles. If your testicles are hit, they may atrophy or become smaller. Ill-nesses such as the mumps can also affect how your testicles function. Diabetics are susceptible to problems ranging from nerve damage in the reproductive tract to epididymitis, an infection or inflammation of the epididymis.

Medications Can Decrease Sperm Count

A number of medications, including some of those used to treat infec-tions, ulcers, and high blood pressure, can influence your sperm count and sex drive. Some of the most familiar ones include:

- Azulfidine (a drug used to treat ulcerative colitis).
- Tagamet (for gastrointestinal problems).
- Ketoconazole (an antifungal medication).
- Antibiotics such as the nitrofurans (nitrofurazone or nitrofuran-toin) and the macrolides (erythromycin).
- Tricyclic antidepressants (Elavil, Norpramin, and Pamelor) can

cause abnormally high prolactin levels, which may lead to sperm damage.

- Calcium channel blockers (verapamil), used to treat hypertension, have been related to fertilization failure with IVF.

Chemotherapy drugs may also lower the number of sperm cells, reduce their ability to move, or cause other abnormalities. A chemotherapeutic drug used to treat arthritis blocks cell division and even in low doses may have an effect on sperm. Colchicine, another chemotherapy agent used to treat gout, is a potent inhibitor of DNA synthesis and

Table 5.1 Commonly Used Medications That Zap Fertility

GENERIC NAME	BRAND NAME
Amantadine	Symmetrel
Chlorambucil	
Cimetidine	Tagamet
Colchicine	
Cyclophosphamide	Cytoxan
Erythromycin	EES and others
Gentamicin	Garamycin
Ketoconazole	Nizoral
Lovastatin	Mevacor
Methotrexate	Rheumatrex
Methyldopa	Aldomet
Metoclopramide	Reglan
Mustine	
Neomycin	
Nifedipine	Procardia, Adalat
Nitrofurantoin	Macrodantin, Macrobid
Phenytoin	Dilantin
Prednisolone	
Propranolol	Inderal
Sulfasalazine	Azulfidine
Sulpiride	
Trimethoprim	Proloprim, Septra, Bactrim
Verapamil	Calan
Vincristine	

arrests cell division. If you are about to undergo chemotherapy, talk with your doctor about sperm banking.

Men exposed to diethylstilbestrol (DES) in their mother's womb may have low sperm counts, decreased sperm motility, and abnormal sperm forms, as well as testicular and epididymal abnormalities.

To make sure your doctor knows all your medications, vitamins, and supplements, pack them in a paper bag and take them to your next doctor's visit. This will help him make sure that you will not have a drug-drug interaction that may result in infertility. Also ask him to check the dates to make sure they are not expired. Check out Table 5.1 for medications that may zap fertility.

Erectile Dysfunction

Erectile dysfunction, or impotence, affects more than 50 percent of men aged forty to seventy worldwide. This breaks down to *one out of every ten* men in the United States, yet only about 5 percent of those affected get treatment for their problem. With the aging of America, this problem is only going to skyrocket as baby boomers and busters enter their middle age and senior years. Even though sexual dysfunction is reported in about 20 percent of infertile men, research shows that an estimated 90 percent of those suffering with erectile dysfunction do not seek medical help.

Impotence, which is simply the consistent inability to maintain an erection to satisfy sexual performance, is a frustrating condition that may have psychological, medical, or physical causes. Nonetheless, many types of sexual dysfunction may be confused with impotence. Impotence does not mean premature ejaculation, low sex drive, or infertility. It is not caused by masturbation or too much sex earlier in life. While impotence is common with most men at some point in their lives, it is not normal and can be easily treated.

Many varied causes of erectile dysfunction affect your arteries, veins, nerves, or hormones in a manner to deactivate your erection. Nerve problems may occur after injuries, in diseases such as diabetes mellitus and multiple sclerosis, and with other common medical problems. Antidepressants, tranquilizers, antianxiety drugs, and lithium can all cause erection problems, as can medications widely used to control hypertension. Narrowed arteries can also result in erection problems by impeding blood flow to the penis. This common problem is frequently associated with aging. If the veins don't close off effectively, the blood cannot stay in the penis long enough to cause the erection. (The anxiety and frustration of infertility testing can also cause erectile dysfunction!)

While medical therapy with the drug Viagra may be helpful, this drug should not be considered a cure-all and should be avoided in men with high blood pressure.

Damage or Obstruction Blocks Conception

Tubal obstruction accounts for about 10 percent of male infertility. Half of these men may have been born with abnormal or missing ducts, while the other half usually have blockages from STD infections such as chlamydia or gonorrhea. No matter what the cause, obstructions occur at different points in your reproductive system and keep sperm from coming out.

If you had a hernia repair in the past, there is a chance the vas deferens may have been damaged, blocking the normal flow of sperm during ejaculation. This is a common occurrence in about 15 percent of boys who have had hernia repair. Past surgeries, some medications, or even nerve damage from diabetes mellitus can result in retrograde ejaculation, in which the sperm go in a totally opposite direction and end up in your urine instead of in the ejaculate.

Some men experience infertility because their testicles did not descend during puberty. This may occur because their body temperature is too high and can affect both the quality and quantity of sperm production. Other men may be born with abnormal or missing ducts, such as an absent vas deferens or an abnormal epididymis. Vasectomy is another common cause of infertility. In this surgery, a piece of the vas deferens is cut out and the cut ends are tied off. Thus the semen produced by vasectomized males lacks sperm. Although a repeat reversal procedure could be considered, it is probably better to consider another option. IVF with sperm injection may be performed successfully, but sperm aspiration procedures where sperm are drawn directly from the epididymis or testis are usually avoided. Donor sperm is also an option.

Baby Booster

If you are seeking a sterilization reversal, be sure to select a surgeon who has experience and a high success rate. Ask about the number of cases handled per year. Be cautious when the success rate sounds too good. Possibly even seek a second opinion for comparison. Usually general or spinal anesthesia is required for this procedure, so inquire about all costs, and if it is outpatient or day surgery. The success rates should be more than 50 percent and sometimes near 90 percent.

Is It in Your Genes?

It's important to know your family history, especially if there has been any male-factor infertility. The capacity for normal spermatogenesis rests on the short arm of the Y chromosome. Abnormalities in specific genes of this region are associated with markedly reduced sperm counts. Previously, men with such abnormalities were diagnosed with idiopathic infertility, meaning infertility with no identifiable cause. Today fertility is a possibility, even though there is no treatment for the genetic problem.

Klinefelter's syndrome in men is characterized by an extra X chromosome (XXY) and is thought to occur in about 1 out of 1,000 births. Signs of Klinefelter's include tall stature, long legs and arms, female fat distribution, sparse sexual hair, and very small testes. Gonadotropin levels (LH and FSH) are very high, suggesting gonadal failure, and intellectual functioning and social behavior may be altered. Most men with Klinefelter's have few or no sperm present and are sterile. The good news is that assisted reproduction may be used successfully for conception.

Another genetic condition is the congenital absence of the vas deferens, which is related to the cystic fibrosis gene. Even if you do not have cystic fibrosis, it can still be in your family history. Androgen-receptor deficiency is a rare condition that is associated with lack of sexual development and complete absence of sperm.

All men with an unexplained absence of sperm should consider genetic testing.

Doctor's Rx

If gonadotropins are low due to hypogonadotropic hypogonadism, the GnRH pump, or injections of gonadotropins, which are used to stimulate female fertility, may be useful. It may take several months of daily injections to make a difference. But generally speaking, the medications are different. In some studies clomiphene citrate (Clomid, Serophene) has been used for low sperm counts, yet the reason for infertility was not addressed and the results were not successful.

Immune Reactions Can Weaken Your Sperm

Fewer than 10 percent of infertile men have immune reactions to their own sperm. In this situation, your immune system produces antibodies that attack and weaken the sperm. In some cases, your wife can even have a reaction to your sperm. Immune problems may occur from the following:

- After a vasectomy, which may complicate reversal
- A history of genitourinary tract inflammation
- Testicular injury

However severe, this autoimmune problem can be successfully bypassed by sperm injection and IVF.

Infections Are Another Cause of Male Factor Infertility

Past or present infections such as mumps in adolescence or adulthood may result in infertility. Other infections of reproductive system structures include:

- **Prostatitis.** An infection of the prostate gland that results in inflammation.

- **Epididymitis.** An inflammation or infection of the epididymis that causes discomfort in the testicle region. It is treated with antibiotic therapy, anti-inflammatory drugs (NSAIDs), and support of the scrotum.
- **Orchiditis.** An inflammation of the testis. There are many causes of inflammation of the testis including infections such as mumps, diseases such as polyarteritis nodosa, or injury.

Sexually Transmitted Diseases (STDs) Lower Sperm Count

According to the Centers for Disease Control (CDC), STDs represent 85 percent of leading infectious diseases reported. STDs such as gonorrhea and chlamydia can lower sperm count and motility and cause infertility through inflammatory obstruction of the male genital tract or urethral stricture. STD infection can be widespread throughout the reproductive system in a situation much like pelvic inflammatory disease in women. But men are lucky, if you can call it that, because the genital tract does not open into the pelvic and abdominal cavity, so STD is usually limited to the reproductive organs.

Some of the most common and serious STDs include:

- **Chlamydia.** A bacterial infection that can frequently go on for a long time without producing symptoms yet can cause infertility in men. As many as 4 million Americans may contract it by contact with infected mucous membranes. When symptoms are present, they include a clear discharge, painful urination, and abdominal pain. Treatment for chlamydia is antibiotics taken several times a day for at least a week. Both men and women must be treated to prevent reinfection.
- **Gonorrhea.** The most frequently reported STD. It is usually contracted through intimate sexual activity, with more than 2 million new cases diagnosed annually. With gonorrhea, you will have a cloudy penile discharge, abdominal pain, and burning with urination. You may experience scarring in the urinary channel or urethra. This STD can also spread through your bloodstream and affect other organs, including your brain and heart. Your doctor will prescribe antibiotics for treatment, and some newer drugs are effective against the once-resistant strains.
- **Genital herpes.** An infection that affects more than 30 million

Americans, with 800,000 new cases each year. Genital herpes is triggered by the herpesvirus, which causes cold sores, chicken pox, shingles, and perhaps even cancer. Type I herpes causes cold sores around the mouth. Type II is transmitted through intercourse, but it can infect the mouth during oral sex. While herpes is not deadly, it is chronic. This means that once you get the virus, it stays with you and continues to break out from time to time. After you are infected with genital herpes, you may feel vague, flulike symptoms, along with swollen glands, pain in the legs and abdomen, sores on the genitals and mouth, and fever. These sores contain the virus. When the sores break out, the infection is gone. Interestingly, genital herpes can be transmitted even when no symptoms are present. There is no cure for genital herpes. It is a viral infection, so antibiotics do not work. Acylovir (Zovirax), an ointment, can help ease symptoms, but it will not wipe out the herpes.

• **Condyloma (genital warts).** Tiny warts that look like growths around the genitals. They are caused by the human papilloma virus (HPV). Genital warts are three times more common than herpes and highly contagious. In fact, cervical cancer in females is said to be associated with genital warts. To get rid of condyloma, you need immediate treatment. Your doctor will remove the warts with surgery or a topical preparation may be prescribed. Keep in mind that the virus may return.

Age Is *Not* Always a Risk Factor

While age itself is not a risk factor for male infertility, with the rise in older men becoming fathers, it is a factor to consider. The good news is that most men remain fertile until age 60. The bad news is that the quality of ejaculate and the frequency of intercourse may be reduced for older dads-to-be.

Just as your partner's body undergoes periodic changes, so does yours. The media keeps us informed on changes for women at menopause. Yet do you know that men undergo a host of physiological changes between the ages of 40 and 70?

• Men lose twelve to twenty pounds of muscle, 15 percent of bone mass, and two inches in height.

- The body metabolism slows, and after the age of 40, the testicles shrink slightly and sperm production declines.
- Thickened connective tissue forms in the prostate gland, leading to problems with urination and ejaculation.
- The functioning of the penis becomes sluggish as the chambers responsible for erection fill with connective tissue and its supporting arteries narrow.
- Testosterone loss is subtle compared with the estrogen decline in women at midlife. However, the levels do drop about 1 percent per year after age 40, resulting in a 30 percent decline in testosterone by age 70.
- Some men experience severe drops in their testosterone levels, resulting in hot flashes and night sweats!

Seek Preconception Counseling

Sometimes older dads-to-be are at greater risk for infertility because of chronic illnesses, medications taken for these problems, or declining testosterone levels resulting in decreased sexual interest. No matter what your age, check out the latest in tests and treatments before you conceive to help you produce that super sperm.

Hormone Problems May Be a Barrier

The production of sperm is primarily regulated by the hormones FSH, LH, and testosterone. While most cases of male-factor infertility are not related to hormone problems, there are some instances when hormones may be a factor. If you have a history of delayed or premature sexual maturation, erectile problems, or loss of libido, your doctor may want to do a hormone evaluation. Hormonal problems that may lead to infertility include:

- Low levels of testosterone
- Low levels of FSH and LSH, resulting in sperm deficiency
- Abnormally low thyroid hormone (hypothyroidism), as well as

overactive thyroid (hyperthyroidism), resulting in lack of libido or impotence, as well as sluggish sperm production

- High levels of prolactin (hyperprolactinemia), which inhibit testosterone and decrease sperm production
- High levels of estradiol, which can lead to breast enlargement in men and decreased sperm production

It's Time to Do a Lifestyle Assessment

While your partner's eggs have been with her since before birth, your sperm are fairly new, developing over a three-month period. Did you know that the mature sperm you have today are ultimately affected by your lifestyle for the past three months? This means if you want to make a healthy baby, you need to do a thorough lifestyle check. If you regularly use alcohol, cigarettes, or recreational drugs, wait three months until your system is purified before you try to conceive.

The following lifestyle issues have been suggested as some of the contributing factors to male infertility:

TOBACCO. Studies suggest there is a 64 percent increase in miscarriage when both partners smoke or when just the man smokes. The problem may not be smoke, but nicotine. Smokeless tobacco may be just as bad. Erectile disorder is common in smokers.

RECREATIONAL DRUGS. Long-term use of marijuana in men results in a low sperm count and sperm that exhibit abnormal patterns of development.

CHRONIC ALCOHOL ABUSE. Alcohol lowers sperm density, sperm motility, and the number of normal-appearing sperm. Studies reveal that beer may especially contribute to infertility. Beer consists of hops that boost the levels of the pituitary hormone prolactin. This appears to decrease secretion of gonadotropin-releasing hormone (GnRH) from your hypothalamus and can result in lower levels of FSH and LH by the pituitary. The result? Reduced testosterone output.

ANABOLIC STEROIDS. Anabolic steroids used to increase muscle mass are clearly dangerous to your health and your fertility. Not only can they kill you, they reduce sperm function and have adverse effects on the male endocrine system in general. Steroids used for bulking up your body or to add sports stamina have serious physiological and psychological repercussions, including:

- Heart problems
- Depression and mood swings
- Testicular atrophy
- Reduction in sperm count and quality
- Sterility
- Psychosis

HOT TUBS AND SAUNAS. Anything that raises the temperature of your scrotum, including overheated vehicles and hot work environments, may decrease the number or quality of sperm. As a rule, stay out of hot tubs, Jacuzzis, and saunas. It is reported that Casanova took long hot showers as a contraceptive measure in his amorous exploits.

ENVIRONMENTAL EXPOSURE TO HAZARDS SUCH AS PESTI-CIDES, LEAD PAINT, X-RAYS, RADIOACTIVE SUBSTANCES, MER-CURY, BENZENE, BORON, AND HEAVY METALS. These can alter the production of sperm and are outlined in Chapter 7. Be careful what you do!

EXERCISE. Excessive exercise may lower your sperm count by producing higher levels of adrenal steroid hormones, which lower the amount of testosterone in the body. When you are deficient in testosterone, your sperm production and libido decrease. Often there are not enough calories taken in to support this level of activity and a chronic state of malnutrition exists. Your body senses that this is not a good time to make a baby. Not enough exercise can lead to obesity, with the same outcome. Keep your running to 20 miles or less weekly.

DIET. Specific deficiencies of vitamins and minerals may contribute to altered sperm function. Studies from the University of California at Berkeley and the U.S. Department of Agriculture conclude that sperm may be harmed when your vitamin C intake falls below 60 milligrams per day. Researchers conclude that increased sperm count, motility, and longevity were found in men who consumed 1,000 milligrams a day. Other studies support the popular notion that oysters are the natural aphrodisiac—fourteen oysters have 182 milligrams of zinc. Testicles need zinc and have the highest concentration of this mineral in the body.

STRESS. Endocrinologist Matthew Hardy at the Population Council

---

Doctor's Rx

Low libido is usually the sign of fatigue, yet may also be caused by depression, obesity, alcohol intake, hyperprolactinemia, and some medications such as cardiac drugs.

---

reports that stress also causes a man's sperm count to decrease. Hardy discovered that stress hormones override the enzymes that help cells produce testosterone (necessary for sperm formation) and have a strong negative effect on the male reproductive system. Definitely not good news for Type A men who are trying to start a family! Success in life does not always translate into success with fertility. Sometimes the harder you push, the farther away the goal will get. Relax!

Idiopathic Oligospermia (Unexplained Infertility)

Idiopathic oligospermia is a case of unexplained infertility when your doctor throws up his hands and says, "I don't know why you can't conceive a child." Some researchers believe that extreme over- or underweight, excessive exercise, or environmental toxins may contribute in some way, but scientific studies are inconclusive. In the future, maybe scientists will uncover the answer.

Combination Infertility Can Happen

At least 30 percent of all couples have combined-factor infertility. Each individually may be fertile enough to establish a pregnancy—if there was not a fertility problem in the other. When both you and your partner have infertility problems, your doctor may use the diagnosis combination infertility. The symptoms could vary from your low sperm count and her irregular menstrual periods to a testicle blockage and POCD.

No matter what infertility problems you have, remember that your overall fertility is often a reflection of your healthy lifestyle and good health. In many cases, if you are a healthy and fit male and avoid negative lifestyle habits or exposures to toxins, the chances are great that your sperm will also be strong and healthy. Of course, there are those cases where you cannot control an inherited disorder, chronic disease, or injury to your reproductive parts. In any situation, call your doctor and talk openly about your infertility because most problems can now be overcome with the new technologies available.

Learn All You Can—Then Take Action!

Understanding the causes of male-factor infertility is the first step in making a baby. Next, get your semen evaluated. If two semen analyses are normal, male factor may not be excluded but it becomes less likely.

Make some positive lifestyle changes that will improve your chances of conception and affect your overall health—today and for the future. After all, your baby will need a healthy father in years to come!

Chapter 6

Midlife Mothers: Misconceptions to Conception

"Why did I wait so long?" said Meredith, age 37. "I'm sure my aunt Phyllis blames feminism for the fact that I, and many women like me, spent the vast majority of my childbearing years giving birth to an accounting career rather than a child. I prefer to thank feminism for giving us that choice. But my career hasn't been the greatest obstacle. More important, I was 30 before I had even met the first—and only— man I could imagine having children with, and then it was several more years before I felt confident that I was up to the task.

"Maybe it took someone like my frank gynecologist to unleash the mother in me. At my annual exam, the year I turned 35, she advised, 'In case you are ever thinking of having a child, your window of opportunity is about to slam shut.' In retrospect, I appreciate the fact that she had no trepidation in calling a spade a spade."

Delaying childbearing is common among many couples today for various reasons. Some women choose to postpone pregnancy because of educational or career goals. Others delay starting a family because of worries about the extra financial responsibility entailed. Still other women do not marry until later in life. Or they may have children from an early marriage, divorce, and then start a second family with a new partner. Unfortunately, some women have had years of erratic infertility treatment and end up with age as a major cause of their inability to conceive. The good news is that advances in medical care and changes in demographics have altered our concepts of old and young. The fact that most women over 35 are in excellent health has helped to make midlife parenting a greater possibility.

"Why didn't someone warn me that I'd be the only 43-year-old mother on the maternity floor?" Sheila should not be concerned that she was the only older mother. In fact, if you are like Sheila and delayed starting a family, you have great company. The March of Dimes estimates that in the year 2000, one in every twelve babies will be born to women age 35 or older. Although the birth rate among women older than 40 has *increased* by nearly 50 percent in the last twenty years, the chance of getting pregnant dramatically *decreases* during a woman's late thirties. Studies show that fertility declines after age 30, with this decline accelerating around 37 to 38 years, and falling sharply after 40 (see Figure 6.1). Your partner's sperm count, motility, and fertilizing potential may slightly decrease with age, yet declines in male fertility are not found until approximately age 60. Even, the Bible contains stories of

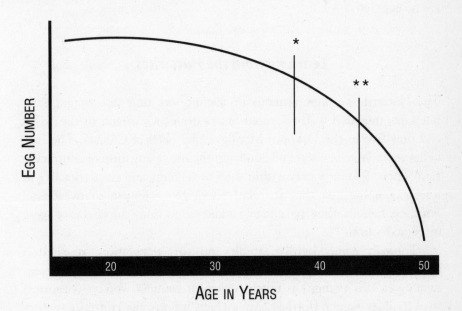

Figure 6.1   Theoretical age-related decline in the oocyte pool
*average age at which the rapid acceleration of oocyte loss begins
**average age at which natural childbearing stops

men in their nineties fathering children. For women, the likelihood of a pregnancy after age 45 is an extremely rare event—without medical intervention.

Blame It on the Dwindling Egg Supply

"So Rick can father children for decades, while I'm cursed with this limited biological capability that takes a nosedive after age 25?" Thirty-two-year-old Lisa was not thrilled with this disparity.

While that is usually the case, you could be in your midtwenties and have difficulty getting pregnant if you have poor quality eggs. Your best friend may be surprised with an unplanned pregnancy at 40-something. Nonetheless, your biological clock does tick away each day as the number of eggs in each ovary decreases by hundreds each month. In fact, the peak number of eggs in the ovaries is actually during fetal life at twenty weeks gestation, when 6 to 8 million are present. Even before you are born, the number of eggs starts to decline until soon after menopause when there are no eggs left.

Learning from the Hutterites

The Hutterites, a monogamous Protestant sect that discourages early marriage, migrated to the United States from Switzerland in the 1870s and now live in the Dakotas, Montana, and parts of Canada. They are believers in large families and condemn the use of any form of contraception. They also marry only within their own group, and since they live in a set geographic area, they are relatively easy for scientists to investigate. For these reasons, they make ideal candidates to study the effects of aging on reproduction.

Through comprehensive studies on this population, researchers found that the fertility rate (the number of women achieving a pregnancy per 100 women) is much higher in younger women (twenties) than in older women (forties). After a baby is born, the Hutterite mother immediately tries to achieve pregnancy again. However, it was noted that the time between pregnancies became increasingly longer with the increasing age of the women studied. The average age at the time of the last pregnancy was 40.9 years among Hutterite women.

Researchers also found that 11 percent of the Hutterite women bore no children after age 34, 33 percent had no children after age 40, and 87 percent had no children after age 44—and this is without any contraception. This corresponds to numerous studies in various populations over several centuries that have shown the last child is born by age 41. Long-term studies of 182,252 pregnancies revealed only three documented pregnancies to women age 50, compared with 52 pregnancies at age 46 and 21 pregnancies between the ages of 47 and 49.

Advancing Age Refers to Egg Quality

Keep in mind that when you read about advancing age in regard to conception, scientists are really targeting the issue of oocyte or egg quality, not your actual age. The longer an egg sits around in your ovary, the more likely it is to develop abnormalities in its chromosomes. If an egg with abnormal chromosomes is fertilized, then the chances are greater that the resulting pregnancy will end in miscarriage. In fact, chromosomal abnormality is the single most common cause of miscarriage. Study after study confirms that more than half of all miscarriages are due to abnormal chromosomes.

Consider the facts: a young woman in her twenties has a 12 to 15 percent chance of having a miscarriage each time she becomes pregnant. But a woman in her forties has a 50 percent risk of miscarriage with each pregnancy. As you realize, not every pregnancy in which the embryo has abnormal chromosomes will end in a miscarriage. Some will continue to develop and even result in the live birth of a baby. These babies, however, may have a host of medical challenges, including mental retardation and birth defects.

Because of the decrease in healthy eggs, reproductive tract injuries, endometriosis or myomas, and also the ovaries' resistance to stimulation, women in their late thirties are about 30 percent less fertile than they were in their early twenties. In fact, the woman's most fertile time is around age 25.

So Many Midlife Misconceptions

"Having a baby was not a reality in my twenties," Liz said. "When I was 25, I was in graduate school and unmarried. Now I'm approaching 37 and we are just now talking about starting our family. Are you saying it is too late?" No, to say that you are too old is a common misconception. Nonetheless, if you are 35 or older, you need to take action—today!

Although the statistics are not in favor of older mothers, there is great hope today for those who have postponed making babies. While the egg quality may have declined, the uterus of a woman in her forties, fifties, or even sixties can still serve as a nurturing womb. With prompt evaluation and aggressive treatment, most infertile older women today can achieve very high pregnancy rates with egg donation.

If you are an older woman contemplating pregnancy, you need to look at both the physiologic and psychological issues; in other words, you need to know the odds you're up against. There are two key realities to consider: it is more difficult to conceive after 35, and it can be more difficult to successfully carry a fetus to term after 35.

Pregnancy Is More Difficult for Older Mothers

As discussed, older mothers are more likely to face issues such as chromosomal abnormalities and infertility. When you are pregnant, your blood volume nearly doubles, increasing the strain on your heart. The extra weight puts extra pressure on your muscles and joints. There are also chronic medical problems to consider such as hypertension, diabetes, or premature menopause. Often, a shortening of the menstrual cycle by two to three days is seen as the beginning of the transition to menopause. Since reproductive function declines significantly before menopause, some researchers hypothesize that the uterus or the hypothalamus is the primary target of aging. Nonetheless, the largest factor of declining reproductive potential is egg quality. Oocyte decline occurs at a steady rate throughout a woman's reproductive life, with an accelerated loss around age 38. Other factors such as surgery, radiation, pelvic disease, or genetic disorders also serve to hasten the loss.

Other concerns older women face include:

- The risk of hypertension during pregnancy, which doubles for women over 35.
- Gestational diabetes, which is two to three times more common in women over age 35 than in younger women.
- The risk of fetal death, which is twice as high as that of younger women, even after controlling for coexisting conditions such as diabetes and hypertension and taking into account improved obstetric care.
- The chance of ectopic pregnancy increases.
- The chance of cesarean delivery increases (about 40 percent higher than a younger woman's).

Nonetheless, if you are in good health and take care of yourself, the chances are great that you can successfully conceive and deliver a healthy baby. The usual recommendation of waiting a period of a year of attempting conception before you have an infertility evaluation does not apply to women age 35 or older. A basic infertility evaluation is suggested for any anxious couple who has been attempting conception for six months if the woman is over 35.

Your 35+ Medical Evaluation

Among the first steps your doctor will take include:

- A thorough preconception medical evaluation.
- A mammogram.
- Laboratory tests for diabetes and heart disease. Diabetic mothers are at greater risk for preeclampsia, preterm delivery, placental problems, or stillbirth. Women with diabetes are also more likely to have a child with poor fetal growth or birth defects.
- Ongoing blood pressure monitoring. Blood pressure normally rises during pregnancy, which can worsen an existing condition, putting you at risk of seizures or stroke.

Even if everything checks out normal and you don't have diabetes or high blood pressure, you still have an increased risk of developing gestational diabetes and pregnancy-induced hypertension (PIH). Both illnesses increase the chances of having eclampsia, a complication of pregnancy characterized by high blood pressure, swelling of your face and hands, and protein in your urine. Eclampsia is very serious and can impair your nervous system function, and also lead to stroke, seizures, or other health problems.

Older Mothers Have More Chromosome Abnormalities

One of the biggest issues for older mothers is the risk of having a child with chromosomal abnormalities. The most common is Down's syndrome, a condition that causes mental retardation and defects of the heart and other organs. While your risk of having a child with Down's syndrome is one in thirty at age 45, at age 49, the risk is one in twenty-one chances. Because of the increased incidence of genetic defects in infants born to older mothers (see Table 6.1), your doctor will discuss such prenatal tests as amniocentesis before conception (see Table 6.2).

Checking Your Infertility History

As discussed in Chapter 2, your doctor will ask questions about your infertility history including:

- Length of time you have been trying to conceive
- The frequency of intercourse
- Menstrual regularity
- Premenstrual problems
- Any prior pregnancies

Table 6.1 Chromosomal Abnormalities Per 1,000 Live Births According to Maternal Age

MATERNAL AGE	DOWN'S SYNDROME	ALL OTHERS	TOTAL
25–29	0.90	1.36	2.24
30–34	1.48	1.72	3.20
35–39	5.56	2.98	8.54
40–44	20.12	7.52	27.64

Table 6.2   Commonly Recommended Prenatal Tests

Amniocentesis
A needle is inserted into your uterus and a sample of the amniotic fluid surrounding the fetus is withdrawn. Usually done within fifteen to twenty weeks of gestation, although it can be performed as early as ten to twelve weeks. The test is 99 percent accurate but carries a 0.5 percent chance of miscarriage.

Chorionic villus sampling (CVS)
Cells are taken from the placenta via your abdominal wall or cervix. CVS is usually done between weeks ten and twelve of your pregnancy. It is about 98 percent accurate and has a 1 to 2 percent risk of miscarriage.

Alpha-fetoprotein screening (AFP)
This blood test checks the level of a substance produced by the liver of the fetus. This level is usually high with some types of birth defects and low when there is Down's syndrome. AFP may be falsely elevated in IVF pregnancy or multiple pregnancy. Since the level changes with pregnancy age, dating may be the problem. Sometimes this test is performed in conjunction with HCG and estriol levels, the so-called Triple Test.

Ultrasound
High-resolution and color Doppler ultrasound imaging are used to identify traits such as shortened thigh bones or gastrointestinal blockage that may be associated with Down's syndrome. Ultrasound is an immensely valuable, noninvasive tool, and with the much improved resolution, even very minor structural abnormalities can usually be identified.

Also important when considering pregnancy is a comprehensive general health evaluation, including a cardiac, respiratory, skeletal, and gastrointestinal review. An FSH and estradiol level (see Chapter 11) are absolutely essential to help determine egg stores. Early in the evaluation an ultrasound should be performed to exclude uterine fibroids. A sono-hysterosalpingogram (SONO HSG) can also be useful to exclude the presence of polyps or other problems of the endometrial lining.

Don't forget Dad! He may have aged, too. A semen analysis should be performed early in the investigation. Be sure to tell the doctor of any medication he is using, as some can have severe consequences on fertility.

If your fertility evaluation is normal, or if the abnormalities have been corrected and you still do not promptly conceive, it's time to take aggressive action.

Stop the Clock!

Unfortunately, no miraculous treatments can turn back the clock on a woman's ovaries. Many physicians use fertility medications that increase the number of eggs that develop in a given month, therefore enhancing the chance that at least one of them might be able to be fertilized and develop into a viable pregnancy. Others have advocated in vitro fertilization (IVF) as a means to achieve pregnancy in such cases. Unfortunately, the pregnancy rates with IVF in women over age forty are very low.

Consider Egg Donation for Age-Related Infertility

Currently, most experts agree that the only consistently successful method to improve pregnancy rates in women with age-related infertility is *egg donation*. The criteria of those women who would benefit most from egg donation include:

- Age over forty
- Persistently high FSH levels at any age
- Poor response to fertility medications at any age
- Poor egg quality IVF
- Age-related recurrent miscarriage with identifiable egg issues (age, chromosomal)

As compared to pregnancy rates of less than 10 percent per cycle for women over the age of forty, egg donation results in pregnancy rates of over 35 percent per cycle. In addition, the risks of miscarriage and Down's syndrome are dramatically reduced. Thus the likelihood of making a healthy baby is much higher. A recent study presented at the IVF World Congress suggested that after four cycles of egg donation, more than 80 percent of women delivered a baby.

Getting the Highest Pregnancy Success Rate

Egg or oocyte donation, particularly using the eggs of a younger woman, gives the highest rate of pregnancy that is achievable with any type of fertility treatment, even for women in their forties, fifties, or sixties. In fact, recent studies show that a success rate of between 35 and 50 percent per cycle can be expected in recipients who are age 40 and older.

Creating the Nurturing Environment

With egg donation, your doctor will prepare your uterus using exogenous estrogen and progesterone to create an optimal environment for implantation. The egg donor then undergoes hormonal stimulation to produce multiple oocytes. These eggs are retrieved with transvaginal ultrasound-guided needle aspiration and fertilized with sperm from your partner. By means of uterine transfer, the fertilized embryos (gametes) are then replaced in your body.

Egg Donation Gives Maternal Benefits

Successful oocyte donation may offer you many advantages over adoption.

1. The sperm is obtained from your partner, and the child is genetically his.
2. Since the pregnancy develops inside you, you have optimal control over such key lifestyle factors as diet, smoking, and drinking during the pregnancy—control you would not have for adoption.
3. You can experience the positive maternal feelings of pregnancy and delivery and can breast-feed—all important moments in establishing a nuturing attachment toward your new baby.

At this time, oocyte donation may be the best option for women over age 40 who have been repeatedly unsuccessful with other fertility therapies, as well as for women with a basal FSH level above fifteen.

If only egg donation were as easy as sperm donation! It is too bad that there are far more recipients than donors. This has dramatically increased the cost of the procedure. Hopefully, in the future it may be possible to obtain large numbers of eggs from donor ovaries that could be placed in an egg bank, just like sperm.

There are several reports in which eggs—not embryos—have been frozen and later thawed to produce a pregnancy. The present success rate is about 1 percent—hardly satisfactory. Yet there are early indications that the procedure holds promise for the future.

What About Cytoplasmic Transfer?

Until now, women whose eggs were defective because of age or other problems could become pregnant only by using a donated egg, which results in offspring not genetically related to the mother. However, in a 1998 study, documented in the British journal *The Lancet*, researchers removed about 5 percent of the fluid from another younger woman's "donor egg" and injected that fluid, along with a single sperm from the older woman's husband, directly into the older mother-to-be's eggs. They did so for a total of fourteen of the woman's eggs, eight of which responded by dividing in laboratory dishes. The four healthiest-looking embryos were transferred into the woman's womb, and one developed successfully. In this study, a healthy girl was born nine months later. (It's important to note that as of this writing, cytoplasmic transfer has had very limited success, and risks to the offspring are unknown.)

You're Never Too Old

Midlife mothers, stand up and be counted! Connie's story should give hope to any woman who is seeking to get pregnant. "When Mac and I got married at age 25, all I wanted was to start a family. We never used birth control pills and knew that nature would take its course eventually. After two years, I was so frustrated that I gave up and applied for a teaching position. We didn't want to go through infertility testing. Our friends were doing that, and Mac was hesitant. Looking back, I can see that we were in denial that we had a problem at all.

"Anyway, I taught school for eight years and loved it. We talked about having kids, but after that many years, we knew that our chances of being parents were slim. Then after Christmas several years ago, I started to feel different: I was queasy for about a week and had a horrible time making it through the day teaching. I just wanted to sleep. I brushed it off as a virus or flu, but it persisted. I felt bloated and my breasts felt so swollen.

"After three weeks of thinking I was dying, I finally got the courage to go to my doctor. During the exam she asked me if I thought I might be pregnant. Of course I never thought that—not after trying for a decade! She ran some blood tests and later confirmed what she knew to be true— I was pregnant. Less than nine months from that time, she delivered our first baby—a healthy boy. It was truly our miracle."

There are millions of stories like Connie's that can give you encouragement. In fact, there has never been a better time than now to get pregnant, especially with breakthrough reproductive technology and the rate of fetal deaths down by more than 70 percent since the 1960s. A host of studies conclude that if you are in good health, have gotten pregnant, and have passed your prenatal screening tests, you are much more likely to deliver a healthy baby than not. Even women seeking to conceive after age 40 have no difficulty in achieving a pregnancy with today's medical breakthroughs, and that's good news.

Chapter 7

Lifestyle and Workplace Causes of Infertility

"Who would have thought that my career was contributing to my infertility?" said Claire, 34. "After having two miscarriages, we were ready to fill out forms for adoption when my husband found some studies on the Internet, alluding to the fact that airline attendants have a higher incidence of miscarriage. While the studies were not conclusive, and my RE said there was probably no correlation, I was willing to try anything to have a baby. I took a leave of absence from the airlines and within five months I was pregnant—and stayed pregnant until the birth of our twins."

You don't think about the detrimental effects of your workplace, home environment, or even lifestyle on your body—until you try to conceive and can't. Then your anxiety levels soar, and your mind starts to race: *Am I having trouble conceiving because of all the alcohol and smoking during college years? Perhaps it was the polluted air I inhaled while jogging after work. What about the electrical generating station down the street, or the paint fumes I inhaled when refinishing that old dresser? Could any of these be contributing to my infertility?*

While each of us is affected differently and much of the research is not yet conclusive, some common environmental and lifestyle triggers may make it difficult to conceive. Think about it. Compared with the lives of those of generations past, our high-tech lives are definitely more complex. Not only do we have multiple stressors juggling careers and commitments, most of us have to deal with longer work hours, compressed workweeks, shift work, reduced job security, and part-time and temporary work. Now add to these stressors a host of toxic chemicals, materials, processes, and equipment (such as latex gloves in health care or fermentation processes in biotechnology), and you can see how your reproductive health may be compromised.

So what are the chances that environmental or lifestyle factors may be hindering your reproductive process? Look at the following questions and mark any risk factors that pertain to you with a yes or no.

____ 1. Do you smoke cigarettes?

____ 2. Do you drink alcoholic beverages?

____ 3. Do you use recreational drugs (anabolic steroids, marijuana, or cocaine)?

____ 4. Do you spend a lot of time out-of-doors or exercise outside during highly polluted times?

____ 5. Do you take medications?

____ 6. Do you spend more than ten hours a month flying on airplanes?

____ 7. Is your diet high in additives such as aspertame?

____ 8. Have you been exposed to chemicals at work or at home?

____ 9. Have you handled toxins found in pesticides?

____ 10. Have you worked a computer for long periods of time?

____ 11. Have you been exposed to lead (paint, varnish)?

____ 12. Have you been exposed to ethylene oxide?

____ 13. Have you been exposed to radiation sources (x-rays or chemotherapy)?

____ 14. Is the air you breathe polluted or does it have an odor?

How did you score? The more questions you answered yes to, the more male or female infertility problems you may have and the more difficult it may be to get pregnant.

You Can Run, But You Can't Hide

So, what's out there wreaking havoc with your reproductive health? Sometimes a wide array of often invisible but deleterious things. The different toxins we come in contact with daily are innumerable. In fact, such toxic chemicals as DDT and PCBs, which were banned nearly two decades ago, are still found in ecosystems, animals, and even humans throughout the United States. Groundwater in many areas is contaminated with metals, pesticides, solvents, or nitrates—all known to be toxic to our reproductive systems, and many of which may act as hormone disrupters.

What about the air you breathe? Now that's difficult to control. Still, did you realize that invisible particles, including radioactive sensors, electromagnetic waves, or air pollutants, may infiltrate the air around you and cause damage? Adding to the air pollution are the billions of pounds of DDT, PCBs, dioxins, alkyphenols, polychlorinated biphenyls, and other chlorine-containing compounds made annually. While you may not see them as poison, they are part of packaging or in metal food-can linings, cosmetics, paint, furniture, and pesticides. Even the residues of these poisons are absorbed daily from drinking water, from the tampons you use, or from the air you breathe. Some types of PCBs can persist in human tissue and blood from one to even twenty years.

If you think this is an overreaction, look at some of your cleaning solvents such as rug or upholstery shampoos, bathroom cleaners, or whitening laundry additives. Now check the labels and read the warnings. The skull and crossbones symbol is there for a reason! If you have ever sniffed drain cleaner or inhaled a soap scum remover in a nonventilated area, you already know those chemicals can wreak havoc with your lungs. Imagine what they are doing to your delicate reproductive system. For example:

- Studies have revealed that pesticides are linked to the drastically declining sperm counts in human males and other species. In one large study involving 15,000 men in the United States and Europe, researchers found that the human male sperm count had dropped 45 percent between 1938 and 1990.
- To these same commonly used poisons are attributed the increase in premature puberty, as well as startling increases in the rates of breast cancer.
- In the last three decades, the rate of testicular cancer has tripled.
- In Great Britain, studies done between 1970 and 1987 report a doubling of undescended testicles and the prevalence of hypospadias (abnormal urethral opening).

Take Control of Your Environment

You cannot deny the studies indicating a link between your environment, lifestyle, and reproductive problems. Everywhere you turn is a possible trigger for infertility. The secondhand smoke of a coworker, the chemicals you touch, the air you breathe, or even the days you spend in front of a computer screen could leave you struggling for months or even years to make a baby. Yet there is good news! If you understand the known environmental and lifestyle triggers and how they may affect your fertility, you can take proactive steps right now to avoid or eliminate these triggers and save your reproductive health.

How's Your Workplace Wellness?

Today, millions of women work outside the home, especially during the young adult years before starting a family. Overall, work before or even during pregnancy is not associated with an increased risk of problems. However, if your career requires prolonged periods of standing or long working hours, these factors may put you at increased risk for preterm birth and the delivery of a low-birth-weight infant. Mental stress at work may exaggerate this risk (see Chapters 15, 16, and 17 for more on coping with stress). For flight attendants, the risk of miscarriage for those who continue to work during pregnancy may nearly double. A number of studies show that flight attendants have many potentially hazardous on-the-job exposures, including increased gravitational forces and increased exposure to radiation.

Electromagnetic Radiation May Zap Fertility

What about the video display terminal where you work? Could it be implicated in causing increased risk of miscarriage? While recent studies cannot confirm these results, some researchers strongly believe women who are exposed to video display terminals more than twenty hours a week may be at higher risk for pregnancy loss because of electromagnetic radiation (EMR).

Your computer monitor isn't the only place where electromagnetic radiation may affect you. EMR and electric fields are present almost everywhere there is development. Electromagnetic radiation emanates from electric power lines, fluorescent light fixtures, and a host of household devices. Even low-voltage appliances such as heating pads, electric blankets, toaster ovens, and clock radios may decrease your fertility by damaging your eggs or upsetting ovulation. Today there is widespread controversy over whether nonionizing radiation (radiation too weak to break chemical bonds) is hazardous to human health and the reproductive system. Nonetheless, questions still remain as to how to measure fields generated by video terminals and other devices to determine how this may affect your fertility. Further studies are planned at the recently formed Video Display Terminal Health Foundation research center at Johns Hopkins.

THE BOTTOM LINE: Reproductive hazards do not affect every woman or every pregnancy. Whether you or your future baby are harmed may depend on the following:

- *How much* of the hazard you are exposed to
- *When* you are exposed
- *How long* you are exposed
- *How* you are exposed

Be Proactive

Video display terminals (VDTs) emit various electromagnetic field (EMF) frequencies. Laboratory tests show that living matter is most sensitive to EMF radiation during periods of rapid cell-splitting, which includes pregnancy/gestation and reproduction-related cycles (sperm development and menstrual cycles). Although the threat of radiation exposure from video display terminals is discounted, there are some actions you can take:

- Increase your distance from the terminal to reduce your potential exposure to electromagnetic fields.
- Make sure you use video display terminals that have the U.S. Environmental Protection Agency's Energy Star label and that

your workplace provides the same. Energy Star monitors emit fewer EMFs because they are not displaying any visual image when in the sleep mode (when you are not using it). Most new terminals are considered safe and have low EMF emissions. However, if you are using an old computer system, ask your employer to update the monitor.

- Limit the use of your microwave if it is old.
- If you suspect a leakage from your microwave, get a home testing kit to see if it is emitting nonionizing radiation.
- Watch television from a distance of at least ten feet to minimize the effect of any nonionizing radiation affecting your fertility.
- Keep your electric alarm clock on your dresser—far from your body.
- Avoid the use of electric blankets or heating pads.

Radioactive Fallout and Infertility

There are well-known negative effects from exposure to high doses of ionizing radiation that may result in menstrual cycle abnormalities. For example, two radioactive isotopes, cesium 137 and 134, have been found throughout Europe since the Chernobyl nuclear plant accident in 1986. In a comprehensive study comparing European and American women undergoing in vitro fertilization (IVF), researchers found detectable amounts of these isotopes in the follicular fluid. Seventy-four European women were undergoing eighty-three IVF cycles and twenty-five American women were undergoing twenty-five cycles. Approximately half the European samples contained isotopes, compared with a quarter of American samples. Researchers also concluded that there was a strong correlation between poor reproductive performance and presence of the isotope cesium 137.

THE BOTTOM LINE: Low-dose, intermittent, or continuous exposure to medical imaging technologies or other environmental or occupational sources have not been studied regarding the potential effects they might have on the female reproductive system. Nevertheless, this is a potential risk factor for infertility that you should be aware of.

The Toxic Effect of Chemicals and Pollutants

There are thousands of chemicals present in the environment and workplace. While you'd like to think you have avoided the most toxic ones, inescapably, more and more of them are a part of our daily lives. Consider those who work in the medical field. Studies conclude that ethylene oxide, a chemical used to sterilize surgical instruments and to manufacture pesticides, may cause birth defects in early pregnancy and has the potential to cause early miscarriage. Along with that, repeated exposure to radiation, such as x-rays, has been shown to affect sperm production and contribute to ovarian problems.

What about the two million tons of pesticides, herbicides, and fungicides introduced into the environment each year, with the United States contributing about 20 percent? While they are suspected to affect reproduction, published reproductive toxicology studies are available on less than 1 percent of these chemicals. In fact, for the vast majority of industrial chemicals, no reproductive toxicity information exists.

Environmental exposure to chemicals is often complex. There may be additive effects, and a high risk of exposure may occur in many occupations. Harmful substances can enter your body in various ways, including:

- Breathing in (inhalation)
- Contact with the skin
- Swallowing (ingestion)

Some known toxic chemicals include:

PESTICIDES AND CHLORINATED HYDROCARBONS. Pesticides such as ant or roach sprays are in widespread use and represent chemicals we may encounter on a daily basis that accumulate in our bodies. Agricultural chemicals including pesticides, herbicides, and fungicides are notorious for this. Some of these chemicals have been found to cause decreased sperm counts and fertility in exposed factory, agricultural, and forestry workers.

These chemicals have been shown to also affect women. For example, menstrual disorders were observed in a population of Japanese women who inadvertently consumed vegetable oil contaminated with polychlorinated biphenyls (PCBs). These chlorinated hydrocarbons are widely used in transformers as heat exchangers. Many chemicals, such as the PCBs and DDT, have become pervasive in nature because of careless disposal, overuse, and their extreme stability. Some studies have revealed that measured PCB levels in adults correlate directly to the amount of fish consumed annually from Lake Michigan. Handling the toxins found in pesticides, such as DBCP, may lead to ovarian problems in women, possibly leading to early menopause.

To determine the presence of chlorinated hydrocarbons (including DDT, dieldrin, PCBs, and hexachlorobenzene), researchers in Germany examined follicular fluid obtained from women undergoing in vitro fertilization. A trend of lower conception rates and numbers of oocytes recovered was noted with increasing concentrations of chlorinated hydrocarbons. One group of women with high levels of PCBs had significantly lower (37 percent) oocyte recovery compared with controls (87 percent). Another study confirmed the presence of chlorinated hydrocarbons in follicular fluids and found as much as twenty times higher concentrations in the cervical mucus of women with unexplained infertility. Perhaps a high concentration of chlorinated hydrocarbons interferes with the function of spermatozoa. There have been a few limited clinical studies suggesting increased rates of miscarriages in the partners of men who are exposed to vinyl chloride and dibromochloropropane.

Many chemical compounds, including DDT, PCBs, methoxychlor, and chlordecone, are estrogenic and can act like estrogens and disrupt progestational events. These compounds may also act like partial or weak estrogen antagonists, and disrupt estrogen-dependent events, or interfere with implantation and tubal transport of the egg.

SOLVENTS AND CLEANERS. In the garment and dry-cleaning industry, there is extensive use of the solvents methylene chloride, trichloroethylene, and formaldehyde. In addition, methylene chloride is a volatile solvent used widely as a paint stripper, degreasing agent, and fat extractant. These suspected carcinogens are known to be harmful to the reproductive system. Menstrual disorders have been documented after exposures to methylene chloride. The long half-life of many compounds may result in cumulative reproductive toxicity; for example, the risk for unexplained infertility among women working in the dry-cleaning industry may be as much as three times higher than in the general population.

Toluene, an industrial solvent widely used in paints, glues, and varnishes, may induce lengthening of menstrual cycles in exposed women. Recently, a comprehensive review of chemicals encountered by firefighters implicated many of the solvents above as potentially hazardous to the female reproductive system.

HEAVY METALS. Many heavy metals, including cadmium, mercury, and lead, have been released into the environment. The most common routes of exposure occur by dermal absorption, inhalation, or diet. Metals enter the food chain often by way of bioconcentration in the environment. Metals are notable for interacting directly with the reproductive system. They have all been implicated in causing infertility. In one study, exposure of workers to mercury vapors in a lamp factory suggested an increasing trend of menstrual disturbances and decreased fertility as well as adverse pregnancy outcome.

More than a hundred years ago, lead was discovered to cause miscarriages, stillbirths, and infertility in female pottery workers. Today, studies show that women with occupational exposures to cadmium, lead, or mercury have an increased risk ratio of 2.9 for unexplained infertility and a 1.7-fold increase in risk for delayed conception. Animal studies reveal that lead ingestion is associated with reproductive problems in adult females. In humans, these problems might appear as menstrual cycle irregularities, abnormal menstruation (either lack of menstrual periods or excessive bleeding during menstrual periods), ovarian cyst development, or delayed sexual maturation. Exposure to lead might appear as decreased sperm counts, low sperm movement, increased prostate gland weight, or impotence for human males.

ANESTHETIC GASES. Women exposed to anesthetics on a regular basis (operating room personnel, dental professionals) often have increased circulating levels of these substances in their bodies and possibly are at greater risk for miscarriages and infertility. Dental technicians exposed to high levels of nitrous oxide (greater than five hours per week) may have reduced fertility and increased rates of pregnancy loss.

THE BOTTOM LINE: Even though studies show a direct correlation between chemicals, toxins, and reproductive problems, it is difficult to prove that exposures at the workplace lead to infertility. Because there are no easy answers, you need to do what you feel is right for your health and reduce any exposure to known toxic substances.

Table 7.1 Chemical and Physical Agents That Are Reproductive Hazards for Women in the Workplace

AGENT	OBSERVED EFFECTS	POTENTIALLY EXPOSED WORKERS
Cancer treatment drugs (e.g., methotrexate)	Infertility, miscarriage, birth defects, low birth weight	Health care workers, pharmacists
Certain ethylene glycol ethers such as 2-ethoxyethanol (2EE) and 2-methoxyethanol (2ME)	Miscarriages	Electronic and semiconductor workers
Carbon disulfide (CS_2)	Menstrual cycle changes	Viscose rayon workers
Lead	Infertility, miscarriage, low birth weight, developmental disorders	Battery makers, solderers, welders, radiator repairers, bridge repainters, firing range workers, home remodelers
Ionizing radiation (e.g., x-rays and gamma rays)	Infertility, miscarriage, birth defects, low birth weight, developmental disorders, childhood cancers	Health care workers, dental personnel, atomic workers
Strenuous physical labor (e.g., prolonged standing, heavy lifting)	Miscarriage late in pregnancy, premature delivery	Many types of workers

Table 7.2 Disease-Causing Agents That Are Reproductive Hazards for Women in the Workplace

AGENT	OBSERVED EFFECTS	POTENTIALLY EXPOSED WORKERS	PREVENTIVE MEASURES
Cytomegalovirus (CMV)	Birth defects, low birth weight, developmental disorders	Health care workers, workers in contact with infants and children	Good hygienic practices such as handwashing
Hepatitis B virus	Low birth weight	Health care workers	Vaccination
Human immuno-deficiency virus (HIV)	Low birth weight, childhood cancer	Health care workers	Practice universal precautions
Human parvo-virus B19	Miscarriage	Health care workers, workers in contact with infants and children	Good hygienic practices such as handwashing
Rubella (German measles)	Birth defects, low birth weight	Health care workers, workers in contact with infants and children	Vaccination before pregnancy if no prior immunity
Toxoplasmosis	Miscarriage, birth defects, developmental disorders	Animal care workers, veterinarians	Good hygiene practices such as handwashing
Varicella zoster virus (chicken pox)	Birth defects, low birth weight	Health care workers, workers in contact with infants and children	Vaccination before pregnancy if no prior immunity

When Temperature Is a Problem

Temperature is an inexpensive and convenient characteristic of ovarian function. Basal body temperatures (BBT) are commonly used to predict ovulation and reflect the possible temperature sensitivity of the female reproductive system. In males, elevation in testicular temperature leads to the decline of sperm and infertility. Hyperthermia in male and female animals also leads to reproductive dysfunction. Although there are no studies examining the effects of heat on the reproductive system in women, a recent study was performed on women exposed to extremely cold temperatures working at a slaughterhouse. Irregular menstrual cycles and work-shift variability correlated positively with extended exposure to cold temperatures.

Proactive Steps You Can Take

"I'm completely distraught. My husband is an x-ray technician, and I work in a fertilizer manufacturing plant. Our city is known to be polluted. Is there any hope for us to ever have a baby?" You can take proactive steps to ensure your own safety. In other words, don't wait for the studies to confirm what scientists already speculate. The National Occupational Research Agenda, which is part of the National Institute for Occupational Safety and Health (NIOSH), recommends the following:

- Store chemicals in sealed containers when they are not in use.
- Wash hands after contact with hazardous substances and before eating, drinking, or smoking.
- Avoid skin contact with chemicals.
- If chemicals contact the skin, follow the directions for washing in the material safety data sheet (MSDS). Employers are required to have copies of MSDSs for all hazardous materials used in their workplaces and to provide them to workers upon request.
- Review all MSDSs to become familiar with any reproductive hazards used in your workplace. If you are concerned about reproductive hazards in the workplace, consult your doctor or health care provider.

- Participate in all safety and health education, training, and monitoring programs offered by your employer.
- Learn about proper work practices and engineering controls (such as improved ventilation).
- Use personal protective equipment (gloves, respirators, and personal protective clothing) to reduce exposures to workplace hazards.
- Follow your employer's safety and health work practices and procedures to prevent exposures to reproductive hazards.

Steps to Prevent Home Contamination

- Change out of contaminated clothing and wash with soap and water before going home.
- Store street clothes in a separate area of the workplace to prevent contamination.
- Wash work clothing separately from other laundry (at work if possible).
- Avoid bringing contaminated clothing or other objects home. If work clothes must be brought home, transport them in a sealed plastic bag.

Don't Let Your Fertility Go Up in Smoke

Hosts of scientific studies have examined the extent to which smoking affects fertility and conclude:

- Smoking decreases fertility in women by delaying time to conception.
- Infertility is more prevalent in smokers than nonsmokers.
- Smoking increases menstrual dysfunction.
- Women who smoke a pack or more a day undergo menopause almost two years earlier than nonsmokers.
- There is a significant decrease in the percent of conceptions in a

given cycle of nonsmokers to smokers (38 percent versus 28 percent, respectively).

- Delays of one year or greater to achieve conception were three to four times as likely in smokers as in nonsmokers.
- Smoking twenty or more cigarettes a day is positively associated with decreased fertility and yielded a relative risk for primary infertility of 1.36.
- Smoking is correlated with cervical factor and tubal disease.
- Fallopian tube motility is decreased by cigarette smoking. This may result in altered transport of gametes, delays in blastocyst implantation, and therefore decreased chances of conception.
- Smokers have increased incidence of tubal ectopic pregnancies and spontaneous abortions.
- Smoking may interfere with the ability of the embryo to implant or, alternatively, decrease uterine receptivity to successful implantation.
- The chemical thiocyanide, which is found in cigarettes, has been isolated in the cervical mucus of smokers and is believed to inhibit sperm motility.
- Women whose mothers smoked during their pregnancies may be 50 percent less fertile, on average, requiring a longer time to conception. Even prenatal exposure may lead to decreased fertility.
- Men who smoke are much more likely to have erectile dysfunction.

THE BOTTOM LINE: All studies point to this one truth: Cigarette smoking has a profoundly negative effect on your reproductive system. Still, these negative effects of smoking appear reversible, as ex-smokers regain normal conception rates. The trend toward decreased unassisted fertility and IVF success suggests that couples receiving infertility care should be advised to stop smoking and limit exposure to passive smoke.

Heavy Drinking Is Linked with Decreased Fertility

The number of women at childbearing age who are classified as heavy drinkers (greater than two drinks per day) is estimated to be 5 percent in the United States. While some studies suggest acute alcohol exposure in women apparently has little effect upon gonadotropins or sex steroids, other research suggests an increase in sex steroid levels and reduced gonadotropin levels.

Chronic or long-term alcohol exposure has been associated with the following:

- Infertility
- Inhibition of ovulation
- Menstrual disorders
- The onset of premature menopause

Plus, animal studies show that alcohol induces atrophy of female sexual organs, inhibition of the midcycle LH surge, reduced estrogen and progesterone levels, decreased fertility, and absence of corpora lutea. The following studies confirm what you must know to increase fertility—avoid alcohol!

- Researchers from the National University Hospital in Denmark evaluated 430 Danish couples (ages 20 to 35) who were trying to conceive a child for the first time. The reported results confirmed that women who did not drink at all had the highest chance of conceiving in that menstrual cycle, followed by those who drank one to five alcoholic beverages per week. Women who consumed ten drinks or more had only one-third the chance of conceiving compared with the nondrinkers. In this study, alcohol did not affect male fertility.
- While scientists know that alcohol can damage the fetus after conception, they are unsure about the actual mechanism that triggers lower fertility in those who drink alcohol. In a study reported in the *British Medical Journal* (August 1998), scientists speculated that even low doses of alcohol may increase miscarriage.
- In another study from Johns Hopkins School of Medicine, women who consumed any alcohol and more than one cup of coffee per day achieved 10.5 pregnancies per 100 menstrual cycles compared with 26.9 pregnancies per 100 menstrual cycles achieved by women who did not consume any alcohol and less than one cup of coffee per day. Scientists reported an overall 50 percent reduction in conception for women who consumed any alcohol. Evidently, while consuming coffee did not

directly affect fertility, it worked to enhance the negative effects of alcohol (*Fertility and Sterility*, October 1998).

• A study at Harvard University has linked moderate drinking to irregular ovulation and other physiological changes that may interfere with conception.

Illicit and Recreational Drugs Block Conception

It is estimated that upwards of 10 percent of women of childbearing age are using illicit drugs on a daily basis. In fact, 37 percent of those older than age 12 admit to having used drugs at one time in their life. The numbers are staggering: 72 million people have been exposed to illicit drugs during their lifetime and 14 million have used them within the past four weeks. The potential for infertility from drug abuse depends on a number of factors, including:

- Multiple drug usage
- Poor compliance
- Tolerance
- Inadequate medical care
- Poor nutritional habits

Associations with harmful effects on the reproductive and endocrine system are often difficult to assess. Because of this, conclusions regarding drug use and fertility are drawn from mostly epidemiologic studies as well as a few case reports and isolated, small, limited clinical studies.

THE BOTTOM LINE: The available evidence suggests most of the harmful effects of illicit drugs upon the reproductive system may be temporary and reversible. This means that if you stop using drugs, the chances of fertility potential increase. Of course, exposure to these illicit drugs prepubertally or during puberty may cause more lasting and potentially permanent damage, as the drugs interfere with physical maturation. Because of the potential for reproductive system damage caused by illicit drugs, discuss any past or present drug use with your doctor before getting pregnant.

Marijuana Inhibits Ovulation

Marijuana and cannabinoids have well-documented negative effects on the reproductive system by inhibiting ovulation and causing menstrual cycle disruption. Chronic treatment of rats with THC results in delay of pubertal development, specifically with delay of first ovulation. A study compared twenty-six women who smoked marijuana at least four times per week with age-matched controls who had never smoked marijuana; the results showed significantly shortened menstrual cycles and shorter luteal phases in the marijuana users. The disruption of ovulatory function by marijuana may be the cause of the increased risk for infertility. According to one study, a relative risk of 1.7 for infertility was seen compared with nonusers. The greatest risk was observed in women who had smoked within one year of attempting pregnancy (relative risk of 2.1). Marijuana also has been associated with reduced sperm count and sterility.

THE BOTTOM LINE: Don't smoke marijuana!

Detox Your Body

While there is still much information to be gathered on thousands of untested toxic chemicals, you can work with your doctor now and take a thorough environmental exposure history. After you list those workplace and lifestyle factors that may affect your reproductive health, make changes in the ones over which you have control. For example, while you cannot change what you were exposed to as a child, you can stop smoking cigarettes today or move away from the coworker who smokes at work. You can quit using alcohol during your childbearing years, and use only natural products for household cleaning purposes. If you are exposed daily to x-rays, radiation, pesticides, or chemicals at work, talk to your employer about a temporary change in your job responsibilities until you complete your family.

Chapter 8

Taking the Mystery
Out of Miscarriage

"I had been told by a doctor in New York that my uterus was tipped, which is why we were having trouble getting pregnant," said Kristin, age 33. "I decided to check that diagnosis with another doctor just to make sure there wasn't another problem. This doctor did a hysterosalpingogram. It proved inconclusive, so he did a laparoscopy. From it, he determined I have a bicornuate uterus—a condition where the uterus is effectively split into two separate horns (almost two distinct, small uteri). He said I could try to get pregnant, and we'd just watch the development carefully. I became pregnant that summer, but didn't realize it. I had severe cramping and some heavy bleeding, so I called the doctor's office. One of his nurses told me it was probably just a reaction from the surgery, and I should ignore it. I went on a business trip and the bleeding got worse. When I returned home, I went to the doctor. He said I was at the end of a miscarriage and should be thrilled to know I could get pregnant. Thrilled? Ron and I were devastated."

If you or someone you love has experienced miscarriage or pregnancy loss, you know all about the devastation it can cause. In the past, couples who experienced miscarriage would numbly move on with their lives, pretending as if the pregnancy never existed. Today, the deep emotional impact of pregnancy loss with the resulting feelings of distress, loss, and grief is fully acknowledged. Yet in the midst of the heartache you feel, you should try to understand all you can about miscarriage—what it is, why it happens, and how, in some situations, it may even be prevented.

In the midst of your grief, don't be surprised if your doctor is less concerned about your miscarriage than you are. Doctors often interpret the biological meaning of miscarriage—that it's a natural process that will happen in a certain percentage of pregnant patients. Doctors also see miscarriage as an encouraging sign because a pregnancy has occurred.

Miscarriage Is a Common Occurrence

Pregnancy loss or miscarriage (medically referred to as spontaneous abortion) is an extremely common event that occurs in more than 25 percent of known pregnancies. Some recent studies report as many as 50 percent of women miscarry, with many not realizing they were pregnant until the pregnancy is lost. While the normal gestation period for fetal development is considered to be forty weeks, a miscarriage or pregnancy loss is the termination of a pregnancy before twenty weeks' gestation.

As your pregnancy progresses, the risk of miscarriage decreases. That's because 75 percent of miscarriages occur during the first twelve weeks. Although it varies from state to state (because of reporting regulations), a baby born dead after the twentieth week of pregnancy is usually classified as a stillbirth. In fact, the risk of pregnancy loss increases with each successive pregnancy loss. For example, in a first pregnancy the risk of miscarriage is 11 to 13 percent. In a pregnancy immediately following that loss, the risk of miscarriage is 13 to 17 percent. The risk to a third pregnancy after two successive losses nearly triples, to 38 percent.

Recurrent Pregnancy Loss Is Challenging

For most couples, the risk of having a second consecutive miscarriage is only around 15 to 20 percent. Yet there are couples who continue to lose pregnancies. This recurrent spontaneous abortion is a common complication of pregnancy with no known cure. While the experience of losing one pregnancy is physically and emotionally challenging, when this occurs repeatedly, these feelings are greatly magnified.

Table 8.1   Types of Miscarriage

Blighted ovum   A pregnancy that has implanted but has failed to develop past the point where the embryo can be identified on ultrasound scan. Although evidence of a gestation is seen by ultrasound, the lack of fetal parts is often called an empty sac. These pregnancies are uniformly believed to have a genetic or endocrine reason for their poor outcome. May or may not require intervention with dilation and curettage (D&C).

Complete(d) abortion   Expulsion of the entire pregnancy: the embryo's fetal parts and membranes/placenta. The cervix is left closed. Usually completed abortion requires no intervention.

First-trimester miscarriage   Pregnancy loss within the first twelve weeks after last period. Often hormonal and/or genetic in origin, especially before six to eight weeks.

Incomplete abortion   Expulsion of only a portion of the pregnancy. The cervix is usually left open. Bleeding and pain are common. Usually requires surgical removal of the retained portion of pregnancy with D&C.

Inevitable abortion   Bleeding and pain, usually with cervix dilating.

Missed abortion   Embryo or fetal death at any stage, without expulsion of the pregnancy.

Recurrent (habitual) miscarriage   At least two, some define as three, consecutive undesired pregnancy losses.

Second-trimester miscarriage   Loss before twenty weeks. Less often genetic and more often anatomic (abnormal uterus), immunologic, or due to maternal disease.

Septic abortion   Pregnancy loss due to infection. Also used to describe infection associated with abortion without direct cause and effect. In the past, a common complication of elective terminations performed under nonsterile conditions.

Spontaneous abortion (SAB)   Unplanned pregnancy loss before twenty weeks.

Therapeutic abortion (TAB)   Abortion performed electively for medical reasons. Also used to describe elective or voluntary interruption of pregnancy (VIP) for any reason.

Threatened abortion   Bleeding with or without cramping, cervix is closed. Outcome is uncertain.

Fertility Treatment May Increase Chance of Miscarriage

Miscarriage rates may be slightly higher with pregnancies achieved after infertility therapy. Just as with pregnancies conceived without therapy, first trimester losses are most common. A part of this reported increased risk is that the pregnancies may have gone unrecognized outside of the close monitoring of an infertility treatment cycle. Generally, it is believed that it is the woman who is at risk and not the therapy that is the cause of pregnancy loss. Women with borderline reproductive capacity would naturally be thought to have a greater chance of pregnancy loss. The rate of pregnancy loss drops by at least half when the beating heart is seen on ultrasound at six to eight weeks, and the rate of loss is even much lower after a heartbeat is detected by a Doppler stethoscope.

Signs and Symptoms of Miscarriage

The symptoms of miscarriage are bleeding from the vagina and cramping of the uterus. In first-trimester miscarriages, you may not even realize you are pregnant. Usually there are no warnings until you see a brownish discharge when you go to the bathroom or have a cramping pain in the lower abdomen. Bleeding can range from a few drops to a heavy flow with clots and tissue. A miscarriage later in the pregnancy may involve tremendous cramping and profuse bleeding, with solid material passing along with blood. If your body does not expel all of the placenta and embryonic tissue, your doctor may have to do a dilation and curettage (D&C). This is a surgical procedure that removes any remaining tissue, which may be used in determining the cause of the miscarriage.

Sometimes Bleeding May Be Normal

Although vaginal bleeding during the first trimester is a key sign associated with the risk of miscarriage, not all women who experience bleeding suffer pregnancy loss. In fact, up to 25 percent of all pregnant women have bleeding at some point in pregnancy, and of these women, about half will have a miscarriage. In any case, your doctor should be notified immediately if you have any unusual bleeding or cramping—just to be safe.

Often bleeding is due to normal cervical changes. During pregnancy, the cervix softens and the surface may easily bleed with even minimal trauma, such as an exam or intercourse. Bleeding or spotting can also occur when the embryo implants (burrows) into the wall of your uterus and the placenta forms.

Bleeding and Cramping May Signal a Threatened Pregnancy

A general rule is the greater the amount of bleeding and the more cramping that is present, the greater the chance that the threatened abortion will turn into an inevitable or completed pregnancy loss (see Table 8.1). The inevitable pregnancy loss is indicated when your cervix dilates and is usually accompanied by pain and bleeding. At this point, most doctors believe that there is no chance the pregnancy can be saved. After the pregnancy is completely lost, an abortion or miscarriage is said to have been completed. Sometimes only a portion of the pregnancy is lost, resulting in an incomplete abortion. A sign of a completed pregnancy loss is often a marked reduction in bleeding and cramping.

After three (some authorities say two) consecutive pregnancy losses, diagnosis of recurrent or habitual pregnancy loss is made. Every pregnancy loss is associated with an emotional scar, yet there are few couples who have more despair than those who experience repeated losses. Most are unsure whether or not they could withstand yet one more loss in their lives. The best news is that even after three successive losses, the chance of an uneventful successful pregnancy is generally greater than 70 percent.

The Danger of Ectopic or Tubal Pregnancy

An ectopic pregnancy refers to any pregnancy that implants outside the uterine cavity. Approximately 1 percent of all pregnancies are ectopic, and about 1 percent of ectopic pregnancies are outside the fallopian tubes. Ectopic pregnancies in the fallopian tubes are usually called tubal pregnancies, while those outside the tubes are called abdominal pregnancies. The problem is that once you've had an ectopic pregnancy, the risk of having another one increases significantly.

Who's at Risk?

Those at risk include people who have suffered from the following:

- Previous ectopic pregnancy
- Previous pelvic/abdominal surgery
- Known or suspected PID
- Previous tubal sterilization/reversal
- Previous or present intrauterine contraceptive device
- Infertility

What Causes Tubal Damage?

The most common reason for tubal damage is a previous tubal infection, and the most common cause of this is a sexually transmitted disease (STD). You may not even know you had the infection, as many are silent. The larger the number of sexual partners, the greater the risk that there has been an infection. Other causes of an ectopic pregnancy are previous abdominal or pelvic surgery, especially surgery on the fallopian tubes to remedy infertility. Abdominal pregnancies may result from fertilization and implantation outside the tube. Or, in many cases, abdominal pregnancies are thought to rise from a normal or tubal pregnancy that was aborted through the tube and then secondarily implants in the abdomen.

Signs and Symptoms

The initial symptoms are those of an early pregnancy; most often, even a home pregnancy test should be positive. Most ectopic pregnancies do not cause problems until two to four weeks after a missed period (six to eight weeks from the last period). If the test is positive and there are risk factors, call your doctor. There is some degree of pelvic discomfort in most ectopic pregnancies. The onset of pain may be sudden or gradual and mild or severe. Cramping and bleeding is often similar to that of a threatened abortion. Also, the pain is most often felt on one side of the abdomen, but it can be diffuse, or even on the side opposite the ectopic pregnancy. Some ectopic pregnancies may be completely without symptoms and resolve without diagnosis or therapy. Others may turn into serious surgical emergencies. There may be abdominal discomfort or spotting in a normal pregnancy, so do not panic, but do have it checked out.

Making the Diagnosis

Before an ultrasound scan and very sensitive pregnancy tests were available, the clinical diagnosis of an ectopic pregnancy rested on the finding of a pelvic mass, pelvic pain, and a positive pregnancy test. Now with increased awareness and new tools, ectopic pregnancy is diagnosed much earlier and ectopic pregnancy is much safer. Trying to "date" a pregnancy when there is spotting is difficult. Often ovarian cysts, which are common during early pregnancy, will mimic an ectopic pregnancy and make the diagnosis even more difficult.

A critical test is the quantitative hCG level. If this level is less than 5IU/l, pregnancy is very doubtful. In a normal pregnancy, the hCG level doubles every forty-eight hours. A plateau or slower-than-expected rise in hCG raises the possibility of an ectopic pregnancy. A pregnancy should be seen in the uterus on ultrasound scan when the hCG level reaches 1,000 to 2,000 IU/l (about five weeks after the last period). If no intrauterine pregnancy is confirmed, the suspicion of an ectopic pregnancy rises.

Treatment Is Varied

There are several treatment options, and the best depends on the specific circumstances surrounding the pregnancy. In the past, ectopic pregnancies were usually treated by removal of the involved fallopian tube (salpingectomy). This procedure was then replaced by a salpingostomy, in which a small opening was made in the tube and the ectopic pregnancy was removed without loss of the tube. While this increased the risk of an ectopic pregnancy in that tube, there are many documented cases of normal pregnancies after this procedure. The salpingostomy and salpingectomy may be performed by laparotomy, but now are most often performed by laparoscopy because of the quick recovery rate. Most ectopic pregnancies can be treated by laparoscopy even if the tube has to be removed or closed off. Methotrexate, a drug used as cancer chemotherapy, is used to treat ectopic pregnancies, pregnancies of which the site is unknown, and pregnancies that may have been incompletely removed by surgery. The benefit of methotrexate therapy is that the surgery can often be avoided and there may be a better preservation of fertility. Some women will have a tubal rupture or require surgery after medical therapy with methotrexate and the side effects are rough, including abdominal pain, gastrointestinal upset, and mouth ulcers. Serious side effects are uncommon, but blood counts and chemistries must be checked.

When a Medical Evaluation Is Necessary

After successive miscarriages, it's time to dig deeper for the cause with a thorough medical evaluation. In the early stages, this evaluation may consist of nothing more than tracking temperatures, using ovulation detection kits, and testing luteal progesterone levels. Previously, it was thought that more than 50 percent of recurrent pregnancy losses were unexplained. Yet it is now believed that many of these cases are because of subtle hormonal abnormalities.

If you have a history of recurrent pregnancy loss, your doctor may order blood tests and ultrasound examinations long before you experience any symptoms of miscarriage. When the blood tests and ultrasound examinations are normal, the vast majority of bleeding and cramping episodes do not indicate problems with the viability of the pregnancy. In fact, most women go on to later have a normal pregnancy and delivery.

Who's at Risk for Miscarriage?

There are specific environmental and genetic risk factors that may influence miscarriage. These risk factors can be excellent indicators to alert you to the underlying problem, allowing you to change those factors that you can control. After reviewing the following risk factors, talk with your doctor about any tests or treatments that will help prevent miscarriage.

As you read the specific risk factors, you will realize that some cannot be changed, including genetic abnormalities or your age. The good news is that some risk factors can be changed, including treating infections that cause miscarriage, improving your lifestyle by dropping cigarettes and alcohol, getting immunized for the German measles before you conceive, and taking medications to correct a hormonal imbalance.

Genetic Abnormalities Cause Most Miscarriages

Studies show that as many as 60 percent of all miscarriages occur because of either an insufficient number or an extra number of chromosomes. Chromosomes are the tiniest elements of the body that carry all the genetic material that determines your eye color, body type, and overall makeup. A genetic abnormality curtails development of the embryo because the sperm and the egg cannot fuse and divide properly. Pregnancy loss from a genetic problem is nature's way of ensuring good health throughout your unborn child's life. Most pregnancies with genetic abnormalities do not survive to birth. Those that do survive to birth result in less lethal conditions such as Down's syndrome or Turner's syndrome.

Age Increases Your Risk of Miscarriage

Many studies have shown that age is a major factor in infertility, as well as in miscarriage. While a woman in her early twenties has only a 12 to 15 percent chance of having a miscarriage each time she becomes pregnant, a woman in her early forties has a 50 percent risk of miscarriage.

Women are born with all the eggs that they will ever have in their lives (with the chromosomes inside). Men, on the other hand, make fresh sperm continuously, taking approximately ninety days for a sperm to be made and to reach maturity. This is an extremely important difference between the sexes! For example, if a 35-year-old man and a 35-year-old woman try to conceive, they are basically trying to combine a 35-year-old egg with a 3-month-old sperm.

The longer an egg sits around in the ovary, however, the more likely it is to develop abnormalities in its chromosomes. If an egg with abnormal chromosomes is fertilized, then the chances are greater that the resulting pregnancy will end in miscarriage.

Some Infections Lead to Miscarriage

While a minor sinus infection probably won't cause miscarriage, infections that have high fevers may put you at risk. Also, the German measles and Listeria-type infections may lead to miscarriage. Studies show that certain viral infections, including cytomegalovirus and herpes, may be involved in some cases of later pregnancy loss. Toxoplasmosis, caused by a parasite called *Toxoplasma gondii* and found in different forms in raw meat and in cats who eat raw meat and in their feces, is yet another culprit for increased risk of miscarriage. Now if your cat is an indoor cat, the chances are minimal of getting toxoplasmosis. Still, if you have an outdoor cat, ask someone else to change the litter box.

Uterine Abnormalities Interfere with Implantation

Twenty to 30 percent of all recurrent losses are caused by uterine defects. These abnormalities may be in the shape or inner surface of the uterus and sometimes are congenital, meaning you were born with them. A uterus distorted by fibroid tumors (benign masses that commonly grow in the muscular wall of your uterus), or a septum (a wall of tissue that separates the uterus into two halves) can both contribute to pregnancy loss. Or, scar tissue that may interfere with egg transport can affect implantation of the embryo in the uterus or cause abortion. Pregnancy loss due to uterine problems often differs from pregnancy loss due to genetic problems. The pregnancy may survive longer and is more often associated with pain and bleeding. Fetal heart activity is often identified on ultrasound before the loss.

An Incompetent Cervix Opens Too Soon

In a normal labor, the cervix will widen to allow your baby to move through your uterus and into the vagina. With an incompetent cervix, the weakened cervix begins to open early in the pregnancy, possibly resulting in miscarriage. Miscarriage caused by cervical incompetence usually occurs in the second trimester, usually 14 to 16 weeks. You may experience a painless leaking of liquid. Or your doctor may find during a pregnancy pelvic exam a gradual dilation of your cervical opening, with the membranes bulging into the vagina. If diagnosed early enough, there are treatments, such as placing a stitch high up around the cervix to try to keep it closed (cerclage). Newer medications to halt contractions may prevent early labor.

An incomplete cervix is thought to arise from a congenital abnormality of the structural makeup of the cervix. In rare cases, cervical incompetence may occur after extensive cervical surgery such as a cone biopsy.

Hormone Abnormalities Contribute to Miscarriage

Hormonal problems can put you at higher risk of miscarriage. An over- or underactive thyroid or abnormal levels of prolactin are all associated with pregnancy loss. Women with recurrent pregnancy loss frequently have subtle endocrine alterations that suggest poor egg or follicle quality and lower progesterone levels. Although your doctor may call this a luteal phase defect (LPD), there is usually a defect of the follicular phase and egg quality. Treatment involves converting the hormonal imbalance, which will result in normal follicular development. The luteal phase will then correct itself. The first line of therapy is usually clomiphene citrate. Progesterone supplements may also be used.

Lifestyle and Workplace Factors Can Hinder Pregnancy

Sometimes your lifestyle may increase your chance of miscarriage, especially if you drink alcohol or caffeine, and smoke cigarettes. Some prescription drugs used for cancer treatment (chemotherapy), malaria, severe acne, psoriasis, and rheumatoid arthritis have been linked to an increased chance of miscarriage. Some environmental toxins, chemicals, and even radiation exposure—on the job or off—can increase your risk of pregnancy loss (see Chapter 7).

Autoimmune Factors and Recurrent Pregnancy Loss

A competent immune system plays a critical role in our vulnerability to disease. It is also a key factor in ovulation, sperm function, implantation, and pregnancy. All of these processes share components of inflammation and the immune response. A malfunctioning immune system may lead to the development of an autoimmune disease such as arthritis or asthma. With a depleted immune system, the body is at risk of being overwhelmed by invading bacteria and viruses, resulting in cancer or other life-threatening diseases. However certain we are that there is a key role of the immune system in reproduction, scientists are still at a loss for surefire treatments.

At several levels—and in markedly different ways—chemical changes that are directly related to altered emotional states can profoundly influence the immune system. You may know how these emotional states often correlate with life's interruptions or stressors—extended working hours, unhealthy environments, and increasing demands from commitments, careers, and commutes. Science now recognizes that the mind and body are interconnected to an extent far surpassing previous assumptions and that physical health and emotional well-being are closely linked.

Because of the rising research in the mind/body connection or psychoneuroimmunology (PNI), some experts contend that there may be an internal environmental barrier to pregnancy, especially with recurrent pregnancy loss that has no explanation. In years past, miscarriages that couldn't be attributed to chromosomal defects, hormonal problems, or abnormalities of the uterus were labeled "unexplained." Couples would continue to get pregnant, only to suffer time and again as they lost their babies. Today scientists are working to find the missing link.

Normally the cells and proteins (antibodies) of the immune system help your body fight invading viruses, bacteria, and cancer cells, and remove damaged or abnormal tissue. When the receptors sense trouble brewing, they signal to the antibodies and other cells to stop these invaders (foreign materials). Invaders are called antigens and are blocked by the body's protectors (antibodies). Normally, in pregnancy, the immune system is blindfolded to allow the acceptance of the embryo, which has completely different DNA and proteins from its mother. Yet in some cases, the immune system is activated and the host uterus views the embryo as foreign. The embryo is rejected and a miscarriage results.

Comprehensive scientific studies conclude that in as many as 10 percent of recurrent pregnancy losses, immune cells or antibodies attack the developing embryo and cause miscarriage. The scientific community is strongly split on this very controversial area of diagnosis and therapy. Some researchers suggest that as many as 80 percent of unexplained losses may be attributable to immunological factors and propose specific immunologic therapies that may allow most couples with recurrent loss to carry a baby to term.

Making the Diagnosis

Although many doctors do not begin testing for the cause of pregnancy loss until after three successive miscarriages, this may be too long to wait when therapy could have been started much sooner. Because the risk of miscarriage increases to 26 to 40 percent after a woman has suffered two losses, the American College of Obstetrics and Gynecologists (ACOG) now recommends testing after a second loss—especially for women over the age of 35.

Some of the tests your doctor may order include:

ULTRASOUND SCAN. This safe and noninvasive imaging procedure uses high-frequency sound waves that bounce off internal organs and create an image on a monitor. By moving a device called a transducer, either over your abdomen or inside your vagina, your doctor can see if there are abnormalities in the uterus, especially fibroids. Your doctor can also assess the uterine response at the expected time of ovulation and implantation using ultrasound. Ultrasound scan is painless and safe.

HYSTEROSONOGRAPHY (OR SONO HSG). This procedure combines the use of fluid in the uterus with high-resolution ultrasound imaging to find abnormalities of the uterine cavity. It is usually done in your doctor's office. The procedure is mildly uncomfortable, and nonsteroidal anti-inflammatory drugs (NSAIDs) such as ibuprofen or naproxen may be suggested before the procedure. There is a slight risk of infection with this procedure, yet prophylactic antibiotics are not usually used.

HYSTEROSCOPY. Using a small fiber-optic telescope (hysteroscope) and video equipment, your doctor can do an examination of the endometrial cavity of the uterus, checking for abnormalities or fibroids not seen on an ultrasound scan. This procedure may be done in the operating room under general anesthesia (often in association with laparoscopy), or with sedation in the office.

ENDOMETRIAL BIOPSY. In this procedure, a small sample is taken of the uterine lining (endometrium) to see if abnormalities exist. While this was once considered an important test, endometrial biopsy is now used only for very specific circumstances.

BLOOD TESTS. These may include a complete blood count (CBC), thyroid panel (TSH), glucose tolerance test for diabetes, and a biochemical panel. Additional testing may be indicated if specific problems are suspected such as endocrine, autoimmune, or hematologic disorders. The blood tests will help your doctor determine any hormone irregularities, polycystic ovarian syndrome (PCOS), systemic lupus erythematosus (SLE, or lupus), and other problems with antibodies.

KARYOTYPE. This is a test on the amniotic fluid, fetal tissue from the miscarriage, and/or blood from both parents that evaluates chromosome number and configuration and will determine if there is a genetic cause of miscarriage. Only about 5 percent of recurrent loss is thought to be a genetic problem carried by the parents.

Taking Control with Medical Interventions

After extensive testing, studies show that half to two-thirds of recurrent pregnancy losses occur for unknown reasons. Even if an abnormality is discovered, it may not be responsible for the miscarriage. Nonetheless, early prepregnancy counseling may help identify risk factors, and close obstetrician follow-up may permit medical interventions to increase the chances of staying pregnant full term.

Control Chronic Illnesses

Women with chronic diseases such as high blood pressure and diabetes, as well as immunologic diseases, have a higher rate of pregnancy loss. This is probably an abnormality in establishment of the maternal-fetal interrelationship. The best treatment in these cases is making sure that the diseases are under the best control possible before pregnancy is attempted.

Use Hormone Replacement, If Necessary

Replacing deficient hormones such as progesterone, given orally or by intravaginal applications or intramuscular injections, may help your body keep the pregnancy to term. Progesterone stabilizes the uterine lining, reduces uterine contractions, and plays a role in supporting an early pregnancy. Progesterone will not save a pregnancy with a genetic defect, and its use may have the disadvantage of prolonging the time to miscarriage.

Treat All Chronic Infections

Be aware of chronic infections, especially mycoplasma and ureaplasma, which have been identified with a greater risk of pregnancy loss. While there are tests to detect their presence, experts believe it is often easier to treat with a two-week course of antibiotics rather than identify the organism. While the chances of recurrent pregnancy loss due to infection are slim, the treatment is easy.

Consider Medications for Autoimmune Factors

Treatments for autoimmune risk factors include preconception administration of low-dose heparin (an anticoagulant produced naturally by the body), aspirin, and prednisone (a steroid to decrease inflammation). Heparin is used to combat possible clotting problems, while prednisone is given to decrease inflammatory reactions. Aspirin is a prostaglandin inhibitor that can increase blood flow to the placenta by inhibiting the tendency for clotting in women with abnormal levels of autoantibodies. Of the treatments used for women with autoimmune factor, the initial treatment of choice is usually low-dose heparin and aspirin therapy. This is because obstetrical complications, such as preterm birth, premature rupture of the membrane, and gestational diabetes, are more common with prednisone.

Another newer treatment of autoimmune factors is intravenous immunoglobulin (IVIg), a process that infuses the mother with antibodies from thousands of donors in the general population. The basic effect of IVIg is like disarming a large military force (the mother's dangerous antibodies). The army is still present after administering the IVIg, but it is harmless. The donor immunoglobulin keeps the attacking antibodies busy and away from the developing fetus. While IVIg seems effective, it is also quite costly—roughly $10,000 to $30,000 for treatments throughout pregnancy.

Know That the Odds Are in Your Favor

In cases where no cause is discovered and no treatment prescribed, the chance of achieving a healthy pregnancy despite having had several miscarriages is still generally better than 50 percent. Keep in mind that nothing you did caused the pregnancy loss. Lifting, walking, sexual intercourse, driving on a rough road, brief exposures to very hot or very cold weather, or emotional outbursts and arguments have no ill effect on the development of an early pregnancy. Although some doctors advise mothers-to-be to stay off their feet or even stay in bed if there are signs of miscarriage, strict bed rest does not appear to prevent early pregnancy loss. *Knowing this, many experts still agree that bed rest does not hurt!*

Some other factors that may help prevent pregnancy loss include:

- Avoid alcohol and cigarettes.
- Avoid overexercising. Exercise to mild exertion only, taking care to avoid becoming overheated. A light sweat is fine. Soaking your clothes with sweat during exercise or allowing your skin to redden suggests a taxing of the body's ability to dissipate heat and should be avoided.
- Don't take any medications—prescription or over-the-counter—or herbal supplements without first discussing these with your doctor.

Doctor's Rx

The most accurate method of following a pregnancy is by several ultrasound scans. Fetal heart activity is very reassuring.

Be Proactive

Other than these precautions, there are few things that need to be done except to learn all you can about miscarriage and take an active role in deciding on your course of treatment. If you have suffered recurrent pregnancy loss, write down any questions, then talk openly with your doctor about the benefits and the potential risks of any invasive test, medication, or surgical procedure.

Part Two

Drug-Free Conception

Chapter 9

Ten Natural Baby-Making Tips (BMTs)

"After spending a decade using birth control to avoid getting pregnant, we finally let nature take its turn at bat over the course of nine months," said Cal, age 36. "I heard that slow sperm causes infertility, so I'd down a cup of strong coffee right before making love to try to get the sperm to wake up. I even started wearing baggy boxer shorts—which I detest. We tossed out the alarm clock and were awakened each morning by the beep of Stephanie's basal body thermometer. She was, of course, on top of the recent literature on conception, particularly the study that demonstrated that you conceive only during the five days before and including ovulation but not after, so we scheduled our love trysts with increasing precision. Whether I was in a client meeting or on the golf course, whenever Stephanie had an LH surge, my cell phone would summon me home to be promptly amorous."

Even with high-tech methods readily available to treat infertility, the trend toward letting nature take its turn at bat with lifestyle changes has become a popular option. For those who have spent years using birth control pills, condoms, or other methods to avoid pregnancy, the realization that it's not easy to pick and choose the time of conception becomes a grim reality. Yet even though the window of time for conception narrows, there are a host of baby-making tips (BMTs) you can try right now to increase your chances of getting pregnant.

The good news is that there are no great secrets and few rules to getting pregnant. In fact, top reproductive endocrinologists across the nation all agree that the best way to make a baby is to follow the rule of nothing in excess. The bad news is that sometimes the following BMTs may reduce the spontaneity or pleasure of intercourse, so remember to keep everything in perspective. Keep your wits about you, *relax*, and stay informed!

BMT 1. Stop Contraception, Then Start Conception

If you are still using birth control pills, it's time to map out your Baby-Making Plan. Decide when you want to be pregnant, go off the pill, then start trying in the first month off the pill. In the past, doctors recommended a "wash-out" period to allow menstrual cycles to become regular before you were given the green light. During your first few months off the pill, you may find it more difficult to pinpoint when ovulation occurs or to estimate a due date if you do get pregnant. Still, women who will have ovulation problems may be the most fertile during the first several months off the pill. If you do not take advantage of this window of opportunity for a natural conception, it may close.

In the past, it was also believed that the pill could cause birth defects. Because of the many women who have become pregnant on the pill and the information on their babies, it is now believed that the pill has *no* adverse effect on reproduction. In fact, the pill is used in some patients before in vitro fertilization (IVF) attempts to synchronize the cycle and improve egg quality. Of course there may be delayed ovulation, and theoretically, this might slightly increase the miscarriage rate. Still, the trade-off of pregnancies that would not be possible by waiting is probably worth it.

Doctor's Rx

The pill appears to be the best method of contraception to preserve fertility. Pill users usually have a reduced incidence of fibroids, endometriosis, and pelvic inflammatory diseases, and their ovarian function may be better preserved than those women who do not use the pill.

BMT 2. Know Your Menstrual Cycle—
Natural Cycle Tracking

There is no use for home testing—for ovulation—if you do not have regular menstrual cycles. If the number of days between day 1 of your menstrual cycle (counted as any bleeding) until day 1 of the next cycle is more than 35, ovulation is probably not occurring, and you should consult your doctor for an evaluation. Remember, regular periods are no guarantee of ovulation, and that's why it's important to do your homework.

Kimberly knows how important this homework is. She tried every pregnancy test on the drugstore shelf, hoping each time that it would be positive. Kimberly had grown frustrated and was thinking of giving up trying to conceive until a close friend suggested that she learn more about her menstrual cycle. That way she could plan intercourse at the perfect time for conception. Because her cycle was longer than 28 days, she didn't fully understand how to calculate ovulation.

After talking with her doctor, she began to chart the time of ovulation using the BBT for three consecutive months. The fourth month was magic, as she conceived for the first time after two years of trying to get pregnant. She is now the proud mother of 6-month-old Anna.

As Kimberly realized, timing is everything when it comes to making a baby. That's why knowledge of the workings of your menstrual cycle, including ovulation or the release of an egg from the ovary, is critically important.

Ovulation occurs on days 13 to 15 in an idealized 28-day cycle. This is toward the end of the 5- to 7-day fertile period. If your cycles vary within the acceptable 26 to 32 days, the fertile period is from days 11 to 17. If you have intercourse three times during the fertile period, there is probably good exposure. It does not matter if you have intercourse a couple of days in a row, or that several days are skipped without intercourse. The chances are great that over a period of several months, your timing will be perfect. You do not have to play out the sitcoms where the male is called home because ovulation is occurring at that exact moment. Experts all agree that no one ever knows that!

Still, it may help to more precisely determine the time of ovulation to improve your chances. It is best to have mobile healthy sperm waiting

---

Baby Booster

For the sperm to gain the capacity to fertilize the egg, it may need to be in the female reproductive tract for six hours.

---

at the end of the fallopian tube at the time the egg is to be released. The egg, or oocyte, is viable for probably no more than 24 hours. Yet sperm can retain their fertilizing capacity for at least 2 days, and possibly 3 to 4.

Go by the Calendar

If your periods are regular, a regular calendar can show you the most likely time of ovulation. Start by writing down when you first start each menstrual cycle. You may be surprised that you are not as regular as you think.

- Determine the approximate time of ovulation by marking an X when your period should begin.
- Count backwards from 14 to 16 days, and place a second X.
- Now use this calendar as your Baby-Making Cheat Sheet.

Baby Buster

Intercourse every day will drive your partner's sperm count *down*. Intervals of more than three days may not ensure the highest concentration of sperm or it may miss ovulation altogether.

Notice Any Physical Signs of Ovulation

There are two clinical signs signifying ovulation—pain and cervical mucus changes. Some women have both and do not ovulate. Some women have neither and ovulate regularly. Everyone is different.

MIDCYCLE PAIN (MITTELSCHMERZ). Many women know the time of ovulation by symptoms of abdominal achiness, slight cramping, or brief twinges of pain (called mittelschmerz). This pain is usually a good sign! It may last up to several hours and signals that ovulatory activity is taking place. It is not known what causes this pain, but it may come from the rupture of the follicle itself or an irritation as the follicular fluid is released into the pelvis at ovulation. Since ovulation often alternates one side, then the other, the pain may follow this same course. Some women feel ovulation only on one side despite both ovaries taking turns ovulating.

Chart the day, side, and intensity of any pain.

CERVICAL MUCUS. As the follicle containing the egg grows, it produces increasing amounts of estrogen. The amount and consistency of cervical mucus is under the influence of estrogen, and generally speaking, the more estrogen, the more mucus. Some women worry that the mucus discharge could be a sign of infection or lack of hygiene. Nothing could be further from the truth. The presence of midcycle discharge—like midcycle pain—is completely normal.

Mucus tends to increase several days before ovulation, and stops within twenty-four hours after ovulation. The most hospitable mucus for sperm is clear, slippery, and stretchy, similar to raw egg white, and it occurs as you approach ovulation. Immediately after ovulation, the mucus thickens and loses its elasticity.

To check the consistency of your cervical mucus, try the following:

1. Each time you go to the bathroom, wipe the opening of your vagina with a tissue and notice if the feeling is dry, smooth, or lubricated.

2. Check the tissue to see if there is mucus present.
3. If mucus is on the tissue, feel it. Notice its texture, color, and stretchability. Also notice if it has changed from the previous day.

Chart any day-to-day mucus changes.

Recognize Other Common Signs and Symptoms of Ovulation

You may also feel some breast tenderness around ovulation because of the marked and rapid alteration in hormones. While one study has shown that sexual appetite is the highest at midcycle, this is not universal. Many women have less sexual desire because of an increased feeling of fullness. If you have any midcycle spotting, this may be a sign of ovulation or possibly an ovulation. It's important to be aware of this sign, nonetheless.

Chart the days around ovulation that you had sexual intercourse.

Chart any physical events that may be involved with hormones, ovulation, or the menstrual cycle.

Chart any spotting that occurs between periods.

Conception 101

When an egg is not released, you have an anovulatory cycle, which can be normal, long, or short in length. You may experience light or heavy menstrual flow. Your BBT will be erratic and show no thermal shift. There are various causes for an anovulatory cycle including illness, travel, stress, coming off of birth control pills or Depo-Provera, strenuous exercise, and sudden weight loss or gain.

Chart Your Basal Body Temperature (BBT)

Only a small number of women with monthly midcycle pain have charts that do not show a temperature elevation. Usually pain occurs 2 days before the BBT elevation. Ovulation generally occurs 1 to 2 days after the lowest temperature point. A temperature elevation of 0.4 to 1.0 degrees F. is evidence of progesterone production, which is presumptive but not conclusive evidence of ovulation. When there is a clear rise in temperature, this is called the shift. The chart is then said to be biphasic. In a 28-day cycle, the shift should occur on cycle day 13 to 14. In longer or shorter cycles, the shift should occur 10 to 14 days before the next menses. The temperature should remain elevated until just before your menstrual period starts. If the temperature elevation is less than 10 days, or there is a drop after a rise, this is evidence of ovarian dysfunction and possibly a lack of ovulation. If the shift does not occur, the chart is said to be monophasic. In this case, if you put your daily temperature on a graph, you would see a pronounced W pattern, indicating a shift after day 16, or a slow rise in temperature. This may indicate that you have disordered ovulation.

A shortcoming of tracking your BBT is that it tells you that ovulation may have occurred, not that it is going to occur. Many experts believe this to be a poor technique for timing intercourse. It is known that inseminations performed after the temperature shift result in a low pregnancy rate. After the temperature elevation, sexual intercourse or artificial insemination is likely to be unsuccessful.

BBT charting is relatively reliable and cheap, and it offers a model to better understand how your body is functioning. However, keep in mind that most women find tracking BBT a nuisance and just one more daily reminder of infertility that you really don't need! Too often the "lost thermometer" was misplaced or even thrown against the bedroom wall in anguish. These feelings of loss of control or sadness can be diminished if you limit your BBT monitoring to two to three months, which can usually provide you with all the information you will need.

Using a BBT Thermometer

1. Purchase a special basal body thermometer at any drugstore. There are also digital BBT thermometers and those equipped with special minicomputers that store all readings, if your budget permits.
2. Keep the thermometer and a record sheet on the nightstand by your bed.
3. Before you get out of bed in the morning, take your BBT. You must have been at rest for at least six hours to achieve a true basal reading. This test may not be accurate for those who work the night shift.

Chart your BBT before arising each morning for two to three months.

BMT 3. Capture the Moment

Your body normally produces small amounts of luteinizing hormone (LH). Yet just prior to ovulation, there is a rapid increase in this hormone called the LH surge. The LH surge has three functions:

- Resumption of oocyte (egg) development in preparation for fertilization.

- Ovulation.
- Conversion of the preovulatory follicle to the corpus luteum, which produces progesterone. This prepares the uterus for implantation of the embryo.

Ovulation cannot occur without LH. LH is first released into the bloodstream by the pituitary gland and rapidly cleared from the body by the kidneys. While it is not as sensitive as the blood test, urine testing of LH is reliable and much easier. By measuring LH, you can estimate the time of ovulation. In women with 28-day cycles (27 to 29 days), ovulation usually occurs on day 13, 14, or 15. In other cases, ovulation occurs about 10 to 14 days before the start of the next period (menses) cycle. If periods are less than 26 days, or more than 32, there is a greater chance that ovulation is not occurring.

Ovulation Prediction Kits Indicate LH Surge

Ovulation prediction kits (OPKs) use a new technology to cause a chemical reaction and color change when a specific level of LH is reached in the blood or urine. Ovulation usually occurs within 40 hours of this color change. However, there is individual variation ranging from 12 to 60 hours. The OPKs are very sensitive, and they reliably and accurately measure LH. While there cannot be ovulation without LH, LH may be elevated and ovulation still may not occur (false positive). Common reasons for the OPK to result in a false positive include:

1. Some women, particularly those that have polycystic ovarian syndrome (PCOS), have high levels of LH in the blood and urine at all times. This is usually predetermined by blood testing early in the menstrual cycle and is a reason for infertility.
2. Drugs that are used for the induction of ovulation, specifically clomiphene citrate (Clomid, Serophene), work by increasing LH. OPKs will often be positive during use of the medication and for 1 to 2 days after the medication is stopped.
3. There can be a timely secretion of enough LH to cause a color change of the OPK (positive test), yet this may not be enough to stimulate the ovary to ovulate.

Which Kit Is Best?

There are a variety of OPKs available today, and they all work in the same way. Interestingly, while each one claims to be easy, this is far from the truth! All of the kits indicate the presence of LH with the appearance of a colored line, dot, or test area. The intensity of the color change is compared to a reference standard dot or line. Some kits may change color at a lower level of LH, making them more sensitive but increasing the possibility of a false positive test (color change without ovulation).

So which kit is best? A recent *Consumer Reports* study of ovulation predictor kits defined the kit with the best sensitivity as that which provides the most positive test results. However, independent studies have proved that the best sensitivity is the kit which reliably and consistently detects a positive LH surge at the same level each and every time. Your doctor may recommend an OPK, or you may have to experiment with several kits to find the most accurate reading.

Using the Ovulation Prediction Test

If your cycles are 27 to 31 days apart, start testing on the morning of day 11. Day 1 is the first day of bleeding, or spotting. The most accurate evaluation occurs on the second voided sample of the morning. Follow the instructions on the test kit for use.

Timing of Intercourse

There is a relatively brief time during which fertilization must occur. Intercourse on the 2 days prior to ovulation gives you the best chance of making a baby. The timing of intercourse should be for the first evening after a morning color change of OPK. Intercourse should take place again on the following evening, in which the morning color change should be darker.

BMT 4. Try Recreation, Not Procreation

"I know this sounds odd, but we began to hate having sex," Sara said. "We read everything we could get our hands on on how to guarantee conception, including one time when I propped my hips on four pillows. I stayed in that position for two hours and could hardly breathe, but we still didn't get pregnant. It wasn't until we quit trying so hard and began to relax that we finally conceived."

In theory, any position you use to have sex should have no major bearing on getting pregnant—remember, it takes only *one sperm* to make a baby! No intercourse position has ever been shown to be the most likely to make a baby, but it makes sense that the positions that allow maximum contact with the cervix and the deepest penetration are better. These include:

- Face-to-face
- Missionary position
- Rear entry/knee chest position

Since there are many different positions of the uterus and cervix, one position for intercourse may be better for your individual pelvic anatomy. Experiment with different positions. It may add some interest and diversion, especially when you become absorbed with thoughts of fertility instead of pleasure.

Conception 101

Intercourse may be more painful in certain positions. This is because your ovaries, which have the same nerve fibers and sensations as the testes, are being moved or compressed. This is normal. But if intercourse is extremely painful, a medical examination should be sought. Painful intercourse is seldom psychological.

A very common concern is a fear that the sperm may have been lost because of discharge immediately after intercourse. This is highly unlikely. The best quality sperm (the super-sperm) are in the first part of the ejaculation when penetration is usually the deepest. The semen also undergoes a process known as liquefation, during which the semen becomes much more watery. Some semen is almost always lost as the vagina returns to its normal shape.

While you know male orgasm is vital for conception, some new studies show that female orgasm may also play a role. Researchers conclude that the uterine contractions that accompany female orgasm may give sperm an extra boost up into the cervix.

BMT 5. Check Your Lubricants

Most vaginal lubrication is produced as a leakage of fluid (transudate) across your vaginal wall, or mucosa. Vaginal secretions increase markedly during sexual excitement as the blood vessels surrounding the vagina dilate. Unfortunately, and for a variety of reasons, vaginal lubrication can be a problem in infertile couples. This is not a sign of pathology but rather due to lack of appropriate stimulation. Reduction in lubrication can be a sign of estrogen deficiency. Some drugs, especially the GnRH analogs (Lupron), may significantly diminish the amount of lubrication.

Mark and Ashley didn't realize that the lubricant they were using during intercourse was actually blocking conception. Yet when they

---

Baby Booster

If vaginal dryness is a problem, try baby oil. In a study reported in *Human Reproduction* (1999), researchers from the Queen's University of Belfast in Ireland measured the effects of K-Y jelly, baby oil, olive oil, and saliva on sperm movement. These scientists found that all except baby oil significantly hindered sperm—even at diluted concentrations.

Baby Buster

On a cautious note, despite the backing of many ob-gyns who claim that saliva is a safe choice of lubricant, the study reported in *Human Reproduction* concluded that saliva was the *worst offender* and exacted the most damage on the sperm they studied. Also, you should never use a petroleum-based lubricant such as Vaseline.

---

changed to baby oil, Ashley became pregnant within a few months. If you use a lubricant such as K-Y jelly for intercourse, as Mark and Ashley did, you may be defeating your attempts at conception. Many commercial lubricants interfere with sperm motility, making it more difficult for sperm cells to unite with the egg. Speed of sperm movement is an excellent indicator of whether fertilization will occur. Studies show that even low concentrations of certain substances used as lubricants significantly slow the movement of sperm.

BMT 6. Don't Douche

You probably know that the safety of douching has been in question for years. However, it's important to know *why* it's usually unsafe. The cells of the vaginal wall are under the influence of estrogen. Estrogen stimulates the formation of the complex sugar glycogen. Normal bacteria of the vagina use glycogen as nutrition and in the process convert it to lactic acid. The normal acidic environment of the vagina is a barrier to infection. In some cases, an overly acidic environment may be detrimental to sperm. Some physicians have recommended baking soda douches to neutralize the acid, but this has not been shown to be of benefit scientifically and is probably unnecessary. It may even be harmful to your fertility. One company has marketed a douche reportedly for conception, but proof of its effectiveness is lacking.

Douching may alter the normal vaginal environment and make irritation or infection more likely. Studies suggest that the practice may wash microorganisms into the uterus, causing conditions such as pelvic inflammatory disease that are known to have an effect on fertility. Although some doctors may prescribe short-term douching to clear up an infection, usually the recommendation is not to douche. Stick with good hygiene habits, including soap and water while bathing, to preserve your natural fertility. Water does not enter the vagina while you are bathing, and whether you take baths or showers has no effect on female fertility.

BMT 7. Keep It Cool

Heat is clearly damaging to sperm, and most experts will tell you that hot baths, dry saunas, steam baths, or time in a Jacuzzi may decrease sperm production. There is also evidence that the conception rate rises in late fall and early winter, after a cooling-down period. Nevertheless, before you insist on your partner wearing baggy boxer shorts to keep his testicles cool, read on. According to research from the State University of New York at Stony Brook published in *The Journal of Urology* (October 1998), male infertility is *not* linked to boxers or briefs. In fact, semen samples and external and internal body temperatures of ninety-seven men with fertility problems were taken and analyzed, and the results showed no difference in scrotal temperature, sperm count, sperm concentration, or sperm motility from those of other men. Researchers concluded that men who are hoping to father children can wear any type of underwear they choose with no ill effect on their reproductive performance. However, men who have jobs around high heats still should try to minimize exposure. Truck drivers or men who spend lots of time driving may have higher scrotal temperatures. An occasional stretch or break may be in order to preserve fertility.

BMT 8. Modify Your Lifestyle

While earlier chapters underscored the detrimental effect of cigarettes, alcohol, and recreational drugs on fertility, these are factors you can control—today.

• The more one smokes, the higher the risk of damage to eggs, sperm, or embryos.

• Drinking alcohol affects sperm counts and testosterone levels in men and contributes to birth defects. Even in small amounts, alcohol can reduce a woman's chances of conceiving by more than 50 percent.

• Marijuana can suppress reproductive function. Likewise, cocaine use in women is linked to an increased risk of kidney problems in newborns.

• Caffeine intake can increase the risk for fibrocystic breast changes, endometriosis, and possibly male and female infertility. Limit your consumption to 7 grams of caffeine per month.

Caffeine is naturally found in more than sixty plants, including coffee and cocoa beans, kola nuts, and tea leaves. Tea and chocolate also contain ingredients like theophylline and theobromine, which also can stimulate the heart and central nervous system. Watch that chocolate candy bar you eat or medication you take, as many contain caffeine, too.

A number of studies have shown that caffeine increases sperm motility. Whether this is a positive or a negative effect is not known. Scientists know that there is a burst of energy followed by an accelerated sperm death. But before you down cups of coffee before having intercourse, take caution. For every report about the negative effects of caffeine on sperm, there is a report showing *no* effects at all.

• While most food additives are considered safe, others have not been adequately tested. Still others pose a risk of causing infertility.

Doctor's Rx

The risks of alcohol consumption have been much less well documented than tobacco use and are still debated. Moderate to heavy alcohol use probably affects fertility, yet the effects of modest use are unclear. While it is recommended that pregnant women avoid alcohol, a glass of wine on the weekends with friends may help you to relax as you try to make a baby. Perhaps the same can be said for caffeine.

Table 9.1 Foods High in Caffeine

Coffee

Coffee, drip	5 oz.	90–115 mg
Coffee, perk	5 oz.	60–125 mg
Coffee, instant	5 oz.	60–80 mg
Coffee, decaffeinated	5 oz.	2–5 mg
Espresso	1 oz.	50 mg
Flavored	5 oz.	25–75 mg

Tea

Tea, 5 min. steep	5 oz.	40–100 mg
Tea, 3 min. steep	5 oz.	20–50 mg
Tea, green	5 oz.	35 mg
Tea, instant	5 oz.	25–35 mg

Carbonated Drinks

Cola soft drink	12 oz.	45 mg
Mountain Dew	12 oz.	55 mg
Mellow Yellow	12 oz.	50 mg

Chocolate and Cocoa

Chocolate, baking, unsweetened	1 oz.	60 mg
Chocolate, sweet, dark	1 oz.	20 mg
Chocolate bar	1 oz.	30 mg
Hot cocoa	5 oz.	2–10 mg

Medications

Excedrin	1 tablet	65 mg
Vanquish	1 tablet	33 mg
Anacin	1 tablet	32 mg
No Doz (maximum strength)	1 tablet	200 mg
Vivarin	1 tablet	200 mg
No Doz (regular strength)	1 tablet	100 mg

While you may be worrying about the aspartame in the diet drink or the nitrites in your morning sausage, perhaps the th widely used additives—sugar, salt, and caffeine—are of more concern right now.

Sugar not only promotes tooth decay, but it can add empty calories to your diet resulting in poor nutrition and weight gain. While a sprinkle of salt doesn't seem to be harmful, it may contribute to hypertension in some people—and high blood pressure is not something you want to contend with during pregnancy, much less any other time.

BMT 9. Maintain a Normal Weight

Today's society places great importance on physical appearance. Study after study confirms that there is a definite correlation between body weight and infertility. For many women, being at a very low weight or losing too much weight can keep them from making a baby. In mild cases of weight change, your ovaries may still function normally, producing and releasing eggs.

Comprehensive research reveals that maintaining an ideal body weight is most compatible with fertility and normal menstrual function. Rapid weight loss and chronic undernourishment in otherwise normal women can lead to amenorrhea because of lack of ovulation—and again, no baby. In fact, recent studies show that thinner women (and men) may be in a chronic state of malnutrition. A minimum of approximately 22 percent body fat appears necessary to ensure normal ovulation and reproductive competence. When body fat falls below this minimum, altered gonadotropin secretion results from hypothalamic changes. This alteration may be an adaptive phenomenon to prevent pregnancy, a physiologically stressful state, in an undernourished body. Restoration of body fat restores normal gonadotropin secretory patterns and cyclic menses and ovulation.

Don't Tip the Scales

On the other end of the scale (no pun intended) is being overweight, and obesity has reached epidemic proportions. Just as an abnormally low body weight impacts negatively on reproduction, so does an abnormally high body weight. Reproductive disorders may result from hormonal changes caused by increased body fat. Alterations in peripheral gonadotropin feedback can result in increased LH levels, with the resulting ovulatory and menstrual dysfunction. This change in hormones appears reversible. In comprehensive studies, losing weight—as little as 10 percent of body weight—resulted in the restoration of normal endocrinologic and menstrual patterns in obese women who were infertile.

If years of deprivation dieting to stay model-slim have stressed your body, causing an imbalance of hormones and making it difficult to conceive, you owe it to your future family to get off the diet roller coaster. For those who are dealing with added pounds, not only does carrying around extra baggage decrease your fertility, weighing as little as ten or fifteen pounds over your desired weight can exacerbate a heart condition, elevate blood pressure and cholesterol, and even increase your risk of certain cancers. In the midst of the pessimistic fertility outlook for under- or overweight women, there is some good news: While losing or gaining weight can increase infertility, maintaining a normal weight can reduce the risk.

Obesity is defined in terms of excess body fat. Traditionally, height/weight charts gave an accurate portrayal of overweight. Yet now experts believe that your body mass index (BMI) (see page 35) may give a more accurate picture of health. BMI is defined as body weight (in kilograms) divided by height (in square meters). The BMI number or value correlates to your risk of adverse effects on health, with higher numbers showing an increased risk. According to the American Dietetic Association, people with a higher percentage of body fat tend to have a higher BMI than those who have a greater percentage of muscle. It is this extra body fat, not muscle, that may be altering your hormones, leading to infertility.

Balancing the Scale

As you seek to maintain a normal weight, understand that each person is different. While your best friend may be the same height as you yet weigh 10 to 20 pounds less, you may both be at your optimal weight, depending on certain variables, including age, bone structure, and genetics.

The truth is, during the past five years, comprehensive scientific studies have shed light on the impact of deprivation diets on weight loss, and the findings have consistently held true: Diets alone don't work. In fact, if anything, dieting only makes you gain weight by training your body to store fat rather than burn it. Yes, deprivation dieting can help you lose weight. Yet for most people who eat less, a third of this loss is reduction of muscle, not fat—and lean muscle (as opposed to body fat) is what helps burn calories.

Lean on What Really Works

Knowing that deprivation or fad diets don't work, we can lean on research from the experts. The National Institutes of Health (NIH) revealed that true weight-loss success can happen only if you change your eating habits for good—for a lifetime. You already have certain habits like washing your hair or brushing your teeth that you do without thinking twice. Eating a low-fat, healthy diet must also become a natural part of your daily life—a true change in eating habits that will result in your reaching and maintaining a safe, normal weight. Trying to lose weight too fast from crash dieting can drain your body's nutritional stores, which could hurt both you and your baby in the long run.

Yet some women can consume large amounts of food and never gain weight, and others have to almost starve themselves to stay plump instead of severely obese. If you have problems with obesity, sometimes there are no simple answers for losing weight. You may be eating a low-fat, low-calorie diet and exercising regularly and still find yourself at a higher than desirable weight. Don't add to the guilt you may feel; just eat right and exercise to stay healthy, not to stay thin.

BMT 10. Rev Up Your Engines . . . But Not Too Much

The drug-free BMTs would not be complete without addressing the importance of moderate exercise to keep your body running at optimal performance. Studies show that aerobic fitness and reproductive fitness go hand in hand when it comes to making a healthy baby. Yet sometimes too much exercise or the wrong kind of exercise can actually hinder conception. For example, if you exercise intensely to stay thin and fit, you may get more than you bargained for with amenorrhea, or lack of menstrual periods. Men who exercise intensely can reduce sperm count because of the heat that builds up around the testicles during exercise. Those men who ride bicycles may experience impotence from nerve damage caused by pressure from the bicycle seat. Likewise, if your partner enjoys rough sports, the genital area can easily be injured.

Studies on the hidden dangers of overexercising continue to pour in. Experts believe that strenuous exercise leads to increased endorphin levels, which in turn acts on your central nervous system to suppress reproductive function. Increased cortisol and insulin-like growth factor have been observed in elite athletes and dancers suffering from menstrual dysfunction and may limit the metabolic processes that control reproduction.

Overexercising has been linked to menstrual disturbances (delayed menarche, secondary amenorrhea, or shortened luteal phase). In fact, vigorous exercise of one hour or more per day has been highly correlated with infertility. The resulting hormonal imbalances from overexercising can lead to decreases in bone density that may approach 4 percent per year. Studies show that with increasing numbers of women participating in jogging and long-distance running, the prevalence of these disorders is expected to increase. Women with athletic amenorrhea must be provided with hormonal (estrogen and progesterone) and calcium supplementation (1,500 mg/day) to protect against osteoporosis and fractures from bone loss.

While rigorous endurance training may lead to difficulties in conception, the other extreme of no exercise may also increase your chance of infertility. Obesity can hinder reproductive function for both men and women and is often a direct result of a sedentary lifestyle or lack of exercise.

Moderate, routine exercise and an active lifestyle are important to staying at a normal weight and to achieving reproductive fitness. Exercise also offers well-established health benefits, including:

- Increases metabolism to burn more calories
- Improves quality of sleep
- Boosts brain power
- Reduces body fat
- Helps to protect against breast, uterine, ovarian, cervical, and vaginal cancers
- Helps to prevent benign breast disease
- Helps to prevent benign tumors of the reproductive system
- Strengthens your bones
- Boosts endorphins, improving your mood and helping to relieve depression
- Cuts your risk for diabetes, hypertension, and other diseases
- Improves cholesterol profile (increases protective HDLs)
- Enhances your self-image
- Increases your sexual appetite (libido)

If you are athletic and exercise more than one hour daily, talk with your doctor before you attempt to get pregnant. If necessary, consult with

---

Baby-Boosting Activities and Exercises

Biking	House cleaning	Softball	Tai chi
Bowling	Karate	Stair-climbing	Vacuuming
Dancing	Low-impact aerobics	Stationary cycling	Walking
Gardening	Mall walking	Strength training	Water exercise
Golf	Mowing the yard	Stretching	Window
Handball	Qigong	Swimming	washing
Hiking	Rowing	Tae kwon do	Yoga

Different Types of Exercise

Range-of-motion or stretching exercises. These involve moving a joint as far as it will go (without pain) or through its full range of motion.

Endurance or conditioning exercises. These involve cardiovascular forms of exercise such as walking, running, biking, swimming, rowing, or aerobics.

Strengthening exercises. These exercises help to build strong muscles, ligaments, and tendons needed to support your body.

---

a registered dietitian regarding balanced nutritional intake. Be aware of the warning signs of overexercise, including menstrual cycle irregularities. By understanding the benefits and detriments of exercise and activity to your fertility success, you can make healthful choices with minimal risks to your reproductive system.

Start Training for Your Greatest Event

When you consider that you may gain twenty to thirty pounds or more during pregnancy, then have to perform the greatest athletic feat in your life—giving birth—regular exercise becomes increasingly important. While it's hard to say how much exercise is too much, many experts feel that running more than 10 miles per week is considered extreme when trying to conceive. Nonetheless, moderate exercise, alternating between the different types described in the sidebar above, should not affect fertility, especially if you have been exercising regularly. Talk with your doctor about the amount that is best for you—and start now before you conceive to get your body physically fit.

Relax, Relax, Relax!

When all is said and done, probably the best thing you can do is to relax! Sure, you've heard this from your best friend or your mother, but it is important. Change the things you can and seek help for those you cannot change and learn all you can about how your body works. One source of comfort for most people is knowing that you are doing all you possibly can to boost the chances of making a baby. Still, perhaps the greatest source of comfort should be the fact that the vast majority of couples can make a baby over time!

Chapter 10

Making the Food-Fertility Connection

"If only there were a magic fertility food or supplement!" says Judith, age 26. "I know I could get pregnant. In some countries they eat foods that resemble sexual organs, such as eggs or figs, hoping it will help their internal organs perform better. Or what about an herb like ginseng, or even chocolate? I've read that these are considered to enhance fertility."

Sound familiar? Aren't most of us like Judith in that we hope for a magic food or supplement that will instantly solve our health problems? Whether the problem is fertility, depression, hypertension, or obesity, who wouldn't seek a natural food cure if science proved that it would work?

Yet in the midst of speculation that certain foods or herbs can help you to make a baby, the reality is that researchers have not identified a miracle food to cure infertility. There is no scientific data to support the notion that eating pine nuts, prunes, powdered rhinoceros horn, or even pulverized shark's fin—all rumored to boost fertility—will help you get pregnant and stay pregnant. However, before you skip this chapter, there *are* some amazing food-fertility connections you should know to boost your immune function. A well-functioning immune system fights against any viruses, foreign substances, or potentially cancerous cells and destroys them, preventing infections and disease. When your immune system is working correctly, it allows your body to function at its peak with all the systems, including your reproductive system, working together without a hitch.

In short, eating the right nutrients is an important baby-boosting measure you can take as you play an active role in stopping infertility.

Nutrients are special compounds that support the body's repair, growth, and wellness. They include vitamins, minerals, amino acids, essential fatty acids, water, and the calorie sources of carbohydrate, protein, and fat. Not only can lack of nutrients reduce reproductive health, but the latest research supports the fact that a diet adequate in a variety of key nutrients can actually bolster the immune system and boost your chances of conceiving. While there are no guarantees that these nutrient-dense foods will make you immediately fertile, scientists continue to tout the tremendous benefits of food in healing the body to the point where it can continue to fight off serious illnesses, including hormone-related problems.

Eat to Stay Well

Before you can take advantage of healing nutrients to help boost your immune function and chances of getting pregnant, you must first make some minor changes in your attitude about food.

YOU MUST MAKE A COMMITMENT TO EATING FOR OPTI-MAL WELLNESS. The food-fertility connection is *not* about counting fat grams and calories. While it is important to watch calories and fats to maintain a normal weight, the food-fertility connection focuses on how targeted nutrients work together to help optimize immune function. Comprehensive scientific research concludes that deficiencies of single nutrients can result in altered immune responses even when the deficiency is relatively mild. For those who may have difficulty conceiving because of possible immune problems, eating well may help get your body back on track.

Think of your body as a car. Just as your car needs the proper fuel to make it run, your body needs the exact balance of essential nutrients— vitamins, minerals, antioxidants, phytochemicals, and known and little-known nutrients—to help you stay well. Each vitamin or mineral regulates a specific bodily process. For instance, calcium and iron are two minerals that are especially important during pregnancy. Your calcium intake will help to develop your baby's skeleton and also keep your bones strong. You will definitely need strong bones to carry that extra 25 pounds for nine months! Foods rich in iron are essential for making hemoglobin, which carries oxygen throughout your body and into the placenta for your developing baby. Many women enter pregnancy with marginal calcium and iron stores. The truth is, if you don't consume enough of these minerals, your baby will use the calcium from your bones and the iron in your blood, leaving you feeling fatigued and weak. How can you adequately care for a newborn if your body is depleted? You can't!

YOU MUST REALIZE THAT WHAT YOU EAT NOW CAN AFFECT YOUR HEALTH IN YEARS TO COME. If you're having a baby in your early twenties, you're probably not thinking about heart disease or diabetes. Yet delaying degenerative diseases becomes important as we postpone starting our families until our thirties or even forties. Persuasive research supports the fact that dietary habits play a key role in five of the nation's leading causes of death: cancer, stroke, heart disease, diabetes, and atherosclerosis. A steady diet of highly processed junk foods with empty calories just may be the trigger for heart disease or diabetes at midlife. That is why using the food-fertility connection will help increase your chance of conception and also keep your body functioning at its best so you can stay energetic and well enough to raise that active family.

YOU MUST TRY TO USE NATURAL FOODS TO MEET YOUR NUTRITIONAL NEEDS INSTEAD OF RELYING TOTALLY ON SUPPLEMENTS. The Recommended Dietary Allowances (RDAs) are issued by the Food and Nutrition Board of the National Academy of Sciences as the levels of nutrients thought to be adequate to meet the known nutrient needs of most healthy individuals. In layman's terms, this means that the RDAs will help to prevent deficiency-related diseases such as beriberi or scurvy. The most recent recommendations were published in 1989, before the conclusive data on disease prevention and human embryonic development.

While most women do not meet the RDA of vitamins and minerals by diet alone, national research shows that only 20 to 25 percent of all women of childbearing age take multivitamin and mineral supplements. If you have a long history of dieting and poor eating habits, you may need supplementation. Nonetheless, if you are thinking about making up for years of poor eating habits by taking megadoses of vitamins and minerals, don't do it. Excessive vitamin and mineral intake during pregnancy may have toxic effects on you and your unborn child. Ask your doctor or a dietician about the right level of nutrients for your specific health needs.

Different Types of Supplements

- *Time-released* supplements dissolve slowly in the intestine over a six- to twelve-hour period, thus increasing the absorption of a vitamin.
- *Chelated* minerals are designed to increase absorption in the body.
- *Superpotency* or *therapeutic* supplements contain at least one ingredient in a dose ten times or more greater than the DV (daily value).

You may need to start on prenatal vitamins to prepare your body for pregnancy. These are usually prescription vitamins that contain nutrients at levels recommended for pregnant women, with increased amounts of folic acid, iron, calcium, and vitamin C (improves iron and calcium absorption). Of course, taking additional vitamins and minerals does not lessen the importance of eating a nutritionally balanced diet. Again, talk with your doctor about your specific health needs.

YOU MUST CHOOSE A WIDE VARIETY OF FOODS EACH DAY USING THE FOOD GUIDE PYRAMID. How can you be sure of getting ample nutrients to help you get pregnant and deliver a healthy baby? This is easily addressed by choosing from the foods offered in the USDA's Food Guide Pyramid. For those who are used to snacking on peanut butter crackers and colas throughout the day, this will mean a major change in lifestyle. Now your challenge is to focus on the nutrient-dense foods that will ensure you are getting a necessary amount of vitamins and minerals.

The Food Guide Pyramid (see Figure 10.1) from the United States Dietetics Association gives us an illustration of how we should eat to stay lean and healthy. It recommends plenty of low-fat nutrient-dense foods such as fruits, vegetables, cereal, bread, and pasta, with less emphasis on whole-milk products and high-fat meats. Our diet should be built on the plant foods—fruit, vegetable, and grain products. That does not mean we eliminate the milk and meat or meat substitute groups. You can use low-fat versions of these foods to complement the rest of the plant-based diet. Fats and sweets should be used sparingly, especially by people trying to lose weight, as they contribute extra calories but few nutrients.

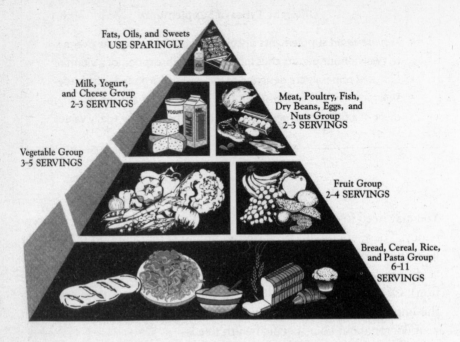

Figure 10.1.   The Food Guide Pyramid

Complex Carbohydrates

Most of your food choices should come from the widest part, or the bottom of the pyramid. These foods include whole grain breads and cereals, pasta and rice, grains, vegetables, and fruits. Carbohydrates are the body's main source of energy or calories as well as a host of vitamins and minerals. Some studies indicate that carbs may promote the circulation of reproductive hormones by promoting a better body-brain connection.

RECOMMENDED DAILY AMOUNT

Starchy foods: 6 to 11 servings
Fruit group: 2 to 4 servings
Vegetable group: 3 to 5 servings

Table 10.1 Food Guide Pyramid Serving Sizes

Bread, Cereal, Rice, and Pasta
1 slice of bread
$^1/_2$ hamburger bun
$^1/_2$ bagel
$^1/_2$ English muffin
$^3/_4$ ounce of pretzels
$^1/_2$ cup cooked cereal, pasta, and rice
1 ounce cold cereal

Fruit
1 medium piece of fruit
$^1/_2$ cup chopped, cooked, or canned fruit
$^1/_2$ cup fruit juice

Vegetables
$^1/_2$ cup cooked
1 cup raw

Milk
1 cup skim or nonfat milk
1 cup nonfat, sugar-free yogurt
$1^1/_2$ ounces fat-free cheese

Meat and Meat Substitutes
2 to 3 ounces of lean meat, fish, or poultry without the skin
1 to $1^1/_2$ cups cooked beans
2 eggs or $^1/_2$ cup low-cholesterol egg alternative

THE BOTTOM LINE. An extra benefit of complex carbs is the calming effect they have on your system. Dr. Judith Wurtman, a nutrition researcher at the Massachusetts Institute of Technology, has found that "persuasive" foods high in carbohydrates, such as breads, cereal, pasta, or sherbet, raise the level of serotonin in the brain. Serotonin is a mood-elevating brain chemical that has a calming effect—pretty important when fertility tests make your stress skyrocket! Studies have shown that by including plenty of foods high in complex carbohydrates in your diet, you can boost the level of serotonin and reap the benefits of a calm feeling throughout the day, along with sounder sleep. Here is a list of some suggested serotonin-boosting foods:

Bagels	Crackers	Potatoes
Bread	Muffins	Rice
Cereal	Pasta	Sherbet

See which ones make a difference in your energy and mood, then incorporate these throughout the day to keep blood sugar and energy levels even.

Milk, Yogurt, and Cheese Group

As you move up the pyramid, it gets smaller, as do the number of servings recommended. Yet if you thought you were drinking enough milk to keep bones strong, wait until you get pregnant. While a nonpregnant woman age 25 to 50 needs 1,000 mg calcium each day, requirements increase during pregnancy to 1,000 to 1,500 mg, or the equivalent of 4 or more cups of milk. Now that's a lot of milk! During the third trimester, most of your calcium is transferred to the fetus, so it's important to have ample stores.

Low-fat dairy products such as low-fat milk, buttermilk, cheese and cheese products, cottage cheese, ice milk, and yogurt will help you maintain a normal weight and keep your bones strong during pregnancy. Studies show that a diet high in low-fat dairy products and fruits and vegetables significantly lowers blood pressure.

RECOMMENDED DAILY AMOUNT. 2 to 3 servings (normal adults); 4+ servings (pregnant women).

THE BOTTOM LINE. While you add more dairy products to your diet, make sure your partner does the same. Infertility researchers at the University of Wisconsin at Madison suggest that consuming 1,000 mg of calcium and 10 micrograms of vitamin D each day may improve men's fertility. Good sources of calcium include low-fat milk (an 8-ounce glass has 414 mg) and yogurt (1 cup has 302 mg of calcium). You'll find vitamin D in milk (an 8-ounce glass has 2 mcg) and salmon (a 3-ounce serving has 8 mcg).

Baby Buster

Avoid soft cheeses such as Brie, blue cheese, Camembert, and feta unless they are heated to boiling stage. These cheeses often have harmful bacteria called listeria, which are linked to miscarriages.

CALCIUM-RICH BABY BOOSTERS

500 milligrams
8½ ounces cheese-filled manicotti
Instant Breakfast drink made with 1 cup milk
1 cup milk
1 fruit yogurt smoothie with ¼ cup powdered skim milk added
1 small cheese pizza

400 milligrams
8 medium sardines, canned with bones
8 ounces of nonfat yogurt
12 ounces of enchiladas with cheese
4 buckwheat pancakes, 4 inches in diameter
1 average chocolate milkshake

300 milligrams
Orange juice with added calcium
Calcium-fortified cereal with ½ cup milk
Cream of broccoli soup made with milk and cheese
1¼ cups of black beans
1 cup of scalloped potatoes with cheese

200 milligrams
½ cup instant pudding made with milk
1 ounce American cheese
1 cup of steamed kale
1 cup macaroni and cheese
1 cup lasagna and cheese

Meat, Poultry, Fish, Dry Beans, Eggs, and Nuts Group

Proteins supply the building blocks that repair and maintain your body tissue and fight infection. They are also the baby-building cell nutrients vital for normal fetal development. Protein is found in meat, poultry, fish, eggs, cheese, milk and milk products, peas, tofu, and dried beans.

RECOMMENDED DAILY AMOUNT. 2 to 3 servings; pregnant women add 10 grams more protein during pregnancy.

THE BOTTOM LINE. Too little protein in your diet may lead to symptoms of fatigue, weakness, apathy, and poor immunity. One ounce of meat, chicken, cheese, or fish provides 7 grams of protein; 1 cup of milk provides 8 grams of protein. If you're not a meat eater, vegetable proteins can make a good substitute for animal protein, if eaten with a complementary starch at the same meal.

COMPLEMENTARY VEGETABLE PROTEINS

Beans and bread   Legumes and grains
Beans and rice   Peanut butter and bread
Corn tortillas and beans   Soy-nut butter and bread

Fats, Oils, and Sweets

Fats supply energy, transport nutrients throughout your body, and help you feel satisfied after eating. Fats fall into three main categories: *saturated* (animal, dairy, coconut oil, and palm oil); *monounsaturated* (canola and olive oil); and *polyunsaturated* (sunflower, corn, soybean, and safflower oil). While fats have been given a bad rap because they cause weight gain, elevate the level of fat in your blood, and are linked to certain cancers, dietary fat is the carrier for the fat-soluble vitamins and for linoleic acid, an essential fatty acid.

RECOMMENDED DAILY AMOUNT. Use sparingly.

THE BOTTOM LINE. While you need a small amount of fat, it supplies more than twice as many calories per gram as carbohydrates or proteins and can quickly contribute to weight gain. The American Heart Association, the American Cancer Society, and the National Academy of Science all recommend that Americans reduce their fat calories to less than 30 percent of total calories.

1 gram of fat = 9 calories
1 gram of carbohydrate = 4 calories
1 gram of protein = 4 calories

YOU MUST CAREFULLY CONSIDER YOUR GOAL OF CONCEPTION IF YOU ARE A VEGETARIAN. Even though under normal circumstances, eating a vegetarian diet is extremely healthful, studies conclude that female vegetarians tend to have an increased incidence of menstrual abnormalities and ovulatory dysfunction, which can delay conception. High-fiber vegetarianism results in decreased serum estradiol levels because of increased fecal estrogen excretion. In two separate studies of female vegetarians, midcycle LH and luteal phase progesterone and estrogen levels were all decreased. These changes were not observed in the respective control groups. If you are a vegetarian, consult with a dietician to see how to supplement your diet to boost fertility.

Boost Your Immune Power

Although genetics probably determine the strength of your immune system, researchers now confirm that specific vitamins and minerals may help boost its function as you focus on optimal fertility health. For example, vitamins A (beta-carotene), C, and E are known as antioxidants and are crucial anti-aging nutrients. Zinc, selenium, folic acid, copper, iron, and magnesium are also involved in the formation of healthy new cells, and your body constantly needs new white blood cells to fight off a host of potentially aging diseases and degenerative problems.

As such, each nutrient may play an important role as a Baby Booster. For example, vitamin E is a major Baby Booster. Studies show this vitamin may help boost reproductive health. Zinc, another Baby Booster, fights against viruses and keeps reproductive health at its peak for men and women. Although the individual properties and functions of each nutrient are important, it is the *sum of their effectiveness together* that may really protect and strengthen your immune system and help to increase your fertility.

Baby Booster 1. Choose Healing Nutrients

As soon as you get pregnant, your body's need for nutrients increases to help your baby develop normally. Some of these nutrients are made by your body (nonessential nutrients); others must come from your diet (essential nutrients). A deficiency of either type of nutrient may lead to illness if left untreated. That's why it's important to start now—before conception—preparing for this physically demanding time in your life.

The baby-boosting nutrients you need to focus on include several important vitamins. Vitamins regulate your body processes, setting off chemical reactions in the cells. Each vitamin performs a specific function in the body, and no single food contains all the vitamins. During pregnancy, your body will require even more vitamins, especially those important for cell division.

Minerals and water are also essential. Minerals are required for normal growth and development and strong bones and teeth.

Water regulates your body temperature and other body processes, carries nutrients to cells, and takes waste material away. You're going to need at least 8 to 12 cups daily during pregnancy, so you'd better start practicing now.

You wouldn't run a marathon if you hadn't spent months getting in shape, would you? Well, the same goes for making a baby. It takes time before you conceive to get your body in top shape nutritionally. You can make sure it's running at optimal capacity by eating foods high in the following baby-boosting vitamins.

Folic Acid

Folic acid is the one vitamin that is a *must* for all women of childbearing age. This B vitamin can significantly lower the risk of neural tube defects such as spina bifida (incomplete closure of the spine) for your baby. Worldwide, it is estimated that about 500,000 children are born each year with anencephaly, meningomyelocele, and, more rarely, encephalocele, with 4,000 of these births occurring in the United States. Neural tube defects occur in approximately one to three of every 1,000 births. The actual incidence is even higher because so many affected pregnancies result in unreported abortion or unrecognized miscarriage.

Infants who have neural tube defects are at higher risk for mortality because of problems resulting from surgical procedures, paralysis, hydrocephalus, bowel and bladder incontinence, and developmental problems. Comprehensive research has found that up to 50 to 75 percent of such malformations can be prevented with proper folic acid intake before and after conception.

Low folate is common among women who do not eat many fruits, green vegetables, and whole grain or fortified cereals, and can lead to:

- Spontaneous abortion
- Preterm delivery
- Small-for-gestational-age infants
- Neural tube defects

Preliminary research also links low folic acid intake with an increased risk of cervical cancer in women. Poor eating habits, alcohol abuse, cigarette smoking, and oral contraceptives have all been linked to low blood levels of folic acid.

RECOMMENDED DAILY AMOUNT. Taking folic acid is a must to protect your unborn child. The RDA for folic acid is 400 milligrams (mg) for all women of childbearing age and *at least 800 milligrams for pregnant women.* (Most standard vitamins contain 400 mcg.)

THE BOTTOM LINE. You must take folic acid!

Doctor's Rx

Other than protecting the health of your unborn child, folic acid has another possible benefit with mood management. In research performed at Massachusetts General Hospital in Boston and the Baylor Research Institute in Dallas, studies are conclusive that people with low folate levels are more likely to have melancholia, a type of depression characterized by sadness and declines in mental and physical activity. The eight-week study of 213 patients also found that those with low levels of folate were significantly less likely to respond to treatment for depression with fluoxetine (Prozac), a common antidepressant medication.

FOLIC ACID BABY BOOSTERS

FOOD	SERVING SIZE	AMOUNT (MG)
Breakfast cereals	$^1/_2$ cup–1 cup	100–400
Chicken liver	$3^1/_2$ ounces	770
Lentils (cooked)	$^1/_2$ cup	180
Chickpeas	$^1/_2$ cup	140
Spinach (cooked)	$^1/_2$ cup	130
Black beans	$^1/_2$ cup	130
Kidney beans	$^1/_2$ cup	115
Orange	1 medium	40
Broccoli (raw)	$^1/_2$ cup	60

Other Key B Vitamins

Several other B vitamins are important to your overall health, as well as for moms-to-be. **Vitamin B_6** is necessary for the metabolism of protein, carbohydrate, and lipids. Some studies reveal that safe doses of vitamin B_6 supplementation may be helpful in treating nausea and vomiting during early pregnancy. One study found that B_6 increases progesterone levels. The recommended daily amounts of B_6 are 2.0 milligrams (mg) for males; 1.6 mg for females; 2.2 mg for pregnant women. Studies show that for many women in the United States, dietary intake of vitamin B_6 is below the RDA. You can get adequate vitamin B through meats, liver, and enriched grains. Vitamin B_6 is one of the few water-soluble vitamins that can be toxic if taken in large doses, so talk to your doctor about the need for supplementation.

Vitamin B_{12}, which is found in animal protein foods such as fish, eggs, meat, and milk, is vital for normal cell division and protein synthesis. Vitamin B_{12} can enhance your partner's sperm count. The recommended daily amounts are 2.0 micrograms (mcg) for normal adults; 2.2 mcg for pregnant women. If you are a meat eater, getting adequate vitamin B_{12} is probably not a problem. Yet vegetarians are at risk for deficiency and may benefit from a daily vitamin B_{12} supplement. Talk to your doctor.

Baby Booster 2. Add Plenty of Antioxidants

Almost nine out of ten doctors endorse the role of antioxidants in fighting disease, according to an informal poll by the *Medical Tribune*, a newspaper for physicians. These essential nutrients help protect your body against life's stressors. New studies from the Male Reproductive Center at Columbia-Presbyterian Medical Center in New York conclude that antioxidants (vitamins A, C, and E) also have a great effect on fertility. Research indicates that vitamin E deficiency can lead to "sluggish sperm," and just 200 milligrams a day may enhance the man's sperm's ability to fertilize an egg by about 10 percent. Men who are diagnosed with male infertility have an increased incidence of an abnormality called lipid peroxidation in their sperm. Adding 500 mg of vitamin C twice each day appears to be helpful in decreasing this type of sperm damage.

Antioxidant food sources are rich in beta-carotene and vitamins C and E. These nutrients are thought to play a role in protecting the body from free radicals, which destroy cell membranes, damage DNA, and may be a root cause of certain types of cancer, heart disease, and even the aging process itself. Using the food-fertility connection to your healthful advantage and to stay disease-free requires a diet rich in antioxidants.

Beta-Carotene

Beta-carotene, found in apricots, carrots, cantaloupe, pumpkin, and spinach, is the water-soluble form of vitamin A. Vitamin A is a fat-soluble vitamin and is found in foods of animal origin such as liver, milk, butter, and eggs. Beta-carotene helps protect the mucous membranes of the mouth, nose, throat, lungs, and reproductive tract, thereby reducing susceptibility to infections. A New York study of 439 postmenopausal women found the highest risk of breast cancer in those women who had low intakes of beta-carotene. Remember, while your goal is to have a healthy baby, she or he will also need healthy parents!

Because of a great deal of media attention, most people think of only beta-carotene as having antioxidant properties, but other carotenoid compounds do as well, including:

- Alpha-carotene (found in carrots, cantaloupe, and pumpkin)
- Beta-cryptoxanthin (found in mangoes, nectarines, peaches, and tangerines)
- Gamma-carotene (found in apricots and tomatoes)
- Lutein and zeaxanthin (found in beets, corn, and collard and mustard greens)
- Lycopene (found in guava, pink grapefruit, tomatoes, and watermelon)

Doctor's Rx

Do not ever take high doses (more than 8,000 international units) of vitamin A. This amount can be toxic to you and your unborn baby. In a study published in *The New England Journal of Medicine,* consumption of vitamin A at or above 10,000 IU was linked to birth defects.

RECOMMENDED AMOUNT. The current RDAs for vitamin A are 5,000 international units (IU) for men and 4,000 IU for women.

THE BOTTOM LINE. The RDA of vitamin A does *not* increase during pregnancy and is easily met by eating a balanced diet. Beta-carotene is in most multivitamin supplements and has not been associated with toxicity. While many people try to get vitamin A and beta-carotene from supplements, using natural foods is best.

BETA-CAROTENE BABY BOOSTERS

Apricots	Mustard greens
Asparagus	Spinach
Beef liver	Squash, winter
Broccoli	Sweet potato
Cantaloupe	Watermelon
Carrots	Yellow corn
Kale	

Vitamin C

Vitamin C (ascorbic acid) is essential for your body's metabolic process. It protects against infection and aids in wound healing. Recent studies indicate that vitamin C is important in women to help the ovaries to respond properly to fertilization. In men, studies show that low levels of vitamin C may produce slow-moving, abnormally shaped sperm, fewer sperm, and sperm that clump together. At the University of Texas at Galveston, researchers reported that men who took 1,000 milligrams of vitamin C daily for two months boosted their sperm counts by 60 percent, and all men who took the vitamin C were able to impregnate their partners.

RECOMMENDED AMOUNT. The RDA for women is 60 mg; 70 mg for pregnant women. Higher doses may cause diarrhea.

THE BOTTOM LINE. Most people get more than the RDA by eating a variety of fruits and vegetables each day. A word of caution: Taking 1 gram of vitamin C, which is commonly done to prevent the common cold, may be toxic for your fetus. If you are a smoker, long-term user of contraceptives, or heavy drinker, taking 50 milligrams of vitamin C each day may be beneficial. Also, because vitamin C has an antihistamine effect in the body, women should be cautious about supplements, as it could dry up cervical mucus.

VITAMIN C BABY BOOSTERS

Broccoli	Papaya
Cantaloupe	Red, green, or yellow pepper
Cauliflower	Strawberries
Kale	Sweet potato
Orange juice	Tomato juice

Vitamin E

Sophisticated research has found vitamin E to be a powerful antioxidant and important to the body for the maintenance of cell membranes. This vitamin, already praised for healthy hearts, has an antioxidant effect that may help prevent breast cancer and delay Alzheimer's disease. In one study at the National Cancer Institute (1997), a derivative of vitamin E called VES blocked the growth of and even killed breast-cancer cells. Vitamin E appears to stimulate the function of T cells, which are considered important fighters in the immune system. This antioxidant may affect the production of prostaglandins, hormone-like substances in the body that regulate different body processes including reproduction, blood pressure, and muscle contraction. Researchers in Israel report an increase in fertility rates by 30 percent in men who took 200 milligrams of vitamin E daily. Other scientific studies report that vitamin E significantly improves sperm motility—vital for making a baby.

RECOMMENDED DAILY AMOUNT. 15 international units (IU) for men; 12 IU for women; 15 IU for pregnant women.

THE BOTTOM LINE. Don't count on your daily diet to provide you with enough vitamin E to make a difference. You ingest vitamin E through vegetables and seed oils, yet you would have to eat 930 almonds to get the benefit of 400 IU of vitamin E—the amount necessary to benefit the heart. Or to get 400 IU from food, you would have to eat about 20,000 calories a day, mostly fat! Some researchers feel that the current RDA for vitamin E—15 international units (IU) for men and 12 IU for women—may be too low for disease protection. Taking 400 IU a day, thirteen times the RDA, appears to lower heart disease risk.

VITAMIN E BABY BOOSTERS

Almonds	Lobster
Cod-liver oil	Peanut butter
Corn oil	Safflower oil
Corn oil margarine	Salmon steak
Hazelnuts	Sunflower seeds

Baby Booster 3. Don't Forget Two Essential Minerals

Iron

Getting the required dietary iron isn't easy for most women, especially during pregnancy. Consider that about 300 milligrams of iron is trans-

---

Doctor's Rx

Most women are borderline in their iron stores. Taking the RDA of iron is vital before you get pregnant to ensure good health. Make sure you talk with your doctor about this during your prepregnancy checkup.

---

ferred to your fetus and placenta and another 500 milligrams are incorporated into the ever-expanding maternal hemoglobin mass. If you don't have enough iron to meet your body's needs, you will certainly know it. Symptoms of iron deficiency include fatigue, shortness of breath, paleness, and iron deficiency anemia.

RECOMMENDED DAILY AMOUNT. 12 milligrams (mg) for men; 15 mg for women; 30 mg for pregnant women. Iron supplements may affect bowels and digestion, so try to balance your iron intake between your diet and supplements.

THE BOTTOM LINE. It is virtually impossible to get the 30 milligrams of iron required during pregnancy from the food you eat. Your doctor may prescribe iron supplements at some point in your pregnancy or even before you conceive to make sure you get the necessary requirements. If your iron-rich food is from a plant source, include a vitamin C source, like orange or grapefruit juice, along with it to enhance iron absorption. Apple juice fortified with vitamin C is also a good source.

IRON-RICH BABY BOOSTERS

Dried apricots   Lentils
Dried beans   Prunes
Enriched or fortified bread and cereals   Raisins
Lean, fat-trimmed cuts of red meat
  (beef, veal, lamb, or pork)

Zinc

Zinc is critically important for proper functioning of the immune system for both men and women. Some recent studies indicate that the more sexually active a man is, the more zinc he will need. It appears that zinc helps to regulate testosterone levels, which dictate a man's sexual appetite. Also, when men exercise regularly and intensely, they may need more zinc. For example, runners have lower plasma zinc levels than controls in scientific studies.

Zinc has been implicated in increasing the number and motility of sperm in some men who are low in this mineral. While a substantial amount of zinc is lost in perspiration, increasing one's calcium intake can inhibit zinc absorption. Foods high in iron also compete with zinc. Zinc is found in eggs, whole grains, and meat. Oysters are high in zinc, yet beware of eating raw oysters, or you may be getting more than you bargained for. In some cases, raw oysters can make you violently ill and can even result in hepatitis, which damages the liver.

RECOMMENDED DAILY AMOUNT. 15 milligrams (mg) for men; 12 mg for women; 15 mg for pregnant women.

THE BOTTOM LINE. Foods high in zinc include seafood, eggs, meats, whole grains, wheat germ, nuts, and seeds; tea and coffee may hinder absorption. Before you begin to stockpile zinc supplements, here's a word of caution: High doses of zinc are toxic and may in fact suppress the immune function. Medications may also interfere with the absorption of zinc in the intestines and cause a deficiency. As with all vitamins and minerals, check with your doctor for what is safe in your situation.

ZINC BABY BOOSTERS

Baked beans	Lean red meat
Chicken	Lowfat milk and yogurt
Eggs	Oysters, shellfish, and other seafood
Fortified cereals	Tofu
Lean pork	Turkey

Baby Booster 4. Eat Your Weedies

Nutritional research reveals that a variety of food choices does more than provide optimal nutrient intake. A varied diet can also provide hundreds of nutrient and nonnutrient compounds that may be vital to disease protection. These compounds found in plant-based foods as a group are called phytochemicals (see Table 10.2) and are essential in boosting immune function and preventing diseases.

Phytochemicals appear in all plants (weedies!). A diet that includes a variety of grains, fruits, and vegetables should provide these substances if you vary your choices and methods of food preparation. Although there are phytochemical supplements and pills, it is better to get your phytochemicals from a varied diet. Because of the wide array of nutrients in foods essential for wellness, including those not yet identified, relying on supplements for good nutrition may limit your intake to just the known compounds. Aim for 5 to 9 servings of fruits and vegetables each day for optimal health.

Table 10.2

PHYTOCHEMICAL	FOOD SOURCES	HEALTH EFFECT
Vegetables, Fruits, and Seeds		
Sulfides (allyl)	garlic, onions, cruciferous vegetables*	cancer prevention, suppress tumor development
Capsaicin	hot chili peppers, Thai peppers, jalapeños	anti-inflammatory, cancer prevention
Carotenoids	carrots, winter squash, sweet potatoes, apricots, spinach, kale, parsley, soybeans, cereal grains, cruciferous vegetables, citrus fruits	antioxidant, heart disease, cancer prevention, improved immune function
Bioflavonoids	most vegetables and fruits, licorice, flaxseed, green tea	cancer prevention
Ellagic acid	grapes, raspberries, strawberries, apples	heart disease, cancer prevention

PHYTOCHEMICAL	FOOD SOURCES	HEALTH EFFECT
Isoflavones	soybeans, legumes	cancer prevention, menopause
Indoles	cruciferous vegetables	cancer prevention
Isothiocyanates	cruciferous vegetables, horseradish	cancer prevention
Limonoids, terpenes	citrus fruits, cumin, caraway seeds, ginger	cancer prevention
Linolenic acid	leafy vegetables, seeds, flaxseed	heart disease, cancer prevention
Lycopene	tomatoes, watermelon, pink grapefruit, guava, red peppers	cancer prevention
Monoterpenes	garlic, parsley, squash, basil, mint, eggplant, citrus fruits, tomatoes, fennel, cruciferous vegetables	antioxidant, heart disease, cancer prevention
Phenolic acids	garlic, green tea, cereal grains, soybeans, fruits, vegetables, licorice root, flaxseed	antioxidant, heart disease and cancer prevention
Plant sterols	broccoli, cabbage, soy products, peppers, whole grains	cancer prevention
Sulforaphane	cruciferous vegetables	cancer prevention

Beans and Grains

Genistein	soybeans and soy products, peanuts, mung beans, alfalfa sprouts	Blocks enzymes that turn on cancer genes, inhibits the growth of new blood vessels needed for new tumor growth, blocks entry of estrogen into cells and testosterone into the prostate; protects against breast cancer and prostate cancer;

PHYTOCHEMICAL	FOOD SOURCES	HEALTH EFFECT
Genistein, cont.		in lab studies, protects against all types of cancer cells including breast, colon, lung, prostate, skin, and leukemia; other compounds in soy may reduce blood cholesterol levels
Phytosterols, saponins	soybeans, dried beans	Suppress the growth of cancer cells in the large intestine and enhance immunity
Protease inhibitors	soybeans, dried beans	Prevent the conversion of normal cells to cancer cells and slow tumor growth
Phytic acid	grains like oats, rice, rye, and wheat; soybeans; peanuts; and sesame seeds	Prevents iron from producing cancer-causing free radicals; may reduce the risk of colon cancer

*Cruciferous vegetables include bok choy, broccoli, Brussels sprouts, cabbage, and cauliflower, among many.

Baby Booster 5. Choose Healing Nutraceuticals

Yes, suddenly food is medicine! In fact, the term *nutraceutical* means "food medicine," and this category includes a host of favorites such as broccoli, garlic, onions, and green tea—each with their own specific healing power. As you eat to boost your immune power, make daily choices from the following healing nutraceuticals:

BROCCOLI. This green tree-like vegetable is full of indoles, isothiocyanates, and sulforaphane—phytochemicals that have been shown to trigger enzyme systems that block or suppress cellular DNA damage, reduce tumor size (in animal studies), and decrease the effectiveness of estrogen-like hormones. In other words, it packs a power punch of healing nutrition! If you really want the highest concentration of these cancer-fighting compounds, get broccoli sprouts at your local health food store. The sprouts have 10 to 100 times more sulforaphane than mature broccoli.

FISH. Pregnant women are urged to eat fatty fish at least two or three times a week to build up reserves of omega-3 fatty acid. This substance in fish is necessary for fetal brain development. Might as well start stockpiling your reserve before conception by eating the following fish and shellfish:

- Anchovies
- Bluefish
- Lobster
- Mackerel
- Salmon
- Sardines
- Scallops
- Tuna
- Whitefish

Baby Buster

Caution: Avoid swordfish, shark, and fresh tuna (canned is fine), which may contain high levels of mercury.

GARLIC. Scientific research claims that garlic contains chemicals that act like ACE (angiotensin-converting enzyme) inhibitors, those prescription drugs commonly given to lower blood pressure and protect the heart. Supplements of garlic reduce blood pressure by dilating blood vessels. In fact, some studies have revealed that ingesting as much as one or two cloves of fresh garlic can lower mild blood pressure an average of 8 percent in one to three months. Researchers have found that garlic and

onions can block formation of nitrosamines. These are powerful carcinogens that target several sites in the body, usually the liver, colon, and
breasts. The more pungent the garlic or onion, the more abundant the
sulfur compounds.

GREEN TEA. Green tea is a powerful antioxidant and may help in
preventing liver, pancreatic, breast, lung, esophageal, and skin cancers.
Some new studies indicate that it may help in preventing osteoporosis,
certainly something for women of all ages to seriously consider. But here's
another surprise: Although scientists do not understand why, researchers
at the Kaiser Permanente Medical Care Program in California found
women who drank at least half a cup of tea a day nearly doubled their
odds of getting pregnant. Researchers also report that a nontoxic chemical found in green tea, epigallocatechin-3 gallate, acts against urokinase
(an enzyme crucial for cancer growth). One cup of green tea contains
between 100 and 200 milligrams of the antitumor ingredient.

OLIVE OIL. Olive oil is a monounsaturated fat that has also been
promoted recently as a heart-healthy oil that is preferable to other vegetable oils and margarine. In Mediterranean countries, olive oil is widely
used both for cooking and as a salad oil. Breast cancer rates are also
50 percent lower in Mediterranean countries than in the United States.

TOMATOES. Preliminary research confirms that the potent antioxidant lycopene, which is prominent in tomatoes, may be more powerful
than beta-carotene, alpha-carotene, and vitamin E. This antioxidant is
associated with protection against heart disease and certain cancers such
as prostate and lung cancer. Cooking tomatoes releases the lycopene and
makes it available for absorption in your body.

Control Is Essential to Optimal Health

No matter how uncertain your future may seem as you wait for the next
fertility test or procedure, eating for wellness is one area you can control
right now. Control is essential to staying well. You cannot control your
age or the hormonal havoc that may be causing your infertility. You can't
control the fact that your partner may have had mumps as an adolescent,
resulting in low sperm count. Nonetheless, knowing that you are doing
all you can to provide your unborn child with a healthy "nest" gives you
a sense of power. It also helps you to cope with the mood swings and

anxiety you may experience during this tumultuous period in your life. Not only will a nutritious diet filled with baby-boosting foods help to increase your chances of conceiving, but women who eat well and avoid known risks during pregnancy tend to have larger, healthier babies and fewer complications. Now that's worth an extra helping of broccoli, isn't it?

Part Three

Breakthrough Medical Solutions to Infertility

Chapter 11

User-Friendly Fertility Tests

*"We tried to get pregnant for two years before seeking further testing,"
said Kristin, age 44. "Daniel went through the sperm analysis with flying
colors, so then it was my turn. After taking my medical history and performing labs, the new RE recommended me for hysterosalpingography
(HSG), an x-ray procedure that uses a dye to show the uterine cavity.
Although there was some cramping, the procedure was not too bad,
and it was done at my doctor's clinic. Yet because the results were
abnormal, my doctor wanted to do further testing. I was immediately
scheduled for an ultrasound test. This confirmed that my fallopian
tubes had some blockage, probably as the result of a long history of
endometriosis. I did not even know I had endometriosis, even though I
had very painful menstrual periods. My RE said there was some scar
tissue in the tubes. Because of my age (late thirties), my RE said we
shouldn't waste any more time and recommended in vitro fertilization.
Within six months, I was carrying twins."*

As with any illness, taking control and reversing infertility starts with
an accurate diagnosis. Using one or more of the tests outlined in this
chapter, your doctor will determine the state of your reproductive health,
then move on with the best treatment—baby-boosting medications
and/or high-tech conception methods described in Chapters 13 and 14.

You should have a proactive, working relationship with your doctor
when discussing which test to order and why. Do not be satisfied with the
"I'm the doctor and I know best" attitude. While your doctor is the
resource who understands human reproduction and infertility, no one

knows your body better than you do. If you still do not feel comfortable with the diagnosis, talk to your doctor and see if more testing may give you peace of mind. Seek a second medical opinion until you feel that your infertility problem is treated correctly. Remember, it's your body and your future family—and for many couples, time and money are important commodities!

Keep in mind that because a person's problem with infertility may vary, there is no "official" order of tests. A study reported in *Fertility and Sterility* (Glatstein, 1998) revealed that although most reproductive endocrinologists agree on the major areas of the performance of infertility testing, there is significant variability in the details of the performance of most testing, especially with respect to the age of your doctor and the area in which he or she practices. While your RE in New York may start testing by ordering an ultrasound, your best friend's doctor in California may do lab work to measure hormone levels. In any case, once the cause of infertility is properly identified, your doctor can move forward with a personalized treatment regime that helps increase your chance of making that baby.

Doctors differ in their policies regarding general preconception blood testing. Some perform a "prenatal" panel; however, little is gained from this general blood testing, especially in infertility patients, who are usually young and healthy. The American College of Obstetricians and Gynecologists recommends that all women considering childbearing undergo testing for AIDS, hepatitis, rubella, and immunity. Once the basic blood work is complete, your doctor may require further testing for your specific situation.

If only one test is performed on a couple to evaluate fertility, it should be a semen analysis (see Chapter 12) to check for sperm quantity and quality. Even if there has been proven fertility in a prior or the present relationship, the test should still be done. In many cases, the semen analysis can be performed and the semen prepared at the same time for insemination. This can be an efficient means of treatment and evaluation at the same time. The diagnosis and treatment of male infertility is discussed in detail in Chapters 7 and 12.

Tests for ovulation can be performed without the help of a doctor. One basic method is charting menstrual cycle characteristics (pain, mucus, temperature changes, monitoring LH surges), which are discussed in Chapter 9. Other means include blood monitoring and ultrasound and are administered by your doctor.

Go FSH!

Certainly if you are over 40 and probably if you are over age 35, the measurement of follicle-stimulating hormone (FSH) level is essential. This blood test should be done at the start of the infertility evaluation and prior to any therapy.

The FSH level indirectly measures the store of follicles (ovarian reserve) and the eggs (oocytes) remaining in the ovary. Higher FSH levels individually also predict the quality of the remaining oocytes. FSH does what it says, it stimulates the development of follicles each month along a path toward ovulation (see Chapter 1). In the body's attempt to maintain normal function, as the number of eggs dwindles the FSH level rises to keep your cycles regular and ovulation occurring as long as possible. In a sense, the body places itself on fertility drugs.

Women who have gone through menopause have very high levels of FSH (and are incapable of becoming pregnant with their own eggs). However, young women who have had an accelerated decline in the ovarian store as a result of diseases or surgery of the ovary may also have high FSH levels. As FSH levels rise, the follicles develop more quickly and your menstrual cycle shortens. Many women think that as they age, menstrual cycles should lengthen, but the reverse is true.

To help predict your fertility, your doctor will measure your FSH levels by drawing blood on the second or third day of your menstrual cycle. The FSH test results will fall into one of three ranges: normal, borderline, or abnormal (see Table 11.1).

Table 11.1

Normal   Gives information on ovarian reserve but not totally predictive of a good response to fertility medication.

Borderline   Suggests poor ovarian reserve and need for prompt, aggressive treatment. In this borderline situation, a short period of time may make a significant difference when using your own eggs.

Abnormal   FSH level suggests poor ovarian reserve and that the chance for a *successful* pregnancy (live birth) with your own eggs is very low.

FSH Levels May Vary

FSH levels will vary from lab to lab, depending on the type of test used in that lab to measure FSH. Understanding this is critical, because results from one lab may indicate your FSH level is normal; while from another lab, an FSH level may fall into the abnormal range. Most infertility practices perform the blood testing in their facility or use a specific reference lab where a given level has been correlated with the response of their patients. Whereas many large independent labs (to which many patients—if they want the testing to be covered—are forced to go by insurance providers) will state a normal range for FSH levels, that may not be predictive of ovarian reserve in infertility patients.

In most labs, an FSH level under 8 is good and an FSH greater than 20 is clearly abnormal. The closer the level gets to 20, the more worrisome it becomes. In many infertility labs an FSH level of 10 to 20 is borderline as a predictor of ovarian reserve and may be associated with much poorer response to fertility drugs.

Estradiol Levels Are Important

Estradiol is the most important hormone in the estrogen family of sex steroid hormones. It does many things to prepare your reproductive system for pregnancy. Along with measuring the FSH level, blood estradiol level should be drawn on the second or third day of your cycle to substantiate the FSH level. If the estradiol level is more than 50, the FSH level may be suppressed. If the estradiol level is more than 50 on cycle day 2 or 3, this could indicate your ovarian reserve is compromised or a cyst has formed. The estradiol level, however, does not seem to be as absolutely predictive as the FSH level. In other words, conception may surprise even your doctor!

In the future, you may be tested for inhibin B, the hormone that is produced by the follicle. Inhibin B directly inhibits FSH production from the pituitary. This may be a more direct test, but at present it is not widely used.

Clomiphene Challenge Test

A further extension of the day-3 FSH level is the clomiphene challenge test (CCT). This test seems to be more sensitive in picking up diminished ovarian reserve, particularly as women get close to 40. For the clomiphene challenge test, your doctor will do the following:

1. Measure FSH and estradiol levels on the third day of the cycle
2. Give you 100 milligrams of the medication clomiphene on cycle days 5 to 9
3. Measure FSH level on day 10

If the FSH level on either cycle day 3 or 10 is abnormal, this suggests poor ovarian reserve. A greater number of infertility patients who are age 40 and older with a normal day-3 FSH and estradiol level will have an abnormal day-10 FSH level.

A modification of the CCT is the same as giving clomiphene therapeutically to induce ovulation with ultrasound and estradiol monitoring of response. This approach may have more practical advantages. It is always encouraging when normal development of a preovulatory follicle is seen on ultrasound.

How Does This Relate to Making a Baby?

In practical terms, an abnormal FSH level usually indicates a very low chance for a successful pregnancy when using fertility medication or in vitro fertilization. A recent study from the large IVF program at Saint Barnabas in New Jersey reported on the outcome of IVF cycles in more than a thousand patients with abnormal FSH levels. The pregnancy rate with IVF in these patients was less than 3 percent, and more than two-thirds of these pregnancies miscarried, resulting in a delivery rate of less than 1 percent. Women who get pregnant with an elevated FSH level have a high likelihood of miscarrying. Some studies have suggested that an abnormal FSH level is associated with a high percentage of genetically abnormal embryos. However, there may be a considerable difference between these women and older infertility patients with elevated FSH levels.

When Does an Abnormal FSH Level
Close the Door to Conception?

Abnormal FSH levels are not absolutely predictive of an inability to conceive. The body continues to try hard to keep ovulating. Most practitioners have treated women with markedly abnormal FSH levels who have gone on to deliver healthy babies.

Nonetheless, fertility is very much age related. Since live birth rates from IVF in women who are over 43 years old are less than 5 percent, and probably less than 1 percent in women over the age of 45, these women may want to consider oocyte donation even if they have normal FSH levels. On the other hand, a woman who is 35 years old with a borderline FSH level would certainly want to consider a trial of IVF with her own eggs before moving on to egg donation. There is some evidence that pregnancy rates with IVF are good in younger women (under 35) even if they do not produce many eggs.

Does the FSH Level Predict IVF Success?

Comprehensive research has found that a basal serum follicle-stimulating hormone level seems to be a better predictor of the outcome of an in vitro fertilization cycle than the patient's chronologic age. In a revealing study by Toner and colleagues, a day-3 FSH level less than 15 was associated with normal pregnancy and delivery rates in IVF cycles in women over 40. No woman with a basal FSH level above 25 achieved an ongoing pregnancy in an IVF cycle. Therefore, a day-3 serum FSH measurement may be very important in evaluating how aggressively to treat women approaching or over age 40, as well as in giving you a realistic idea of the chance of success. As to whether to consider oocyte donation (see Chapter 14), it may become a matter of how you can best apply the limited resources of emotion, time, and money—and whether an IVF program wants to jeopardize its success rate by taking a chance on you. There is really no absolute decision—it's all statistics.

Serum Progesterone Test

Progesterone is a major hormone needed to prepare and sustain the uterus for pregnancy. Most progesterone is produced from the corpus luteum that forms from the ovarian follicle after ovulation of an egg. Progesterone may be measured as an indicator of ovulation or to evaluate the health of a pregnancy. Timing of this test is crucial. A blood sample is obtained 7 to 9 days after ovulation is suspected, or better, 7 days before the next period is scheduled to start. Be aware that the ovary may fail to ovulate and yet produce progesterone as though ovulation did happen. In this case, you and your doctor could be fooled.

Prolactin Testing

The hormone that stimulates production of breast milk is prolactin. Prolactin levels may be elevated outside of pregnancy (hyperprolactinemia) and can interfere with ovulation. A common sign of high prolactin levels is breast secretion (galactorrhea), and this is a major reason why nursing mothers are relatively infertile.

Mildly elevated prolactin levels may result from:

- Drug use
- Anesthesia
- Stress
- Recent breast stimulation
- Breast examination
- Blood sampling around the time of ovulation

All cases of galactorrhea or hyperprolactinemia should be more thoroughly investigated. Prolactin levels should be determined on all women with anovulation or menstrual cycle irregularity. Hyperprolactinemia is often found in women with hypothyroidism, and a TSH level should always be checked.

A blood test for prolactin is best performed in the morning at the beginning of your menstrual cycle. Since elevations of prolactin levels are possible after a breast examination, this is a poor time to obtain the blood sample.

Women with greater than minimally elevated prolactin levels on repeat testing should be referred for magnetic resonance imaging (MRI). This test is safe, involves no radiation, and can be done as an outpatient.

Is the Thyroid-Stimulating Hormone (TSH) Test Necessary?

Thyroid disease is common in women and especially those with a strong family history of bleeding problems or infertility. The problem for those who are infertile is that thyroid disease is proven to interfere with ovarian function. The TSH test is easy, relatively cheap, and can lead to accurate therapy that is also easy and inexpensive and very rewarding.

The TSH level does not vary with the stage of your menstrual cycle or time of day, so the test can be performed at any time. Unless the TSH level returns as abnormal, there is no reason for further thyroid testing. If the TSH is abnormal, then the test should be repeated with a measurement of free thyroxine (Free T4). In most patients, a high TSH (more than 4 to 5 IU/l, depending on the lab) signals an underactive thyroid (hypothyroidism). Suppressed levels of TSH usually indicate an overactive thyroid (hyperthyroidism).

Other Hormone Tests

If your doctor suspects problems with ovulation and especially if polycystic ovarian syndrome is suspected (see Chapter 4), additional hormone testing may be ordered.

Evaluating the Female Reproductive System

The Cervix

While true cervical factor infertility is uncommon, it can occur with previous surgery, congenital problems, or immunologic abnormalities of the cervix. This diagnosis of cervical factor also applies when factors associated with the cervix inhibit sperm function. Most suspected cervical factor is due to problems with ovulation or semen quality. Except in rare cases of severe structural defects, cervical factor should be bypassed relatively easily using various fertility therapies.

The cervix is directly viewed through a speculum. The outward appearance of the cervix provides clues as to possible infection and pathology, and particular attention is paid to the cervix if there has been prior surgery. Your doctor will also note the amount and quality of cervical mucus during the evaluation. If you have not been pregnant, the cervical opening (os) is usually small and round. It becomes slit-like after vaginal delivery. In several studies, researchers have found that women who have an unusually tight (stenotic) cervix have a higher chance of endometriosis. It is easy to imagine how sperm could have a hard time swimming through a tight opening, but in reality, the cervical opening is usually not related to fertility.

The Pap Smear

The Pap smear is a screening test for cervical cancer. A sampling of cells is taken from the interior and exterior of the cervix and sent for evaluation by a cytopathologist. The false-positive rate on Pap smears is about 10 percent.

Annual Pap smears are recommended for women of reproductive age. This test can provide more information than just cancer screening. A Pap smear is a relatively good indicator of infection. Sometimes the infection can be identified and the proper medication can be used to clear it up. Infections commonly found by means of the Pap smear include:

- Candidiasis (yeast infection)
- Trichomoniasis
- Nonspecific vaginal infection (vaginosis)

Occasionally the Pap smear will return as abnormal, with changes suggesting human papilloma virus (HPV) infection. HPV is a family of closely related viruses, with subtypes identified by numbers. These viruses are carried by virtually everyone and are passed through physical contact.

HPV changes are common findings on Pap smears and usually indicate the need for closer observation. The infection also may be transmissible to your partner, but HPV usually has no effect on fertility.

If the Pap smear is abnormal, the next step is to repeat it in several months, treat with antibiotics, or refer for colposcopy and biopsy of abnormal areas, if found. Colposcopy is an outpatient procedure where the cells are examined through a microscope. You are awake and there is pain if a biopsy is taken. Most women consider this only mild discomfort.

Cervical cancer is diagnosed in 15,000 to 20,000 women in the United States each year, with about 7,000 deaths. The average age for diagnosis of invasive cervical cancer is 45; 35 years for localized noninvasive carcinoma in situ. The good news is that cervical cancer has the potential of near-complete prevention with routine pelvic examination. The speed of the progression may vary, but cervical cancer is almost always preceded by precancerous findings on the Pap smear.

Because the human papilloma virus (HPV), which is thought to cause cervical cancer, is a sexually transmitted organism, practitioners now consider cervical cancer as a sexually transmitted disease. Other factors that contribute to this cancer include:

- Age at first intercourse
- Number of sexual partners
- Exposure to viral agents
- Smoking

At the time of a Pap smear, or at an initial examination, some doctors also test for gonorrhea and chlamydial infection by swabbing the cer-

---

Doctor's Rx

Another type of Pap test, ThinPrep, replaces the conventional method by rinsing the cells in a vial filled with a solution that preserves them— a process that improves the quality and is believed to lead to more effective cervical cancer diagnosis and reduction in repeat testing.

vical canal. This can tell if there currently is infection, but does not give clues about past infections. The incidence of current infection is very low in couples who are undergoing infertility investigations, and often these tests are not performed. There have been numerous studies on the testing of chlamydia antibodies to see if they indicate past infections. While you may have chlamydia antibodies, that does not necessarily mean that there has been pelvic inflammatory disease (PID).

Cervical Mucus Tests

For many infertile women, instead of being an excellent indicator of the exact time contraception can take place, their cervical mucus works to hinder making a baby. Abnormalities of cervical mucus may involve both quantity and quality, including:

- Scant, normal mucus
- Thick or cloudy mucus
- Normal-appearing mucus that seems to immobilize or kill sperm

The cervical mucus test, or postcoital test (PCT), is simple, painless, inexpensive, and safe. There is only one disadvantage—it is not predictive. The lack of value of the PCT has been scientifically substantiated in various studies, and while it may confirm sperm and therefore intercourse, it gives little information on sperm quality. When the PCT is not predictive it is usually because of poor timing and lack of ovulation. Seldom does the PCT indicate cervical factor infertility. The reason that the PCT remains a commonly used test is because it is easy and seems logical. Home testing for cervical mucus can be helpful, but it probably is not worth an office visit.

The Use of Endometrial Biopsy (EMB) Is Questioned

Endometrial biopsy has been considered the gold standard for diagnosing luteal phase deficiency (LPD). Yet many experts believe that while there may be a role for endometrial biopsy in evaluating abnormal bleeding when an ultrasound is uncertain, its use in infertility testing is highly questionable.

Luteal phase deficiency (luteal insufficiency, inadequate luteal phase) is a disturbance in endometrial growth in relationship to the day of the menstrual cycle. LPD is implicated in only 3.5 percent of cases of infertility. This test of the lining of the uterus is usually done about 1 to 3 days before the beginning of menstruation. The EMB usually has a similar goal, timing, and purpose as the serum progesterone test. While it does not test the amount of progesterone in the blood, it does assess the effect of progesterone on the uterus. If your uterus receives enough progesterone, usually a healthy embryo can implant.

THE PROCEDURE. Your doctor will carefully slide a narrow catheter into your uterus, and the suction on the end of the catheter will pull cells from the surface. The collected cells are sent to a laboratory, where a pathologist evaluates the progesterone effect.

WHAT YOU MAY FEEL. This test may cause cramping and discomfort, but that can be alleviated by taking medication prior to the procedure.

PRECAUTIONS. Timing is very important, as the test can be misinterpreted if it is done at the wrong time in the cycle. Many experts feel that the endometrial biopsy lacks precision, costs too much, is painful, and usually does not alter infertility treatment. Most women who have an endometrial biopsy have bad memories of the test, and their doctors prescribed the same course of therapy whether they had LPD or not.

Specialized Ultrasound Screening

An essential part of your initial infertility evaluation is an ultrasound scan of the pelvis. Ultrasound is an extremely common noninvasive procedure using high frequency sound waves to reflect body structures and produce a "picture" of internal organs. Many thorough studies have shown that these waves are not harmful to you, your eggs, or your pregnancy. The ultrasound interpretation is based on evaluating the different densities of tissue.

The sound waves pass through each type of tissue with different degrees of difficulty. Bone reflects sound waves and is seen as bright white on the ultrasound screen (echodense). Sound waves pass through water, and the image would be black on the ultrasound screen (echolucent).

A more specialized use of ultrasound involves the monitoring of the progress of a menstrual cycle with the purpose of producing a pregnancy. The follicle containing the maturing egg is followed over several days to watch its growth pattern, to time a medication signal for ovulation, and to confirm that the follicle actually ruptures, releasing the egg. At the same time, the lining of the uterus is followed for appropriate thickness. If the lining is thin, this may indicate a hormonal problem.

Your doctor may do the first ultrasound during menstruation. This is called the baseline scan and is performed during your period because this is the time in which there should be the least cyst change of the ovary and development of the uterine lining. Using this test, abnormalities of the uterus, ovaries, and sometimes the tubes can be identified. Your doctor may find swollen tubes (hydrosalpinx), uterine fibroids, or ovarian cysts, which can be treated after evaluation. The ultrasound can be one of two main types:

TRANS-VAGINAL ULTRASOUND. A transducer probe of less than an inch in diameter is inserted into your vagina. Here it is adjacent to your uterus and ovaries, making the evaluation of the pelvis much more accurate. This type of ultrasound is preferable for most infertility studies and causes little, if any, discomfort.

ABDOMINAL ULTRASOUND. A transducer is passed over your abdomen to view your uterus and ovaries. It is used to view pregnancies after about eight weeks and sometimes may aid in evaluating any pelvic problems. In order for the pelvic organs to be properly seen, the bladder must be full. This allows a "window" between the abdominal wall and pelvic organs to give a clearer picture.

Ultrasound is a powerful tool for examining the ovary and monitoring the number and size of follicles developing during ovarian stimulation (see Chapter 13). Ultrasound also gives vital information on the status of the endometrium, called the endometrial stripe. Cervical mucus secretion can also be an echolucent area in the cervix.

Is Hysterosalpingography (HSG) Cost-Effective for Infertility Screening?

Hysterosalpingography is a screening test for the female reproductive anatomy. This x-ray procedure is used to examine the uterus and fallopian tubes and can help your doctor eliminate structural problems as a reason for your infertility (painful menstruation, heavy bleeding, or amenorrhea). HSG is done a few days after menstruation, when the uterine lining is thin, to avoid the possibility that you may be ovulating or that an early pregnancy is being exposed to x-rays.

THE PROCEDURE. A small tube is inserted into your cervix and a liquid dye is slowly injected into the uterine cavity. The outflow of dye outlines your uterus and fallopian tubes and can be viewed on a screen.

If your HSG is normal, this means that the shape of your uterine cavity is normal, there are no obvious adhesions or scarring in the abdomen, and the fallopian tubes are open so the egg and sperm can move freely. If your HSG is abnormal, the next recommended test may be an MRI scan, an ultrasound test, or hysteroscopy. If the HSG showed that your tubes were blocked, your doctor may want to proceed with in vitro fertilization or surgery to correct the blockage.

The major problem with HSG is that it is *only* a screening test—and it is very costly, painful, and often inconclusive. Many women find this test to be extremely painful. There is a 15 to 20 percent false-positive and false-negative rate. This means that in one out of five cases there will appear to be a problem when there really is not. In an equal number of cases, these tests will be read as normal when an abnormality is actually present. If the HSG is abnormal, a laparoscopy or hysteroscopy is needed for confirmation and treatment. If the test is negative—nothing has been found—it still cannot be trusted, and a laparoscopy or hysteroscopy may still have to be done. It is common for the tube to have muscle spasms during the HSG and appear blocked. Sometimes the tubes may be open, but scarring has caused an abnormal attachment such that egg pickup at ovulation is unlikely.

Still, the HSG can have special value as a diagnostic test and may help you to avoid surgery when an answer to a specific problem is needed. For example, if your doctor questions whether your tubes are open after a procedure has been done to reverse sterilization, the HSG can give the answer. Another positive use is in selective canalization (opening) of the tube(s) where they enter into your uterus. This procedure may be successful by x-ray guidance using the hysteroscope.

WHAT YOU MAY FEEL. Mild to severe cramping is a common side effect. If there are blockages in your fallopian tubes, the pain may be more intense. Try to relax during the procedure. Some of the relaxation techniques in Chapter 17 may help. After the HSG test you may have a small amount of spotting and cramping.

PRECAUTIONS TO TAKE. Be sure to schedule this test prior to ovulation so there is no danger of flushing out a released egg or embryo. Take a nonsteroid anti-inflammatory drug (NSAID), such as ibuprofen or Naprosyn, before and after the procedure to diminish the cramping or discomfort that may be caused. If you have had a previous allergic reaction to shellfish or contrast dye, let your doctor know before the test. Approximately 1 percent of women will develop an infection. Although rare, these infections can be quite serious, requiring hospitalization for intravenous antibiotics. An antibiotic is often prescribed before the procedure to reduce the risk of infection. If you have fever or excessive pain after the procedure, be sure to notify your doctor.

Sonohysterography (sonoHSG) Is Excellent to Evaluate the Uterus

This commonly used procedure is performed in your doctor's office and avoids the use of radiation. It is superior to standard HSG for evaluation

---

Baby Booster

Some women do conceive after an HSG without additional therapy. This is thought to be due to the flushing out of the tubes and the removal of small bits of scar tissue. Some have claimed that using an oil-based instead of a water-based dye can further increase fertility during the months immediately after the procedure. Still, the oil-based medium is associated with some complications, and great care must be taken in its use.

of the uterine cavity and lining for abnormalities such as polyps or fibroids. The drawback on sonoHSG is that it's not a good technique to see if your tubes are open (patent). In this respect, sonoHSG is inferior to HSG with x-ray dye.

Like x-ray HSG, sonoHSG is a screening test, and if a problem is found using sonoHSG, it will need to be surgically evaluated and treated, usually by hysteroscopy.

THE PROCEDURE. Your doctor inserts a very small plastic tube (catheter) through the cervix into the uterus. Water or other substance is passed through this tube while your doctor watches it with ultrasound. Sometimes water can be seen passing through the tubes and accumulating in the pelvis. This is an indication that at least one tube is open. Some prefer using albumin, a thick protein that is more visible on ultrasound, to better check for tubal patency, but the results are not great and albumin is costly.

WHAT YOU MAY FEEL. This procedure may be less painful and the surroundings are more comfortable than the standard HSG. You may have some mild cramping, which can be reduced by taking ibuprofen or Naprosyn before the test.

PRECAUTIONS. This is a low-cost, minimally invasive procedure. If you have a history of PID, your doctor may prescribe antibiotics for you to take. Call your doctor if you have fever after the procedure.

Laparoscopy (LSC) Is a Definitive Diagnostic Tool

Some experts regard the laparoscopy (belly-button surgery) to be the most valuable single procedure in evaluating the female fertility patient. Others, the minority, suggest avoiding laparoscopy with concentration of medical therapy and IVF.

What Can Laparoscopy Do?

Laparoscopy is an excellent diagnostic tool for the causes of infertility. Not only can it let your doctor determine what may be wrong and give her or him a chance to cure the problem, but it also indicates what the prognosis is for your future fertility.

When Should You Consider Laparoscopy?

This procedure should be considered before your doctor tries more expensive or risky therapy, especially if you have experienced the following:

- Pelvic pain
- Obvious abnormalities on ultrasound
- Suspected PID or documented previous infection
- Previous pelvic or abdominal surgery
- Evidence of ovulation and normal semen parameters

If you have been treated with three cycles of clomiphene without success, or have pelvic pain, abnormal bleeding, or if there are specific risk factors that may indicate possible pelvic disease, it may be worth discussing laparoscopy with your doctor. If no other cause of infertility has been found, laparoscopy should be tried.

THE PROCEDURE. Although sometimes performed under conscious sedation (or twilight sleep), laparoscopy is usually done under general anesthesia in an operating room of an outpatient facility. General anesthesia allows a more complete examination and is especially helpful if more thorough therapy is needed. A small incision is made in or just below your navel (umbilicus). A small amount of carbon dioxide gas is placed into the abdomen to allow better visualization and a comfort zone from injury. A slender telescope-like instrument (laparoscope) with a

---

Laparoscopy Can Find:

- Endometriosis
- Blocked tubes or impaired freedom of movement
- Evidence of past infection and pelvic scarring
- Pelvic adhesive disease
- Congenital abnormalities
- Polycystic ovarian syndrome (PCOS)
- Ovarian cysts
- Uterine fibroids

video camera attached is inserted through the incision, and the internal organs are viewed on a television monitor. One to three additional small (about ¼-inch) incisions are made just below the public hair line to allow the instruments to be inserted, manipulated, and operated as required.

Direct evaluation can be made of the uterus, tubes, and ovaries as well as other pelvic and abdominal organs. Under direct observation, blue dye is passed through the cervix and uterus and out the tubes. This is similar to the procedure for HSG, but you are asleep and colored dye is used instead of x-ray contrast to see if the tubes are free and clear.

Practically any fertility problem that can be seen by laparoscopy can also be treated by laparoscopy, depending on your physician's skill level. Laparoscopy may be performed after menstruation stops but before ovulation. This prevents an interruption of an unknown pregnancy. There are reports that the healing process is better during this period. Because the ovary is "quiet," the formation of a cyst is less likely.

Still, some doctors will time the laparoscopy during the premenstrual phase (the week before the next period is due). Others prefer doing this procedure during the periovulatory period when the eggs are ripe. This time allows them to visualize follicular development. A hysteroscopy is often recommended at the time of laparoscopy.

WHAT YOU MAY FEEL. After the anesthesia, you will feel groggy for several hours. You may have mild nausea. Be sure to inform your anesthesiologist ahead of time if there is a history of nausea with anesthesia, as it may alter the medications used. Your doctor will prescribe pain and nausea medication, as necessary. After surgery you will need to rest for 2 to 4 hours, or until the effects of the anesthesia have diminished. Some women complain of a sore throat because of the anesthesia tube. It is not uncommon to have shoulder pain and bloating from the gas for a day or two. You may also notice a change in bowel habits for a few days after the procedure. Spotting is common, but not bleeding. The small incisions are usually closed with stitches that will dissolve on their own. If the incision sites redden, a warm, wet compress will often give relief. You can usually go home the same day and resume normal work in 2 to 3 days. Recovery is usually complete by 7 days after the surgery. If not, call your doctor. Many times experts suggest that you try to get pregnant the same month as your laparoscopy.

PRECAUTIONS TO TAKE. Laparoscopy is considered safe but not risk free. There are potentially very serious risks of damage to the intestine, bladder, or ureter. Luckily these risks are small. As with any surgery, there are risks of bleeding or infection. Complications with the anesthesia are very rare with the new monitoring techniques. When there has been an injury or complication, it may be necessary to make a larger incision in the abdomen for investigation and treatment.

Fever is rare, as is excessive abdominal swelling, pain, or nausea after 24 hours. If you experience these, call your doctor.

Laparotomy Has Passed Its Prime

Laparotomy is a major surgical procedure performed through an abdominal incision under general anesthesia, usually by two surgeons. Because everything can essentially be done with laparoscopy today, this invasive procedure is rarely performed. Not only does laparotomy require 1 to 4 days of hospitalization and a recovery period of 3 to 4 weeks, the risks are great, including infection, hemorrhage, damage to the intestine or bladder, and anesthesia complications. There may be special situations when only a laparotomy will allow proper evaluation and therapy.

The Mini-Laparotomy May Still Be Useful

Sometimes the small incisions for laparoscopy are too restrictive, yet a major laparotomy is not necessary. The mini-laparotomy (mini-lap) may be a good compromise. This procedure is usually immediately preceded by laparoscopy in which the pelvis is evaluated and the stage is set for the procedure. Most of the procedure can be performed through the laparoscope, but a small incision is considered safer or more efficient. Mini-laps may be most useful for removal of fibroids or reversal of sterilization, or if there is an inability to treat a bleeding pregnancy through the laparoscope.

Tests You May Need After Recurring Pregnancy Loss

While the previously discussed user-friendly fertility tests are indicated for women trying to conceive, once you do get pregnant yet experience recurring pregnancy loss, your doctor may recommend a series of tests to identify why miscarriage occurs. Some of these tests are described below.

Immunological Testing

Tests for anti-phospholipid antibodies, anti-cardiolipin antibodies, or lupus anticoagulant, among others, may help to diagnose some auto-immune problems related to this syndrome and pregnancy loss in the second trimester. In the phospholipid antibody syndrome, small blood clots form in the blood vessels of the placenta. Normal development of the placenta is retarded because of insufficient blood flow. This often coincides with marked elevation of the mother's blood pressure.

Less well documented is the hypothesized pregnancy loss in the first trimester due to alloimmune response. Tests proposed to evaluate the alloimmune response include levels of natural killer cells, embryo-toxicity, and leukocyte antibodies.

The relationship of the antibodies above to infertility is very controversial among infertility specialists. Some experts from very successful programs believe that every woman having assisted reproductive technology (ART) cycles should be extensively tested for a group of antibodies that might affect fertility. Other practitioners believe that this might be helpful if a woman has had previously unsuccessful ART cycles. Still others feel that the testing is completely worthless. There have been a number of scientific reports that conclude that women with and without antibodies achieve pregnancy at the same rate without treating the patients shown to have antibodies. Clinics involved in the controversy have similar pregnancy rates. If antibodies are determined to be present, treatment is even more controversial. Although testing only involves drawing blood and is not risky in any way, the treatment for antibodies can carry a risk. Certainly the immune system has a key role in reproduction. While it is unclear why there are so many discrepancies, look to the future for greater scientific clarity on the role of the immune system in recurrent pregnancy loss.

Genetic Testing

KARYOTYPE. Karyotype is a photographic record of a person's chromosomes. Cells are obtained from a blood sample, amniotic fluid, or other tissues, then are cultured and allowed to multiply. The process is stopped when the chromosomes are the most visible. The chromosomes are stained with material that makes them visible under the microscope. A photograph is made and enlarged. Karyotypes are sometimes performed in women with marked alterations in ovarian function, but the most common use is in the evaluation of fetal tissue or blood sample from the male or female partner as part of the investigation into pregnancy loss.

PREIMPLANTATION "GENETIC" DIAGNOSIS (PGD). The main purpose of PGD is to determine, prior to implantation in the uterus, if a certain abnormality exists or could be present in the embryo. Using this test, abnormal or possibly abnormal embryos are not placed in the uterus; only normal embryos are transferred. While PGD gives the correct determination more than 90 percent of the time, it is not yet perfect, and errors do happen. This is due to the fact that the techniques that are used are not always perfect in differentiating between embryos that do or do not have a certain gene or chromosome.

A potential use of PGD is when women 37 years old and older are having ART cycles. In this case, PGD is used to determine which embryos contain the proper number of chromosomes. Then the ART clinic knows which embryos can be transferred with the best chance for the couple to achieve pregnancy and can avoid transferring embryos that could potentially result in an abnormal fetus. PGD is also used when a couple knows of an inherited disease in one of their families and wishes to avoid passing the disease to their children. Many inherited diseases can now be detected, and new tests for such diseases are being developed all the time.

PGD is not recommended for "family balancing," and most centers will not perform the test for this reason.

Your doctor will use in vitro fertilization prior to PGD. The embryos developed in the laboratory are each biopsied, which means one or two of the cells are removed; then PGD testing is performed on those cells. The lab reports back to the clinic which embryos are the ones to transfer and which probably have an abnormal gene. PGD is very expensive if it is not covered by insurance, and there are only a certain number of centers capable of doing PGD at this time. The risks of PGD would be the same as IVF, plus the remote possibility of the test being wrong.

Chapter 12

Not for Women Only:
Tests He May Need

"Even though Ben was near 50 with grown children when we got married, we were determined to have our own child," said Lisa, age 38. "We knew that the first thing we had to do was untie the knot—reverse his vasectomy. No mean feat, we knew, given that his vasectomy was performed in a small town, twenty-five years earlier.

"The surgery was scheduled, then after an afternoon of preop testing, we returned to the hospital at the crack of dawn for the big event. Although Ben never saw him, our expert pulled me out of the waiting room to announce gleefully that his scope had revealed 'sperm heads' peeking out. I assumed this was good news, though even in my primitive state of knowledge, I felt sure we needed bodies as well.

"When Ben awoke, I stood by while a resident inspected the dressing. When asked if he had actually performed the operation, he said just a little of it. After all, he explained, the vas deferens is no wider than vermicelli, and at this point, he was no Chef Boyardee."

Whether to untie the knot, check for infection, or test for mobile sperm, it's your turn to see the doctor. The thought makes you nervous? You're not alone—don't worry! Most men are gun-shy when it comes to seeing a doctor. According to a recent survey, just 60 percent of the nation's men had a physical exam in the past year. Compare this statistic with 76 percent of women. It's revealing that these same studies show that while men have the tendency to worry more about diseases than women, overall, men have less knowledge than women about personal health.

Since the male evaluation is much quicker and easier than the female, what are you waiting for? Certainly you will be relieved when your doc says, "All is okay." If not, you would have probably been here sooner or later anyway, so why postpone the inevitable?

Male Factor: Checking It Out

There is no reason for any man to postpone tests and treatment for infertility, especially if your female partner is over age 35 and her biological clock is limited. In that regard, you don't mess around with Mother Nature! Infertility must be dealt with quickly and effectively. The good news is that by using new methods such as intracytoplasmic sperm injection (ICSI), the majority of cases of male factor infertility can now be treated. Whether you will need ICSI or just a simple antibiotic to clear up a hidden infection, your doctor will have the answers.

As you read in Chapter 5, male factor infertility can happen for myriad reasons. For example, laboratory tests that analyze your semen, urine, and blood can reveal information about sperm quantity, quality, and abnormalities, as well as crucial hormone levels. Treatment may involve abstaining from such known sperm blockers as alcohol and cigarettes, keeping your testicles cool by avoiding hot tubs and overexercise, and boosting your intake of vitamins C and E, and zinc. Or you may benefit from new medications to balance hormone levels. If there is an obstruction blocking sperm from being released or a problem such as trauma to the testicles followed by atrophy or shrinking, your doctor can use simple tests to diagnose the exact cause, then treat it quickly.

As your doctor evaluates your situation, your personal medical history may begin to give clues as to the cause of male factor infertility. This will allow the doctor to discern between reversible and irreversible causes. Some common questions you may be asked include:

REPRODUCTIVE AND SEXUAL HISTORY

- Have you ever fathered a child with your partner before?
- Have you ever fathered a child in a previous relationship?
- Have you been investigated for infertility in the past year?
- When you were born, were both testes descended into the scrotum?

- At what age did you start to shave?
- How long have you been off birth control?
- How long have you been trying to conceive?
- Do you have difficulty in achieving or maintaining an erection?
- Do you believe that you ejaculate completely?
- Do you think that either you or your partner may have a sexual problem?
- How frequently do you have intercourse? (Too frequent intercourse could deplete sperm reserve.)
- Have you experienced erectile dysfunction?
- What type of lubricants do you use for intercourse? (Some lubricants are spermicidal.)

MEDICAL HISTORY

- Have you ever been hospitalized? Had surgery?
- Did you have mumps as a child?
- Have you had any past surgeries or injuries to the groin or testes?
- Have you had hernia repair?
- Have you ever noticed blood or pus in your urine?
- Are you presently under the care of a physician for medical conditions?
- What medications do you take?
- Have you ever been diagnosed with diabetes, high blood pressure, thyroid disease, chronic respiratory infection, or cancer?

FAMILY HISTORY

- Is there a history of infertility or long spaces between pregnancies?
- Is there a history of pregnancy loss or birth defects?
- Is there a history of cystic fibrosis?
- Are there diseases that run in your family?

SOCIAL HISTORY

- What is your occupation and major leisure activities?
- Have you been exposed to high heats, solvents, chemicals, or radiation?

- Do you use any medications? (Remember to bring these with you to your visit.)
- Do you use tobacco of any sort? What kind? How much? How long?
- Do you drink caffeine beverages? How many daily?
- Do you or have you used recreational drugs (i.e., marijuana)?
- Are you more than 10 percent over or under your ideal weight?
- What do you consider your stress level to be?
- Do you take long hot showers or saunas?

Table 12.1   Guidelines for Regular Examinations and Preventive Measures for Men

EXAMINATION	FREQUENCY
Physical exam	Every three years from 20 to 39
	Every two years from 40 to 49
	Every year after 50
Blood pressure	Every year
Tuberculosis	Every five years from 20 to 39
Blood and urine tests	Every three years from 20 to 39
	Every two years from 40 to 49
	Every year after 50
Electocardiogram	Every three to five years after 50, or after 30 if at high risk from heart attack
Tetanus booster	Every 10 years
Rectal exam	Every year after 40
PSA blood test	Every year after 50; if you are at high risk, have this exam every year after 40
Hemoccult	Every year after 40
Sigmoidoscopy	Every three to four years after 50
	If you're at high risk, you should have a colonoscopy at age 40. If you have a family member (father, mother, brother, sister) with colon cancer, you should have a colonoscopy every three to five years. Check with your doctor.

The Physical Examination

During the minimal physical examination, the focus will be on your external reproductive organs and secondary sex characteristics. Your doctor will pay attention to the size of your testes and the presence of varicocele.

In a more comprehensive examination, special attention is given to your weight, blood pressure, degree of male hair growth, muscle bulk, breast enlargement, an abdominal exam for an enlarged liver, the external genitalia, and a rectal exam to evaluate your prostate and associated glands.

The Search for Super Sperm

"Well, I had the physical exam, then had to give a semen analysis (SA). I thought sperm was just that—sperm. I didn't realize it took a super sperm to fertilize the egg." Mark was taken aback when his urologist told him his sperm was not adequate to fertilize his wife's egg.

"We had tried for two years to have a baby. Then our new RE suggested that I have a physical and semen analysis to see if I had a problem. After giving a sperm sample, I watched the lab technician check it out under the microscope, then do a high-tech computer analysis of it."

Mark's story illustrates the need for an early evaluation of semen. Think about the amount of emotional trauma in those many months with little chance of pregnancy and possible expensive and painful therapy of the female partner. And—perhaps even more important— Mark and his wife realized that not all sperm are created equal. It's not only the number but also the quality that determines if super sperm can fertilize the egg. While conventional semen analysis cannot guarantee fertility, it can go a long way toward assessing the problem.

A semen analysis (SA), an assessment of a freshly ejaculated semen sample, is a vital part of every infertility exam. This laboratory test measures the number and activity of the sperm, as well as the color, shape, and form. The sample is also examined for any white or red blood cells that could indicate inflammation or infection.

Semen Is Made Up Of:

- Sperm (as many as 120 to 600 million per one ejaculation)
- Water
- Simple sugars (to give sperm energy)
- Alkalis (to protect sperm from the acidity of the male urethra and the female vagina)
- Prostaglandins (substances that cause contractions of the uterus and fallopian tube)
- Vitamin C
- Zinc
- Cholesterol

Because such factors as fever, medications, unusual stress, or any injury to the testicles can affect the quality of your sperm, talk with your doctor about any of these before giving the semen sample. Sperm motility (or the percentage of sperm with forward movement) appears to be a key factor in determining if your sperm are capable of fertilizing your partner's egg. Even with a low sperm count, many men with highly motile sperm are still fertile. Again, it takes just one! But with any negative report, your doctor will want to do the SA again. Sometimes the semen analysis can be done in conjunction with a natural or clomiphene cycle, adding therapy to the diagnosis.

In assessing sperm motility, technicians look for a number of factors, including:

- **Volume of the semen.** Low volume could indicate a partial obstruction or infection.
- **Sperm concentration (the amount of sperm in a certain volume of semen, also known as sperm density).** If there is no sperm, the condition is called azoospermia; if the count is low, it is called oligospermia.
- **Sperm morphology (size, form, and shape).**
- **Sperm motility (percentage of actively moving sperm).** Problems with motility are referred to as asthenospermia.

- **Sperm viability (whether or not they are still alive).**
- **pH.** Alkalinity is necessary for sperm survival. A low pH may suggest a problem with the man's prostate gland or seminal vesicles.
- **Liquefication.** If the semen stays thick (viscous) or does not liquefy, it may be a problem of the seminal vesicles.
- **Fructose.** Sugar produced by the seminal vesicles serves as food for sperm. If the person's fructose level is low, there may be a blockage of the ejaculatory duct or congenital absence of the seminal vesicles.
- **Leukospermia.** When white blood cells are in the semen sample, leukospermia is reported, which may be a sign of infection requiring antibiotic therapy.
- **Agglutination.** If sperm are stuck together in clumps, they are agglutinate, which is a sign of infection or sperm antibodies.

For the complete evaluation, you may need to give several semen specimens several weeks apart. The best results are obtained when you *abstain from sexual intercourse for three days* before producing the sample. Your doctor will give you instructions on how to provide a semen sample. You will masturbate into a sterile plastic specimen cup in a private room in your doctor's office. Or you may choose (as most men do) to ejaculate into a special condom during intercourse with your partner in the privacy of your home. The condom has no spermicide, and the sample must be kept warm (hold it under your armpit) and delivered to the laboratory quickly for best results (usually within one hour or less).

If the results of your SA are unclear, there are further types of analysis your doctor may do.

HIGH RESOLUTION SCROTAL ULTRASONOGRAPHY OR VENOGRAPHY. This ultrasound helps identify varicoceles that are too small to be accurately felt by the physician during a physical examination. It also provides your doctor with an accurate means of studying the accessory sex glands, prostate gland, and seminal vesicles, as well as the ejaculatory duct, which if blocked or damaged can impair sperm quality and cause lack of sperm in the ejaculate.

ENDOCRINE TESTING. This is usually confined to testing LH, FSH, and testosterone, with possibly TSH and prolactin (see Chapter 1). This testing can be indispensable in determining whether the problem is one of sperm production or outflow. Normal levels may be misleading.

GENERAL MEDICAL TESTING. There are no routine tests other than a semen analysis. If in reviewing your medical history a risk factor is identified, other general or specific tests may be needed to optimize your health.

Special Studies of Sperm Function

POSTCOITAL TESTING. PCT has been shown to be of little value overall except if there are sperm present—it will tell you that there *are* sperm present!

ZONA-FREE HAMSTER EGG SPERM PENETRATION ASSAY (SPA, OR HAMSTER TEST). This test places sperm with hamster eggs that have had the protection of the zona pellucida removed. While it sounds odd, the capacity of human sperm to fertilize hamster eggs is generally related to the capacity to fertilize human eggs. The test can be a valuable resource tool and has been useful in determining the source of no fertilization during assisted reproduction cycles. SPA is also very expensive. Men who fail the SPA may still achieve a pregnancy either spontaneously or more likely through ICSI.

HEMIZONA ASSAY. The zona pellucida from unfertilized donor eggs are used to assay the binding capacity of the human sperm. Half of the zona is used for the male partner and control donor sperm are used on the other half. Some believe this to be a clever, tricky, and expensive test that has largely been replaced by sperm injection.

SPERM ANTIBODY TESTING. In some cases the immune system fails to recognize foreign substances in the body and can attack its own tissues. Sperm antibodies are chemical substances in the semen, cervical mucus, blood, and other body fluids that may attach to the sperm's head or tail, making them ineffective or immobile. The most widely used test is immunobead testing. Here, the degree and position of sperm binding to small glass beads coated with immunoglobulin is measured. The test is run in parallel with donor sperm. If a high percentage of sperm bind, it is suggestive of antibodies. The test, although relatively accurate, is poor at predicting fertility. If antibodies are found, there is no effective treatment except for IUI or other assisted reproduction techniques (see Chapter 14).

VIABILITY. Special stains can be used that identify dead sperm. Most often the number is as expected based on semen parameters.

ACROSOME STUDIES. The acrosome is a small enzyme-laden cap on the sperm's head. Special studies can be obtained to evaluate how many sperm have this cap or have been activated in preparation for fertilization. Sometimes on routine semen testing, a skilled observer can find globospermia, a condition where the sperm head appears more rounded due to the absence of an acrosome.

SURGICAL EVALUATION. This includes a scrotal exploration and vasography. Some obstruction may be cleared by canalization with injections into the vas and the path followed to the bladder.

TESTICULAR BIOPSY. If the FSH level is normal, suggesting testicular failure has not occurred, a testicular biopsy may be in order. A biopsy examines the testes for the number of sperm, stages of development, and other pathologies like internal scarring. Doctors now think that if this procedure is performed, it should be in conjunction with therapy so that any sperm obtained can be used for fertilization. A consideration should be made about combining biopsy with assisted reproduction therapy or at least an attempt at cryopreservation of the sperm. This small needle biopsy can usually be done at your doctor's office with local anesthesia.

VASOGRAPHY. This x-ray uses a dye to reveal any blockage or leakage of sperm within the duct system, from the testes to the prostate gland.

Are Your Sperm Stressed Out?

The central theme in the biology of sperm function involves a process known as oxidative stress. Just before the sperm dies, there is a sudden burst of energy. This same process occurs just before fertilization and is probably necessary. A group of chemicals called reactive oxygen species (ROS), or free radicals, are produced by sperm membrane damage, which is more likely in damaged or dying sperm. Bacteria also produce ROS. Increased ROS is associated with decreased motility and egg membrane fusion. The seminal plasma contains antioxidants, such as vitamin E. It scavenges for ROS and neutralizes them. Nicotine clearly increases oxidative stress, and this may be its major negative action on fertility.

Presently there are no tests outside the research laboratories that evaluate ROS or oxidative stress.

When Impotence Is the Barrier

Other tests might be ordered by your doctor to gauge arterial blood supply to the penis or to test the nerves or the veins. Or if you have impotence (erectile dysfunction), you might be asked to take a test measuring erections during sleep called nocturnal tumescence and rigidity (NPTR). Because normal men of all ages have erections during the dreaming (rapid eye movement, or REM) stages of their sleep, the NPTR test will measure these erections. If no nocturnal erection occurs or if the erection is hampered, the cause of your erectile dysfunction is likely to be physical. If you have a normal NPTR yet have erectile dysfunction during sexual intercourse, it may stem from a psychological cause.

Solving the Problem of Male Factor

After your doctor has determined the cause of male-factor infertility, treatment will vary, depending on the initial problem that is found. Studies show that up to 75 percent of men with male factor have treatable or identifiable conditions found that affect their fertility. Nearly *all* men with male-factor infertility are treatable with assisted reproductive techniques (ARTs).

It's worthwhile to remember that up to 1 percent of men with subfertility have a potentially life-threatening condition associated with their fertility problem, such as a tumor of the testis. In that light, you can see how important an evaluation is—not only for getting pregnant but perhaps to save your life!

If low-tech methods to increase fertility fail, your doctor will point you and your partner toward the high-tech treatment methods (see Chapter 14) to help you conceive. Or your doctor may find that insemination with your own sperm that has been treated may be an option. Intracytoplasmic sperm injection (ICSI), a new procedure for those with severe sperm problems, may be used. ICSI involves injection of a single sperm captured in a thin glass needle directly into your partner's (or donor) egg.

You're Not Alone, and There *Are* Answers

No matter what the problem, you're not alone. But more important, your doctor has the resources to find out how to best treat your specific problem. Although infertility is a complex situation, if you utilize experts in the field, you and your partner will be able to overcome the hurdles and quickly move to your ultimate goal of making a baby.

Chapter 13

The Latest Baby Boosters

"Because our pre-RE IUIs had been amateurishly timed, Dr. Peters suggested one last insemination as our next step," said Candy, age 41. "This time we combined IUI with Clomid, the most basic infertility-fighting drug on the market. Clomid induces ovulation in some 80 percent of anovulatory women, frequently causing more than one egg to release per cycle. Though I was certain I was ovulating normally without it, Dr. Peters convinced us that anything that would push our chances up a percentage point or two would be worthwhile. Despite the horror stories of Clomid side effects I found on the Internet, I noticed no changes of any sort. Well, there was a bit of a rise in, er, sexual appetite, but perhaps this was due to the increased optimism that Dr. Peters had inspired in us.

"This IUI was timed to the hour with the help of ultrasounds that assessed egg growth and HCG (human chorionic gonadotropin) to ensure egg maturation. HCG is administered by intramuscular injection exactly 35 hours before the procedure, which means an evening shot. Needles appealed to neither of us. Fortunately, I had a nurse friend who agreed to help out in a pinch ... so to speak."

You've finished the battery of tests, and your doctor finally has a diagnosis. So, you think, let's skip the baby-boosting meds and move right to the high-tech conception. After all, it makes sense that if the infertility treatment is more complex, invasive, and expensive, it has to work best, right? Not necessarily. Working closely with your doctor, the chances are great that you will start the least invasive treatment options—fertility medications—first. Let's go back to the basic premise of what it takes to make a baby:

- A sperm
- An egg
- The proper anatomy for the two to meet and be nurtured

To get the egg, you must first ovulate—the disorders of ovulation are the most common cause of female infertility and arguably the most common cause of infertility in general. Baby-boosting drugs take direct charge of ovulation or are directed toward improving the ovarian environment to let ovulation occur naturally. In the old days (ten years ago!), there was controversy about using ovulation-promoting agents without a clear diagnosis of anovulation (failure to ovulate). More recently, and perhaps because the other therapies are invasive or expensive, most infertility treatments begin with at least several cycles of clomiphene citrate before moving on. The key word here is *several*. Infertility investigations should not stay static for too long. If one therapy isn't working, your doctor needs to look to another until you find the one that enables you to successfully make a baby.

Baby-boosting drugs are extremely effective, and millions of couples who rely on these safely get pregnant and stay pregnant—without surgery or depleting their savings on assisted reproduction.

For many women, this "boost," called controlled ovarian hyperstimulation, or COH, is all they need to get pregnant. The major problem with fertility drugs is the Goldilocks phenomenon. It is sometimes hard to get it just right! Too little, and there is inadequate response, and too much can lead to potentially serious hyperstimulation.

Before you read about the latest in baby-boosting medications, let's dispel several myths you may have:

MYTH: Fertility drugs are risky because of the proven side effects such as cancer.

TRUTH: According to the latest studies, ovarian cancer is relatively common. The fact is that some women will develop ovarian cancer—whether or not they take infertility drugs. Backed by the results of several comprehensive studies, the American Society of Reproductive Medicine issued a statement rejecting the proposed relationship between fertility drugs and ovarian cancer.

Many of the fertility drugs have been used safely and successfully for more than thirty years. While there is always a risk of side effects with any treatment, trust your doctor to outline the risks involved and do preventive cancer checks after you have conceived.

MYTH: Fertility drugs cause birth defects.

TRUTH: In multiple studies, this claim has never been substantiated. In fact, there is no proof that any fertility therapy is related to an increased incidence of birth defects. There is a good chance that miscarriage rate is slightly increased after fertility-promoting agents have been used. It is clear that if you ovulate late in your cycle, the risk of miscarriage increases. Likewise, the risk of miscarriage is thought to be higher in women with polycystic ovarian syndrome, whether they use fertility drugs or not.

MYTH: Fertility drugs guarantee multiple births.

TRUTH: The chance of twins is 5 to 10 percent with clomiphene, and the chance of triplets and above is quite rare on this medication. Gonadotropin injection gives a 20 to 25 percent chance of twins and about a 5 percent chance of triplets and above. Unlike many other high-tech solutions, such as in vitro fertilization, ovulation induction has rates of multiple pregnancy similar to those of IVF. With IVF, the number of pregnancies is limited to the number of embryos transferred. With ovulation induction there is not much control. While avoidance of multiple pregnancies should be one of the main responsibilities of your supervising physician, they do still happen.

MYTH: Fertility drugs are dangerous.

TRUTH: Clomiphene rarely causes serious cyst formation, and it virtually never causes ovarian hyperstimulation syndrome (or OHHS). Clomiphene can cause cyst formation, and most cases of painful cyst formation occur in the second month clomiphene is given and involve a cyst already there to stimulate. This is a reason for a thorough check before each trial of clomiphene. The injectable drugs can cause the formation of cysts, and it may be difficult to determine in advance who may have a problem. The condition can be dangerous. Certainly women with polycystic ovarian syndrome are at increased risk. Excessive weight gain or pain after any fertility drug use should always be reported to your doctor.

MYTH: Fertility drugs are outrageously expensive.

TRUTH: This can be true, but it depends on which drug. Clomiphene, the most commonly prescribed fertility medication, costs just

$30 to $150 per cycle. The injectable drugs are much higher ($500 to $2,000) per cycle, but the pregnancy rate is really quite good (10 to 40 percent).

MYTH: More clomiphene is better.

TRUTH: Once it's clear that you are ovulating, increasing the dose of clomiphene to improve your chances does not work. Also, one of the most common mistakes made in infertility therapy is the prolonged use of clomiphene. There is virtually never a reason to use more than six cycles of clomiphene. Most pregnancies occur in the first three cycles.

MYTH: Previous use of birth control pills decreases your chance of getting pregnant.

TRUTH: Use of the pill does not increase your chances of infertility or problems with ovulation. In fact, it may protect your body from many female problems that would have occurred if the pill was not used. The use of the birth control pill reduces the incidence of polycystic ovarian syndrome, ovarian cysts, uterine fibroids, endometriosis, heavy bleeding, anemia, pelvic pain, PMS, and ovarian cancer. There is a 40 percent reduction of ovarian cancer in women who are long-term pill users. Birth control pills are sometimes used in infertility therapy to regulate or synchronize the menstrual cycles.

First Ask About Antibiotics

Before you fill your prescription for baby-boosting medications, ask your doctor about trying a newer antibiotic to help treat a hidden infection. Perhaps this sounds too simple, but recent studies from the University of Maryland show that uterine infections are a common cause of infertility and may be quickly eradicated with a few weeks of antibiotics.

Find the Fertility Drug Best for You

Both types of drugs used for ovulation induction—clomiphene and gonadotropins—work differently but have the same objective: to facilitate ovulation. They create a situation in which an extra push is given for follicular development. Each month there is a relatively large group—say, 5 to 20 follicles—that are recruited from the resting pool of follicles. From this group, several are selected to continue their growth while the others degenerate. From this small group, one follicle achieves dominance over the others and progresses to ovulation. The symphony is conducted by the gonadotropins released from the pituitary gland.

Both clomiphene and injectable drugs increase the stimulation of the ovary by increasing the concentration of gonadotropins. Clomiphene causes a release of the body's own gonadotropin stores and indirectly stimulates the ovaries, while the injectable gonadotropins stimulate the ovaries directly.

One of the drawbacks of all fertility drugs is that they tend to work in only one cycle (month). However, the developing follicle may take as long as three months (cycles) to go through the entire process of growth and maturation. For some women, such as those with PCOS, this means that the follicle and its egg have progressed through their early stages of growth in an abnormal hormonal environment that may contribute to poorer egg quality despite aggressive stimulation.

Clomiphene Citrate (CC)
(Clomid, Serophene, Milophene)

Clomiphene citrate (CC) is a relatively inexpensive and effective synthetic medication that affects the way in which you ovulate. This medication is also used to treat low sperm counts in men, but with limited success.

How Does It Work?

CC is taken in pill form daily and signals your pituitary gland to make more of the follicle-stimulating hormones (FSH) that trigger ovulation. Because CC is not a hormone, but a synthetic anti-estrogen, it fools your body's regulatory mechanisms into perceiving that more estrogen is needed. By stimulating the hypothalamus in your brain to release more GnRH (gonadotropin-releasing hormone), the clomiphene citrate prompts the pituitary to release more LH and FSH. The result? The ovary is stimulated and produces a mature egg that is possible for fertilization.

The Upside

If you usually ovulate, clomiphene can produce extra mature eggs, or theoretically improve the maturation of the eggs released. Clomiphene can also help you overcome lack of ovulation. CC is less expensive than other treatments, and it has a lower multiple pregnancy rate. The success rate of CC is high, with more than 70 percent of pregnancies achieved during the first three months of use. During the first three cycles, an expectation of pregnancy of 5 to 25 percent is reasonable; after that, there is generally reported to be a cumulative pregnancy rate of about 30 percent expectation after six cycles.

The Downside

- This anti-estrogenic action is a double-edged sword, extending to other target organs such as the lining of your uterus (endometrium) and cervix.
- CC retards endometrial development and may decrease the possibility of implantation of the embryo.
- CC may decrease the amount and quality of cervical mucus, thus impeding sperm transport.

Limitations

Except under very specific circumstances, CC therapy should not be used for more than six months. The lowest dose of CC that results in ovulation should be used. The "more is better" rule does not apply here, because higher doses of CC increase the negative anti-estrogenic effects. The dose may need to be adjusted according to your weight. After several cycles, a wash-out period may be useful.

How Is It Taken?

CC is usually begun on cycle days 2 through 5 and continued for five days. Your doctor will have a personal preference in using CC, and there is no conclusive evidence that one regimen is superior to the others. The dose is usually started out at 50 mg daily until ovulation is achieved. Success is limited in doses over 150 mg (three tablets per day).

CC is sometimes combined with injectable medications, such as hCG, human menopausal gonadotropins (Pergonal or Humegon), or an oral steroid like dexamethasone. For those women with PCOS who are otherwise unresponsive to ovarian stimulation, there is some evidence that a ten-day trial at 50 to 100 mg may be effective.

Side Effects

Because of the anti-estrogenic effects, some women have hot flashes while using CC. Other possible side effects include headache (about 29 percent), blurred or double vision, moodiness, and breast tenderness. When the drug is finished, these symptoms disappear quickly. One study reports that there is an increase in ovarian cancer in patients who have used twelve or more cycles of CC. Still, it is believed that the cancer is more likely a result of already existing infertility and ovarian dysfunction than of the drug itself.

The risk of twins is 5 to 10 percent with clomiphene use, supposedly due to the increase in the number of mature eggs available. Triplets and greater are uncommon (less than 1 percent) when used in the prescribed way. Ovarian hyperstimulation is also uncommon and may be more related to stimulation of residual cysts from the previous cycle rather than multiple cystic development in a current cycle.

Precautions to Take

Have a baseline ultrasound scan performed before the first CC cycle. This will help your doctor exclude ovarian cysts and other pelvic abnormalities that may complicate therapy or make it less effective. Each time you take CC, your doctor should perform some form of exam, ultrasound or manual (pelvic), to check the number and size of the resulting follicles.

In some cases, the use of CC can alter the ovulation detection kit by causing it to show a false positive on the first day of use because of elevated LH.

Human Menopausal Gonadotropins (HMG)

If CC does not work for you or if you are getting ready to undergo a cycle of IVF, your doctor may prescribe gonadotropin therapy. These medications contain both follicle-stimulating hormone (FSH) and luteinizing hormone (LH), or just FSH alone.

Gonadotropins stimulate the ovaries to produce hormones and to prepare eggs for release. In men with male-factor infertility, gonadotropins are also used to treat undescended testicle problems, low sperm count, and abnormal hypothalamic activity.

How Does It Work?

Follicles are constantly in a partially mature holding pattern awaiting instruction from gonadotropins. Early in each menstrual cycle, FSH secretion from the pituitary rises in response to the drop in progesterone at the end of the previous cycle. The FSH does what it says—it stimulates the growth of the follicle. With follicle growth comes increasing amounts of estradiol. It's not clear what triggers the sudden release of LH, the LH surge, but it must be present and strong enough to cause follicle release. If the follicles are not sufficiently mature, ovulation will not occur. This is often the case when there are multiple follicles of different sizes. The single lead follicle may set the pace and ruin it for a larger number of smaller follicles (those that need more time to reach their peak development).

Gonadotropins supercharge your body's normal process of follicle development. The chances of pregnancy are increased by causing multiple ovulations and giving the tubes a better chance at egg pickup and the sperm a bigger target at which to shoot. This is a time when more—but not too much—is better.

How Is It Taken?

Gonadotropins must be given by injection. HMG (Pergonal, Humegon, and Repronex) are injected deep into the muscle in the upper leg or buttocks either once or twice daily. A self-administered route in the thigh using a smaller needle may be tried. There are no studies to suggest that twice daily is better than once daily.

Recombinant gonadotropins (Gonal F, Follistim) are given subcutaneously. This injection is much like an allergy or insulin injection, with a very small needle.

The injections typically start on the second or third day after menses. The first day of bleeding is counted as day 1. Usually any bleeding counts as a period, but call your doctor if you have a question. When GnRH analogs are used, the cycle start day is less strict.

Cycle Monitoring

Usually you will be seen for injection instructions, ultrasound, and possibly blood work on either days 1, 2, or 3. You will take 4 to 6 nights of medications, depending on your history and the amount of medications used. From that time until the follicles are mature, you may be seen daily or every other day for vaginal ultrasound and estradiol levels. The ultrasound will determine the number and size of the follicles. (The estradiol level tells about their activity, and indirectly, their health. Sometimes an LH level will be added to the blood test or you will be asked to do a home ovulation predictor kit to detect the presence of an early LH surge.) As the cycle progresses, the endometrium grows. The uterine lining on ultrasound is called the endometrial stripe. As ovulation nears, the stripe is usually over 8 mm and has a halo appearance. This suggests appropriate development. When several follicles reach the 16 to 20 mm range, you are ready for the hCG injection. Usually this is an intramuscular injection, but the subcutaneous route is possible. IVF follicle aspiration is usually performed 34 to 37 hours after the hCG. Artificial insemination (IUI) timing may range from 12 to 40 hours after injection. Sometimes a second smaller booster of hCG may be given. If there is any hCG remaining from the first injections, put it in the refrigerator for safekeeping.

How Much Is Enough?

The amount of gonadotropin to be given is determined by your expected and previous response. The amount of drug necessary may be hard to predict in advance. Low dose stimulation is considered 1 ampule daily; high dose is 4 to 6 ampules daily. Most ovulation induction is performed with 2 to 3 ampules. The lower dose has a greater chance of cycle cancellation due to poor response; the larger dose, a greater chance of hyperstimulation.

STEP-UP. In the step-up method, you start low, then increase as needed to stimulate follicle growth. Often this method is prolonged and may not change the overall number of preovulatory follicles.

STEP-DOWN. In the step-down approach, the doses are decreased once a good response has been mounted.

Some REs start and stay at the same dose for a complete cycle and go up in the next cycle if the response has not been satisfactory. Gonadotropin therapy is used for a total of 6 to 12 days.

The Upside

Clomiphene is not terribly strong to start with, and there can be significant negative anti-estrogenic effects on the cervix, uterus, and possibly ovary. Using clomiphene is like driving with one foot on the accelerator and the other on the brake—at the same time. Gonadotropin is the gas. Multiple follicles are brought forward with increased chances of pregnancy.

The Downside

Gonadotropin injections have three major disadvantages:

1. They are injections, and therefore inconvenient.
2. They cost from $40 to $100 per ampule, and usually 5 to 40 ampules are used in each cycle.
3. They carry a significant risk of ovarian hyperstimulation and multiple pregnancies, with the rate of twins at about 20 percent, and larger order pregnancies occur in about 5 percent of cycles.

Ovarian Hyperstimulation Syndrome (OHSS)

The condition known as ovarian hyperstimulation syndrome (OHSS) is different than the overstimulation that occurs through medical treatments. While the cause of OHSS is unknown, it seems to be a discrete disease process associated with altered permeability and leakage of fluid from the small vessels of the ovary. Mild hyperstimulation is common with polycystic ovarian syndrome. The syndrome is usually said to be mild when there is abdominal swelling, ovarian enlargement with cysts up to 5 centimeters, and discomfort. Most pregnancies are also associated with mild hyperstimulation, while multiple pregnancies increase this risk.

In severe ovarian hyperstimulation syndrome, there is marked fluid in the pelvic and abdominal cavities. The greatest concern is that there is a concentration of blood cells and the possibility of clot formation. Because of this, in some cases, hospitalization is necessary for treatment.

Human Chorionic Gonadotropin (hCG)
(Profasi, Pregnyl)

HCG is a hormone that is naturally produced by the human placenta. The drug is used during controlled ovarian hyperstimulation cycles with gonadotropin injections or clomiphene. HCG mimics the action of luteinizing hormone (LH) to signal or trigger egg maturation and release. This drug is also used to treat problems with undescended testicles, low sperm count, and abnormal hypothalamic activity in men with male-factor infertility.

Side effects include headaches, irritability, depression, and pain at the site of the injection. When hCG is used with gonadotropin injections in superovulation, the risk of hyperstimulation is significantly reduced, but ovulation does not occur and the cycle is of no therapeutic value.

When the ultrasound indicates that follicles are of appropriate size and estradiol level is adequate, an injection of hCG (5,000 to 10,000 units) is given intramuscularly. Ovulation should occur approximately forty-eight hours after taking the hCG injection. You'll be sent home to have sex or scheduled for an intrauterine insemination within 1 to 2 days. HCG injections are sometimes used to support the luteal phase by stimulating progesterone production.

Gonadotropin-Releasing Hormone (GnRH)
(Factrel, Lutrepulse)

GnRH is the hormone that is secreted by the hypothalamus, the pacemaker (pulse generator) of the endocrine system. GnRH controls the release of gonadotropins (LH and FSH) from the pituitary gland. It receives signals from throughout the brain and body, translating them into short bursts (pulses) of releasing hormones. This pulse frequency is altered by drugs, such as clomiphene, and in cases of ovarian dysfunction, for example polycystic ovarian syndrome.

To be effective, synthesized GnRH must be administered in a pulse-like fashion mimicking the normal cycle. You wear a small pump attached to your belt, much like a diabetic wears an insulin pump. Every 90 minutes a small amount of GnRH is released either through a small needle placed under the skin (subcutaneous) or by an indwelling IV catheter.

GnRH therapy is most useful if you have a low output of hormone, such as with hypogonadotropic hypogonadism. It is less useful in hypergonadotropic conditions such as polycystic ovarian syndrome. Your doctor may recommend GnRH when clomiphene and gonadotropin injections have been unsuccessful in stimulating the ovary. This therapy is very natural and is associated with development of a single follicle. However, it's difficult to use and relatively expensive, costing more than $2,000 per month. If used with intravenous therapy, the IV sites have to be changed routinely, and infection or inflammation may complicate therapy.

GnRH Analogs

GnRH analogs share some of the properties of the natural GnRH but have prolonged effectiveness and are up to sixty times as powerful as the natural hormone. There are two types of analogs—agonists and antagonists. Antagonists directly block the action of GnRH. While there are several of these under development, their release for use in the United States has been hampered by undesirable side effects of histamine release.

Agonists first stimulate the release (a flare) of GnRH, then block it. There are three agonists used in the United States—Lupron, Zoladex, and Synarel. While they have the same action, they differ in administration: monthly to tri-monthly injection, implant, or daily nasal spray. By blocking GnRH and subsequently LH release, the follicle growth is inhibited and estrogen and androgen production is markedly reduced.

Gonadotropins given to stimulate the ovary in order to produce the larger numbers of mature follicles represent a double-edged sword. They may improve a disordered ovarian function and increase the number of follicles. They may also produce a group of follicles in various stages of growth and maturation. Some IVF programs use GnRH analogs in conjunction with gonadotropin injections, with Lupron as the principal drug. Lupron blocks the release or surge of LH, which is associated with less chance of pregnancy. The major disadvantage of Lupron is the same as its advantage—ovarian suppression. This may lead to more days of injections and a higher number of gonadotropin ampules needed for stimulation. In some cases (less than 5 percent), LH is not fully suppressed. In other situations, the suppression may be so strong as to block the development of follicles. In controlled ovarian hyperstimulation, Lupron is used for a short time (several days to several weeks) and has few, if any, side effects. As soon as the ovary is suppressed, gonadotropin therapy is started and any side effect of Lupron is reversed.

If used for a long time, GnRH creates a reversible medical menopause. This may happen in a 3- to 6-month regimen for the treatment of endometriosis. GnRH robs the endometriosis lesions of estrogen, which is their food for growth. The lesions regress, resulting in less endometriosis, less pain, and improved fertility. When used for PCOS, ovarian androgen production is reduced. The side effects of long-term use are more pronounced and similar to those of menopause, including hot flashes and reversible reduction in bone density. These negative effects can be reduced using estrogen and progestins.

Conception 101

FOLLICLE. Each egg is enclosed in a small fluid-filled sac called a follicle. The egg has very limited capacity to fend for itself, and the follicle provides a micro-incubator to care for and nourish it. The follicle that will ovulate starts its development about 3 months prior to ovulation. Up until 10 days prior to ovulation, the follicles are too small to be seen without the aid of a microscope. It is about this time that they start to produce estradiol. When the follicle reaches about 6 to 8 millimeters (the size of a small pea), it can be seen for the first time by ultrasound. The follicle grows rapidly as ovulation nears. In the natural cycles the follicle is about 20 to 23 mm when it ovulates, the size of a silver dollar.

ENDOMETRIAL STRIPE. On ultrasound the endometrial lining is called the stripe. The lining thickens from 3 to 4 millimeters at the start of the cycle to 8 to 16 millimeters prior to the LH surge. It is considered that the lining should be at least 8 millimeters. In addition, the appearance of the lining changes from a homogeneous white line to a characteristic three lines (also known as a Type I or A or trilaminar appearance) prior to ovulation. The subsequent release of progesterone further changes the appearance of the lining as the halo fills in.

CORPUS LUTEUM. After the follicle ovulates, it is converted into a mostly solid structure, the corpus luteum (CL). The CL makes large amounts of both estrogen and progesterone, providing support for continued endometrial development in preparation for supporting the implanting embryo. The CL has a finite life span of about 12 days, and if it is not rescued by pregnancy, the CL will degenerate, progesterone will fall, and a period will result.

Prolactin-Inhibiting Agents
(Parlodel, Permax, Dostinex)

Excess prolactin inhibits ovulation. These drugs (taken orally or as a vaginal pill) correct this by suppressing hypothalamic activity and reducing the output of the hormone by the pituitary gland. Women with ovulation problems caused by a pituitary adenoma (a benign tumor), or a condition called hyperprolactinemic amenorrhea, may benefit from these agents.

You may experience side effects such as nausea, nasal stuffiness, dizziness, low blood pressure, drowsiness, and headaches. The first few days of treatment can be very uncomfortable, but the side effects usually resolve. Cabergoline (Dostinex) is taken only twice weekly and may have significantly fewer side effects than bromocriptine (Parlodel).

This treatment is considered safe even if it goes on for several years. Studies show that up to 90 percent of women will ovulate if they continue taking these medications, with as many as 65 to 85 percent conceiving. Usually the medication is stopped when you get pregnant, but there are no studies suggesting that the drug is harmful. Let your doctor know if you have been taking this drug.

Progesterone
(Crinone, Prometrium)

Progesterone, the hormone produced by the corpus luteum following ovulation, plays an important role in embryo implantation and the maintenance of early pregnancy. Progesterone supplementation, usually given by injection or vaginal suppository, is often administered during the luteal phase of assisted reproduction cycles. It is certainly known that Lupron can inhibit progesterone production, but it is not thought that ovulation induction alone has any adverse effect.

Although the FDA has never approved the administration of progesterone in pregnancy, many studies have demonstrated the efficacy and relative safety of progesterone supplementation in these circumstances. Understand that progesterone is the same substance the ovary would normally make. Progesterone levels after controlled ovarian hyperstimulation are often many times over what could be obtained by progesterone administration. There has never been and there will never be a report of a detrimental effect of progesterone on pregnancy.

An oral progesterone preparation (Prometrium) was introduced in 1998. While less potent, the natural preparation may have theoretical benefits over the synthetic progestins. Prometrium may be given as a boost to luteal function in infertile women or in early pregnancy, but it should not be the total supplementation after GnRH, or with oocyte donation. It may not be well absorbed or provide adequate blood levels for total luteal support. Prometrium may be used like progestin to bring on a desired period.

Side effects of progesterone include lethargy, mood swings, depression, and/or breast soreness. It may cause pain or irritation at the site of the injection when given intramuscularly or it may cause irritation of the vagina when given intravaginally.

Progestins (Progestogen)
Medroxyprogesterone (MPA) (Provera, Cycrin, Amen)
Norethindrone Acetate (Aygestin)

Progestins mimic the action of progesterone. They are not fertility boosters but are used to regulate menstruation. In fact, it is not the progestin itself, but its withdrawal, that results in menstruation. The most commonly used agent is medroxyprogesterone acetate (MPA) (Cycrin, Amen, Provera). A regimen of 5 to 10 milligrams for 10 to 14 days every 1 to 3 months is used to normalize bleeding. Aygestin can be used at 5 milligrams daily in a similar regimen.

For a progestin to work, your uterus must first be primed with estrogen. In some women with PCOS, the estrogen levels are not sufficient for the progestin to have an effect. If a progestin alone does not induce bleeding, a regimen first using estrogen, then progestin, may be tried. Progestins are sometimes used in ovulation induction or IVF cycles to regulate bleeding and as an attempt to get off on the right foot. This may be useful if you have irregular cycles. The safety of synthetic use in pregnancy has not been confirmed, and its use should be avoided.

With the exception of a limited use in treatment of endometriosis, the long-acting depo form of provera probably has no role in reproductive medicine. Menstrual cycle disturbance is very common after its use.

Estrogen

Although estrogen supplementation for fertility purposes is controversial, your doctor may recommend this therapy to enhance uterine lining development and possibly increase the implantation rate and reduce the chance of miscarriage. Some REs advise using estrogen in the follicular development phase, then resuming this 4 to 5 days after the surge or trigger. Normally, the estrogen drop follows the surge and slowly increases during the luteal phase. This regimen has not been proven, but it probably does no harm.

Estrogen, either orally or by transdermal (skin) patch, is important in the cases of programming the uterus to be receptive to the embryo, either as a donor cycle or in a thaw cycle. There are various regimens that differ among centers. Although the package insert is scary, it has nothing to do with the reason the estrogen is being used in this case. In the amounts given, a normal physiologic level is reproduced.

Insulin-Altering Drugs

Insulin-altering drugs are a potential monumental breakthrough in the treatment of PCOS. They actually treat the disease rather than overpower it. There is still much to be learned about these medications, but reports so far are very encouraging. Remember that they do not work for everyone and that a diagnosis of insulin resistance should be made before they are instituted. They are not FDA approved at present for treatment of PCOS, but keep tabs on these drugs.

Metformin (Glucophage) was approved in 1994 for the treatment of insulin resistance and Type 2 (insulin-resistant) diabetes that cannot be controlled by diet alone. This drug enhances the body's sensitivity to insulin and inhibits glucose production from the liver without the risk of hypoglycemia. It does not lower blood glucose levels below normal, but acts to improve the body's sensitivity to insulin without affecting insulin secretion. Some patients on metformin have experienced weight loss, improved lipid profiles, lowering of blood pressure, the return of menstruation, and pregnancy.

Metformin appears to have an excellent safety profile and is generally well tolerated. Gastrointestinal upset and a tendency toward looser stools or more frequent bowel movements are the most common side effects, and can be experienced after eating a fatty meal or dessert. Lactic acidosis, a rare and potentially fatal condition, has been associated with use of metformin (3 out of 100,000 patients using the drug for one year), but most cases were with older patients with other chronic illnesses. The usual dose is 500 mg three times daily, 850 mg twice daily, or 1000 mg twice daily with meals.

Troglitazone (Rezulin) is an anti-diabetic agent not related to either the sulfonylureas (DiaBeta, Diabinase, Tolinase) or metformin (Glucophage). It was introduced in 1997 for treatment of Type 2 diabetes and appears to work by directly affecting insulin production. Blood glucose is lowered by improving the body's response to insulin. Troglitazone is better tolerated than metformin, with less gastrointestinal distress. While many patients on Rezulin do not lose weight, their overall metabolism improves and insulin levels are universally lowered. The FDA has strongly warned about the potential of liver damage, so liver function testing must be followed closely. The usual dose is 400 to 600 milligrams once daily.

Aspirin/Heparin/Prednisone

Baby aspirin, heparin, and prednisone are sometimes used to help obtain and/or maintain a pregnancy and may be helpful for women with the following:

- Endometriosis
- Salpingitis isthmica nodosa
- Hashimoto's thyroiditis
- Raynaud's disease
- Lupus
- Rheumatoid arthritis
- Other autoimmune disorders

The latest studies show that women undergoing in vitro fertilization (IVF) are more likely to become pregnant if they take low doses of aspirin in conjunction with drugs that stimulate ovulation. In a study published in *Fertility and Sterility* (May 1999), researchers compared 149 women who ingested a daily dose of 100 milligrams of aspirin while taking ovulation-stimulating drugs to 149 control women undergoing the same IVF treatment who did not take aspirin. They found that 45 percent of women in the aspirin group became pregnant, compared with 28 percent in the control group. Researchers conclude that low-dose aspirin treatment significantly improves ovarian response, uterine and ovarian blood flow velocity, implantation rate, and pregnancy rate in women undergoing IVF. Despite this study, aspirin has not been widely adopted yet.

The side effects of these medications may be serious. Long-term heparin exposure is associated with increased bone loss. Because pregnancy is a bone-losing situation, the heparin only adds to the loss, and calcium supplementation does not appear to reverse the effect. The risk of a bone fracture is thought to be as high as 15 percent. The fracture could be as slight as a stress fracture in the hand or foot, or as serious as a vertebral crush fracture as seen in elderly postmenopausal women. Another side effect may be a drop in circulating platelets. Blood platelets help initiate clotting and block small holes in the vessel walls. If the platelet count drops, the heparin has to be discontinued and some other medicine considered. Heparin can also create bruises and welts at the injection site, which can become infected.

Prednisone induces bone loss, in addition to weight gain, hypertension, sleep and mood disturbances, glucose intolerance, and aseptic necrosis of the femoral head (hip).

Despite possible risks involved with this therapy, the benefits are that you may conceive and give birth to a healthy child. You can work with

New Hope with Viagra?

Some new studies reveal that Viagra, a drug used to treat erectile dysfunction in men, may also help some infertile women. In an article in the *Journal of Human Reproduction* (April 2000), Dr. Geoffrey Sher, an infertility specialist from the Sher Institute for Reproductive Medicine, reported that three out of four infertile women in a small study became pregnant after using Viagra.

Before taking Viagra, the women had thin uterine linings that prevented the embryo from attaching to the lining and developing. Researchers believe that Viagra may increase blood flow to the uterus, helping the uterine lining to thicken and allowing the fertilized egg to implant. Although the results are preliminary, they do offer new hope for those with this infertility problem. More studies will have to be made to see if any harm is done to mother or the developing fetus. Ask your doctor for an update.

your doctor and decide if the trade-offs are worth the risk and if this therapy is something that you would pursue.

Intravenous Immunoglobulin (IVIG)

Intravenous Immunoglobulin (IVIG) is basically a treatment administered as a liquid directly into a patient's vein. The liquid is comprised of a certain type of antibody that has been pooled together from thousands of human blood donors. IVIG has been used for years to treat various types of diseases thought to be related to problems with the immune system. Recently, scientists have hypothesized that some couples may have infertility or recurrent pregnancy loss that is due to immune problems and have offered IVIG as a possible solution. Specifically, attention has been focused on women who have been through a number of IVF cycles with presumably good embryos but have never achieved pregnancy. This implantation failure (failure of the embryos to implant into the wall of the uterus) has been attributed by some to an immunologic abnormality treatable by IVIG. There are other women who appear to get pregnant often but frequently or always miscarry the pregnancy. Some studies over the years have suggested that these women may have immunologic problems treatable by IVIG.

There have been 5 RCTs (retrospective controlled trials) studying IVIG for recurrent pregnancy loss. Some showed a difference, some did not. When they are combined and analyzed, it seems that IVIG does *not* reduce the risk of miscarriage. For implantation failure, no one has even attempted to do a study.

Ask Questions

No matter what fertility medication your doctor recommends, it is important to ask questions. Be sure you understand:

- What the medication is
- How to take it
- What its potential side effects are and how to manage them
- What its potential for interactions with other medications is
- How long you will need to take the medication
- What the next steps would be if the medication does not work

Remember, just as with any chronic illness, knowledge is power with infertility. The more you understand your body and how it is being treated, the more in control you will feel.

Chapter 14

Works of ART

"Sensitive to our financial concerns, Dr. Miller suggested one try at IVF without injectable drugs, which can reduce the cost of an average cycle by $1,500," said Jess, age 34. "So it began as just another month on Clomid with some extra ultrasounds and blood tests added in. Not too big a jump in time demands, though a significant jump in psychological energy expenditure.

"Once again I produced three eggs, which were harvested at the appropriate time. With the ultrasound inserted, Mac was able to observe Dr. Miller's extraction of the eggs on the monitor. As I'd been warned, the plucking process was momentarily painful, but certainly tolerable. I think Mac hurt more, watching it on the screen.

"Dr. Miller worked latexed hand in latexed hand with an embryologist who was responsible for the actual fertilization part of the process—adding Mac's sperm to the eggs.

"We were fascinated by the science of it all, and were even granted a look at both sets of players under the microscope. Two days later, the call came. Though Mac's sperm were still swimming, they hadn't managed to crack the shell of my eggs. We joked that I always have been a tough egg to crack, but that didn't make the blow any easier to take. I could tell that even Dr. Miller felt bad. After another period of mourning—and a forced one-month rest period for my body—we moved to the big drugs and another trial of IVF."

Avast array of assisted reproductive technologies (ART) are now available. The high-tech choices for conception are many. Even the list of abbreviations is bewildering—IUI, IVF, ICSI, GIFT, ZIFT, and AID. So which will help you to make a baby?

Many breakthrough treatments are touted to help couples make a baby, but many factors must be considered in understanding and choosing the type of treatment. After your doctor assesses you and your partner's medical records, including test results and fertility history, you need to discuss the effectiveness, complexity, and cost of the various high-tech methods in detail with your physician. Some of the key factors you will consider before approaching treatment include:

- Cause and length of infertility
- Age
- Personal, religious, and emotional preference
- Cost and insurance coverage
- Access to a successful fertility clinic
- Prognosis for success

ART or Science?

Assisted reproductive techniques (ART) have been used in the United States since 1981 to help women achieve pregnancy. ART is a broadly defined term that could mean any method to improve reproduction. Most commonly, ART refers to the transfer of fertilized human eggs into a woman's uterus, or those procedures that use some form of in vitro fertilization. This would include IVF, GIFT, and ZIFT, and associated procedures such as ICSI (intracytoplasmic sperm injection).

While many clinics report successful ART treatments, your chances of becoming pregnant and having a live birth by using ART are directly related to key factors outside of the fertility clinic's control, including:

- Your age
- The cause of infertility
- The number of children you already have

Intrauterine Insemination (IUI)

Intrauterine insemination (IUI), the process of placing sperm directly into the uterus, is probably the simplest form of ART available. Although artificial insemination (AI) has been performed for a very long time, it was not until the techniques of sperm preparation were refined from IVF technology that IUI became popular. IUI now replaces other types of insemination procedures such as intracervical and placing the sperm in the vaginal pool.

IUI is used in cases of male-factor infertility to improve the number of sperm reaching the site of fertilization. It may bypass the cervix, which is the main site of sperm antibody production. It is used in conjunction with fertility-promoting agents to increase their effectiveness. IUI is also an effective semen analysis. Rather than discarding the semen sample after it has been analyzed, why not add an insemination to combine therapy with diagnosis?

How Does It Work?

Before IUI is performed, sperm have to be removed from the seminal fluid and concentrated. This process of sperm preparation is called washing. The seminal fluid, which includes prostaglandins and other chemicals, must be removed. During the washing, the sperm are activated, so their capacity to fertilize the egg is immediate. But this also means that they will not live as long in your body, so timing is critical.

IUI must be performed near ovulation. Often insemination and ovulation are synchronized either by the LH surge, as determined by an ovulation predictor kit, or by an injection of the hormone hCG. You may be instructed to have intercourse the night before IUI and after the insemination to increase the amount of sperm available.

The semen sample is usually obtained by masturbation. If this is not possible, there are condoms specifically designed for collection. The sample must have about 30 minutes to liquefy. This allows the specimen to be produced at home if you live within 30 to 60 minutes of the clinic. After being spun, the semen is then mixed with a nutrient medium and placed in a centrifuge. The fluid is taken from the top and discarded and the pellet of sperm is again mixed with a medium for a second centrifugation. This time the sperm pellet is suspended in a drop of medium and the insemination is performed by passing a small plastic catheter (a tube about the size of a ballpoint pen refill) through the cervix and into your uterine cavity. An ultrasound scan may be used before the insemination to check for follicle and endometrial development. At the time of the insemination, the amount and quality of cervical mucus is recorded. There is no advantage to lying down or limiting activity after the procedure. Unlike conventional insemination, it is highly unlikely that the sperm will escape. You may have some discomfort during the procedure and afterwards because the cervix tissue is soft. There may be slight bleeding or spotting. In any case, report any fever or excessive cramping or bleeding to your doctor immediately.

In other alternative methods, sperm are concentrated and allowed to swim into the medium, rather than washed. This is gentler and selects only the most motile sperm, but the sperm yields are considerably smaller. This procedure is more labor intensive and time consuming, and therefore more expensive. It has not been shown to be superior to the washing method for IUI.

Combined Treatment May Be Best

Combining artificial insemination with hormone treatments appears to give infertile couples a better chance of pregnancy than either method by itself. In a study in *The New England Journal of Medicine* that assessed 932 couples, researchers from the University of Rochester and Baylor College of Medicine in Houston found that women who received hormones with artificial insemination were three times more likely to become pregnant than those who received the equivalent of no treatment and twice as likely to become pregnant as those who received only one form of treatment.

THE UPSIDE. IUI is safe and easy. It allows your evaluation around the time of ovulation, as well as that of a semen sample. It gives the sperm a head start toward fertilization. It avoids the potential hostile mucus of the cervix and cervical stenosis. It may improve pregnancy rate, especially when used with fertility drugs.

THE DOWNSIDE. Timing is critical. The natural reservoir of sperm in the cervix is bypassed, so the sperm don't have the same lasting power. IUI without fertility drugs is of questionable therapeutic benefit. The procedure costs $100 to $500; with fertility drugs another $200 to $1,500. IUI itself does not increase risk of multiple pregnancies, but fertility drugs do.

THE BOTTOM LINE. It is worth a go on one or two cycles in most infertile couples. Starting with IUI may help you avoid more aggressive and costly therapy.

In Vitro Fertilization and Embryo Transfer (IVF-ET)

IVF is the oldest and most widely used assisted reproductive technology. With IVF, the retrieved eggs are mixed with your partner's sperm outside your body in a laboratory setting (see Figure 14.1). The fertilized eggs (embryos) are transferred back into your uterus through the cervix.

IVF-ET represents the flagship of assisted reproduction. Despite the technological explosion in the new reproductive technologies, tubal damage/blockage still represents a common and undeniable reason for IVF-ET. IVF-ET may even be preferable to surgery to reconnect the tubes after previous sterilization in some cases. This avoids major surgery with its prolonged recovery period and the increased risk of ectopic, or tubal, pregnancy. The reasons IVF-ET is used have expanded past tubal infertility to include many types of both male and female infertility. Besides its utilization as therapy, IVF-ET may now be used as a diagnostic tool. IVF-ET no longer can be considered an experimental procedure. The American Society for Reproductive Medicine states "in vitro fertilization for infertility, not solvable by other means, is considered ethical."

In theory, the IVF-ET procedure is simple. An egg is taken from the ovary, and healthy sperm are selected from a sample produced by the male. The egg and sperm are mixed together in a culture dish where fertilization takes place. The resulting embryo is transferred into the uterus about the time it would arrive there in a natural conception. Sounds easy, does it? Wrong!

In actual practice, IVF-ET demands a high level of expertise and

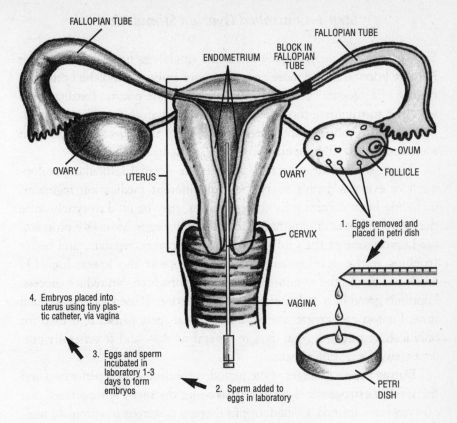

Figure 14.1 Diagram of the IVF Process

attention to detail, as well as a precisely coordinated effort between you, your partner, and a large IVF-ET team. IVF-ET is a very emotional experience. It seems to focus all your hopes and fears about fertility and pregnancy into a procedure. That's why an understanding of the actual steps involved will help you maintain a feeling of control.

There are five stages in the IVF-ET process:

1. Controlled ovarian stimulation
2. Follicle aspiration
3. In vitro fertilization and culture
4. Transfer of embryos
5. Implantation support and monitoring

Step 1. Controlled Ovarian Stimulation

Each month a woman usually releases a single egg from the ovary. For IVF, we know that the more eggs, the more embryos, and the better the chance of a pregnancy. To obtain more than one oocyte, fertility drugs are given to stimulate the ovary, so that more than one preovulatory follicle develops. Usually the drugs involved are the injectable ones, but some centers use clomiphene for selected patients.

There is some degree of disorder in the normal follicular development of every woman's ovary. Several different medication regimens, including birth control pills and progestins, may be used to synchronize the ovary in hopes of obtaining the best quality eggs. Most IVF programs use Lupron, one of the GnRH analogs, to suppress, regulate, and better synchronize the development of follicles. Lupron also lowers high LH levels and blocks the natural LH surge, both of which can reduce success. Lupron is given by a daily subcutaneous injection. If used for an extended time, Lupron can create a reversible medical menopause. It is used for only a short time—several days to several weeks—and it generally produces few, if any, side effects.

During the early stages of the period, a baseline scan is performed and the level of estrogen is assessed to make sure the ovary is suppressed and no cysts have formed. Gonadotropin therapy is started to stimulate multiple follicles to develop. Ultrasound scan and estrogen level tests are then used to monitor follicle growth and response to stimulation. When the follicle(s) are judged to be mature, both by size (16–22 mm) and estradiol level (above 400 μg/ml), an injection of human chorionic gonadotropin is given to allow the follicles to complete their last stages of maturation.

Step 2. Follicle Aspiration

The follicle aspiration, in which the eggs are removed from the ovary, is scheduled about 36 hours after the hCG is given. By that time, the egg has separated and is floating in the follicle. A needle is passed through the upper vaginal wall, and with the use of vaginal ultrasound, fluid is removed from the follicles under gentle suction. The procedure may last from 5 to about 30 minutes with few exceptions. Centers vary in the levels of sedation that you will receive, from a pain pill to general anesthesia. You will have from minimal to moderately severe pain, but the procedure is generally considered very tolerable.

Immediately after aspiration of a follicle, the oocyte is isolated from the follicular fluid, placed in a culture dish containing nutrient media, and then transferred to the incubator. Shortly before or after the aspiration procedure, the sperm are isolated from the semen obtained earlier. During this procedure, the most active sperm are selected and transferred to a culture dish for completion of the changes necessary for fertilization.

Step 3. In Vitro Fertilization

Oocytes and sperm are placed together in a culture dish kept inside an incubator. They are left undisturbed until the next day, when they are examined for fertilization. Over the next day the 1-cell embryo will divide into a 2-cell embryo, then 2 cells into 4, and 4 cells into 8. At about this time, the embryo is ready for transfer (unless an extended culture has been selected).

Step 4. Transfer of Embryos

On the second or third day following follicular aspiration, you will receive the embryo(s). The transfer takes only a few minutes, and the procedure involves placing a speculum into your vagina and transferring the embryo(s) via a small plastic tube placed through the cervix into the uterine cavity. No anesthesia is required and usually only minimal, if any, discomfort is felt.

Step 5. Implantation Support and Monitoring

It is unknown when implantation takes place or what can be done to ensure the best chance of implantation. Because of the extreme manipulation of the ovaries that has taken place, your body will receive additional supplements of hCG and/or progesterone to provide the optimum environment for implantation. Hopefully, a pregnancy test is positive at the time of your expected period.

Although many pregnancies are established in the first cycle, the chance of pregnancy appears to be equal with each try through the first four attempts. It's important to know up front that the average couple will undergo two to three IVF attempts before either a successful pregnancy occurs or they abandon therapy altogether. Once established, a pregnancy after IVF-ET is no different from a pregnancy established without fertility therapy and is not considered high risk.

Success Rates

With IVF-ET, using multiple drugs for ovarian stimulation, a realistic expectation for delivering a baby from any cycle is 25 percent. This is almost equal to the natural fertility rate in fertile couples having unprotected intercourse. This rate is highly dependent on the mother's age and the reason for IVF. Still, most REs agree that the issue of success rates with fertility centers has gotten out of hand. In other words, more is not better. Centers have been known to misrepresent themselves by changing statistics to their benefit. The costs must be considered, as well as the experience and success rate of the RE performing the ART.

THE UPSIDE. IVF-ET works, and the success rate with this procedure exceeds those of almost all other infertility therapies. IVF can also serve simultaneously as a diagnostic procedure as well as a treatment. For instance, a woman who has a poor response to fertility medications often has little chance for achieving success. During the stages of IVF, it is possible to inspect the eggs under the microscope for abnormal-looking eggs. The failure to see successful fertilization after the addition of sperm may identify a previously unknown problem with the sperm/egg interaction. Finally, abnormalities in the development of the embryo after fertilization could reveal the cause for infertility.

THE DOWNSIDE. It does not always work, and the procedure comes at a high physical, financial, and emotional cost. There is a substantial risk of multiple pregnancies. Hyperstimulation of the ovaries, especially if a pregnancy is established, is common and can lead to serious short-term complications. For women over 40, pregnancy rates drop and miscarriage rates rise with IVF. Even though several embryos may be transferred for implantation, the chance of producing one full-term baby ranges from 18 to 25 percent each time embryos are placed in the uterus.

THE BOTTOM LINE. IVF is the central therapy in present infertility practice and unites many different causes of infertility into a single treatment.

Blastocyst Culture

With conventional IVF-ET, embryos are cultured to the 8-cell stage of development before they are transferred to your uterus. This stage of development is usually reached on the third day after aspiration. The term *blastocyst* refers to the stage of embryo development just prior to implantation; it is reached after approximately five days in the culture. By extending the culture period, the best embryos can be selected; theoretically, pregnancy rates improve while the possibility of multiple gestations decreases. With the development of new types of media, embryos can be cultured for longer periods of time in the laboratory.

THE UPSIDE. There are improved pregnancy rates and reduced chance of multiple gestations with blastocyst culture. You can know that you will be pregnant without having to wait for a period.

THE DOWNSIDE. Your uterus may still be a better incubator than the laboratory. Some pregnancies may be lost by extending the culture period and delaying the transfer. There will be fewer embryos for cryopreservation due to the need to keep all embryos in culture to see which ones continue to develop.

THE BOTTOM LINE. This represents an important scientific advance, but the practical advance in success is much less clear.

Assisted Hatching

The zona pellucida (ZP) is a protein halo that surrounds the egg and later the embryo. The ZP may serve to prevent the embryo from attaching to the wall of the tube as it travels down to the uterus. Once the embryo is in the uterus, the ZP dissolves and the embryo "hatches." There are several studies suggesting the ZP is abnormally thickened in some infertile women, and this may prevent proper hatching and implantation. If you are over age 35 and have had failed fertilization, unexplained infertility, or repeated IVF cycles with no success, you may be at risk.

Assisted hatching is a selective thinning of the zona pellucida either mechanically, by puncturing the ZP, or chemically, by using an acid solution to partially dissolve the ZP. Some excellent fertility clinics swear by this technique. Other centers with equally good success rates condemn the procedure as unnecessary.

THE UPSIDE. It may improve the chances for pregnancy and is one more theoretically advantageous procedure that can be done with expected low success rates.

THE DOWNSIDE. It is more costly and the procedure may destroy the embryo.

THE BOTTOM LINE. The procedure has not consistently shown itself to be effective in all centers.

Embryo Cryopreservation

Most doctors will only implant three or fewer fertilized embryos during an IVF-ET cycle. Because there may be more follicles harvested than can be used during a single cycle, cryopreservation is a viable option.

After fertilization has been confirmed, early embryos are chosen for the freezing process. The day embryos are frozen varies. Sometimes one group is frozen as soon as fertilization has been confirmed. Other times they are cultured until the day of transfer to make sure the best are available. Usually the earlier embryos are frozen, the better they survive. The freezing process involves placing the embryos in a special protective medium to diminish the shock of freezing and then gradually lowering the temperature, using liquid in a device especially designed for this purpose. The embryos are then stored in liquid nitrogen ($-276°$ C) in small straws that have been individually labeled. The chance of a mix-up, while not nil, is slim. There is *no* evidence that freezing has an adverse effect on pregnancies once established after cryopreservation.

If your cycles are very regular and ovulation occurs, the embryos can be transferred in a natural cycle with medications. In some cases, your menstrual cycle may be suppressed with the GnRH analogs, followed by hormone replacement using estrogen and progesterone. An exact replica of a normal cycle can be re-created using hormone supplements.

One to three days before the transfer, the embryos are thawed and placed in the same environment as a standard IVF would be. Usually about 50 percent of the embryos survive the thawing process. This varies by the quality of the embryos frozen.

The thaw cycle is a breeze compared to the IVF cycles. No shots; no aspiration; just the transfer. The success of thaw cycles varies greatly between centers. Sometimes the best-quality embryos are not frozen, but have been transferred in the original cycle. Still, an expectation of success is at least 50 percent of the center's IVF success rate.

THE UPSIDE. This procedure is ethically better than destroying healthy embryos. Cryopreservation allows additional chances of pregnancy with one stimulation cycle. The chances of multiple gestations are reduced.

THE DOWNSIDE. The success rate is not that great. This creates a possible ethical problem of what to do with the frozen embryos.

THE BOTTOM LINE. Cryopreservation is a legitimate method of managing the surplus of embryos that is sometimes available with IVF, allowing reasonable chances of pregnancy.

Gamete Intrafallopian Transfer (GIFT)

GIFT is generally done when you have at least one normal fallopian tube and no hint of male-factor infertility involved. In the GIFT procedure, follicles are aspirated during laparoscopy, and the unfertilized oocytes are placed in the fallopian tube along with a sample of unprepared sperm. Some centers may use ultrasound-guided aspiration followed by the laparoscopic egg/sperm placement. This allows fertilization to occur naturally inside your body (not outside), the way a normally fertilized egg would start its journey to the uterus for implantation. Any remaining eggs following the GIFT transfer may be inseminated with sperm in a laboratory dish, and the resulting embryos can be frozen.

It used to be thought that this environment might be preferable, since the fallopian tube is the place where fertilization and early embryo development normally occur. However, it is now known that the better pregnancy rate initially seen with GIFT was due to the fact that the patients who underwent GIFT were better candidates for achieving pregnancy overall. When studies were done comparing IVF to GIFT using two groups of equivalent patients, there was no difference in pregnancy rates.

THE UPSIDE. One of GIFT's major advantages over IVF is that the technique relies to a far greater degree on your body's natural processes to produce pregnancy, as the conception takes place in your body.

THE DOWNSIDE. Even though it is usually an outpatient procedure, GIFT requires general anesthesia and more invasive surgery (laparoscopy), which adds to the risk and expense. With IVF, the advantages of knowing that fertilization has occurred and that transport through a possibly abnormal tube is not necessary may have important diagnostic, prognostic, and therapeutic consequences. These are not available with GIFT.

THE BOTTOM LINE. If you have an abnormal cervix, which makes it difficult or impossible to place the embryos in your uterus, or if you have a personal objection to a standard IVF procedure, GIFT may be the high-tech method for you. You must have normal fallopian tubes, and your partner must have adequate sperm for success. With a recent increase in the success rates and relative ease of the IVF-ET procedure, GIFT is probably on its way out, as indicated by dropping numbers of GIFT cycles.

Zygote Intrafallopian Transfer (ZIFT)
Tubal Embryo Transfer (TET)
Pronuclear Stage Transfer (PROST)

The above techniques all combine the potential advantages of GIFT with IVF and possibly sperm injection, hoping to increase the pregnancy rate. The capacity to see if fertilization has occurred and select early embryos with the greatest potential for development overcomes a major objection of GIFT. With ZIFT, TET, and PROST, fertilization is confirmed before the transfer. Several centers in the United States have performed transfers directly into the tube by going through the cervix and uterus using hysteroscopy, but this requires considerable skill on the part of the surgeon.

THE PROCEDURE. Oocytes are obtained by transvaginal follicle aspiration, fertilized in the laboratory, and transferred into the tube via laparoscopy on a subsequent day. Procedures such as ZIFT, TET, and PROST are all modifications of GIFT/IVF protocols but differ in the stage of development at which transfer into the tube takes place. Success rates with these procedures is reported to be superior to conventional IVF-ET.

THE UPSIDE. The chief advantage of these techniques is thought to be the ability to ensure that fertilization has taken place before placement of conception. Success rates are relatively high.

THE DOWNSIDE. The cost is also extremely high, and laparoscopy is still necessary. If you have abnormal fallopian tubes, this technique will not work. Also, because your eggs must be harvested and transplanted, two procedures are required (follicle aspiration and laparoscopy for transfer).

THE BOTTOM LINE. These are effective ART procedures, but the high cost has caused them not to be chosen by many.

Intracytoplasmic Sperm Injection (ICSI)

ICSI was introduced in 1992 and has since led to successful pregnancies among couples in which the male has an extremely low sperm count. Procedures are performed on sperm and eggs under controlled environmental conditions using specialized equipment with high-powered magnification. The equipment is designed to allow the embryologist to perform very intricate movements. One glass tool (the holding pipette) is used to stabilize the egg while a second glass tube containing sperm (the injection pipette) is used to penetrate the zona pellucida and egg membrane. Thus a single sperm is deposited into the egg cytoplasm. An enzyme (hyaluronidase) is used to aid in removing the cells and to better visualize the oocyte. Sperm are suspended in a second chemical (polyvinyl pyrolidone, PVP), which improves the handling of the sperm with the injection pipette. After injection of the sperm, the oocyte is released from the holding pipette and washed in a drop of fresh culture medium.

The oocyte is checked for evidence of fertilization the morning following the ICSI procedure. Fertilized eggs are cultured for 1 to 4 additional days. At the end of the culture period, normally developing embryos will be either transferred to the uterus or cryopreserved.

Success with ICSI should equal the clinic-specific IVF-ET rate for couples not using ICSI. Success rates when sperm aspiration is used is about 50 percent of the ICSI rates without sperm aspiration in the same age groups.

THE UPSIDE. ICSI works well. It bypasses many forms of male infertility and offers success which would be impossible with other procedures.

THE DOWNSIDE. This treatment is expensive and can possibly damage healthy oocyte or sperm during the procedure. The sperm usually need to be collected from the testicle using a microscopic needle or surgical biopsy. ICSI must be used in conjunction with IVF with the added expense of that procedure.

THE BOTTOM LINE. If male-factor infertility is your problem, ICSI may work.

Sperm Aspiration
Percutaneous Epididymal Sperm Aspiration (PESA)
Microsurgical Sperm Aspiration (MESA)
Testicular Sperm Aspiration (TESA)

There are many reasons for azoospermia (lack of sperm on ejaculation), as described in Chapters 5 and 12. In the case of total lack of sperm production, there is no treatment other than donor sperm. Yet even if there is no sperm in the ejaculation, there may be sufficient sperm in the testis or epididymis to provide a sufficient quantity for ICSI.

Sperm aspiration is especially useful when there is an anatomic obstruction of the male reproductive tract, but the sperm are still functioning normally. A particularly good reason for PESA is failed vasectomy reversal, or a vasectomy and female infertility. The female blood tests for LH, FSH, and testosterone can help sort out the difference between sperm production and obstruction. Because of the low numbers of sperm aspirated, this treatment must be used with ICSI.

ICSI is used with aspiration of sperm directly from the testis or the epididymis by percutaneous epididymal sperm aspiration (needle biopsy) (PESA) or through a microsurgical incision in the epididymis or testis (MESA, TESA). Both of these procedures are performed as an outpatient and just before the follicle aspiration of eggs. Pain is often less than that of a sterilization procedure, and swelling, while common, resolves in a few days. Local anesthesia and mild pain medications are all that is usually necessary for the PESA procedure.

THE UPSIDE. This treatment gives new hope for previously "no cure" cases.

THE DOWNSIDE. It's expensive and has less chance of success than ICSI. There is also temporary discomfort.

THE BOTTOM LINE. Technology had to wait for ICSI to be effective. Continued development is now expected.

Ovum Donation (OD)

Ovum donation (OD) is the process of placing younger eggs in older mothers. Although the average age at menopause is 51, many women experience a decline in egg numbers and quality as young as age 35. In fact, it is very rare for older women to get pregnant, and when they do, they are at high risk for miscarriage and for having babies with abnormalities such as Down's syndrome.

A woman is first identified as a donor. She takes fertility medications in order to stimulate the development of multiple eggs. When the eggs have developed or matured, they are removed from her ovaries. Typically 10 to 20 eggs can be obtained. Once they are outside her body, they can be fertilized with sperm from any source (such as the older woman's husband or a sperm donor). The fertilized eggs are matured further in the laboratory.

In the meantime, the older woman has taken hormones (estrogen and progesterone, which are normally produced from the ovaries) to prepare the uterus for the acceptance of embryos. The uterus doesn't know or care where the embryos come from. Finally, the embryos are transferred into the older woman's uterus. She continues to take hormones to support the lining of the uterus after the transfer. If a pregnancy occurs (that is, the embryo implants into the lining of the uterus and continues to develop), then the older woman continues the hormone treatment for the first trimester of the pregnancy. This allows the baby's placenta to develop and eventually take over the production of hormones. The success rates for egg donation far exceed those for regular IVF. This is probably due to the fact that the donors who provide the eggs are young and don't have fertility problems themselves. In addition, the risks for miscarriage and babies with chromosomal abnormalities are also reduced, since they are dependent on the age of the donor, not the recipient.

THE UPSIDE. This procedure allows women with ovarian failure or the potential to pass on genetic defects to carry and deliver a child who has their husband's genes. The paternal investment can be sizable. Even though there is not a combination of the couple's genes, the woman is able to experience birth.

THE DOWNSIDE. The baby has no genetic ties to the recipient. The procedure is also very expensive. There may be unknown or unreported problems with the donor, with the same concerns as sperm donation.

THE BOTTOM LINE. This is a very important technology that has provided the chance for more natural parenting to many couples.

Donor Cytoplasm

There is a theory that some eggs may not be capable of producing a pregnancy because they "run out of energy." All cells, including eggs, are made up of two principle components: the nucleus, which contains most of the genetic material, and the cytoplasm, which contains most of the machinery for making a cell work. The cell derives its "power" from small structures in the cytoplasm called ribosomes. The theory states that if you transplant cytoplasm from a young healthy egg cell into an older or unhealthy egg, you may induce the older egg to work better and therefore be more likely to produce a pregnancy. In fact, a couple of pregnancies have occurred in women whose eggs were treated this way. It is not known, however, whether the pregnancies occurred because of the treatment or in spite of it. Therefore, further study is necessary to determine if it works or not.

THE UPSIDE. The procedure offers new hope using breakthrough scientific methods.

THE DOWNSIDE. Donor cytoplasm is extremely expensive, with a very low success rate to date.

THE BOTTOM LINE. Donor cytoplasm should not be considered a viable option at this time.

Donor Embryos

If you are considering the use of donor eggs or donor sperm, you may also want to consider donor embryos. Embryo donation involves the use of eggs from a donor that have been fertilized with either sperm from the donor's partner or donor sperm. Surplus embryos arise from many IVF programs that perform cryopreservation—and most do. Often these embryos come from couples who successfully had a child and don't want more. These couples may object to destroying the frozen embryos and choose to place them up for "adoption" instead. They sign a release and relinquish all rights, legal and otherwise. This should stand up in courts, as sperm and egg donation have, but this area is more complex and has not been legally tested. Generally these donations are anonymous. Embryo donations are usually completely altruistic, and the donors do not expect or receive payment, other than possible reimbursement for cost of the embryo storage.

With donor embryos, you would pay for the professional and laboratory charges associated with embryo transfer. The offspring will not be related genetically to you or your partner. Success rates for previously frozen embryos are lower than if fresh embryos are used. There must be documentation for the release of embryos from the donor to the recipient. Laws concerning this procedure vary from state to state.

You will undergo treatment to prepare your uterus in the same manner as during oocyte donation.

THE UPSIDE. You will be able to carry and deliver a child. There is the potential for superior obstetric care and prenatal nurturing. There is much less legal red tape than with adoption. The procedure should be very cost effective.

THE DOWNSIDE. It's hard to find information about the donors, and they probably will not be screened as well as the oocyte donor. The child will not have your DNA (genes).

THE BOTTOM LINE. This is a very ethical and successful form of final disposition of the large number of embryos that remain frozen in IVF laboratories around the world.

Surrogacy

Remember the three essential requirements for reproduction: an egg, a sperm, and the uterus? The first two can be substituted for by egg or sperm donation. The last requires surrogacy. A surrogate is a woman who carries a pregnancy for another woman. While the barriers in surrogacy are not medical, they are social and legal.

There are two types of surrogates.

1. The first type is called a *gestational surrogate* or *carrier*. This woman carries a pregnancy that is the product of an egg and sperm of two other individuals. This process involves the use of IVF, and the fertilized egg (embryo) is implanted in the surrogate's uterus. The gestational carrier is not related genetically to the child because she did not provide the egg.
2. The second type of surrogate is the *traditional surrogate*. This procedure does not involve IVF because the surrogate is inseminated with sperm from the male partner of the infertile couple. The child that results is genetically related to the surrogate and also to the male partner, but not to the female partner of the infertile couple. The female partner or couple must legally adopt the child after the birth.

THE UPSIDE. The child will be your offspring.

THE DOWNSIDE. In most states and by the American College of Obstetricians guidelines, the birth mother has the legal right to the child. Natural instincts make it difficult for a mother to give up a child that she has carried. The legal ramifications of surrogacy are staggering, and programs are very limited in number.

THE BOTTOM LINE. If you can get over the legal hurdles, the success rates are high.

Semen Banking

Short-term semen cryobanking is the depositing, freezing, and storage of sperm at a cryopreservation facility (usually an IVF center), for less than one year. Cryobanked sperm is then used in artificial insemination, in vitro fertilization, and other assisted reproductive procedures.

Short-term semen cryobanking is recommended in the following situations:

- To preserve semen for deferred inseminations when an intimate partner is temporarily absent
- In cases of oligospermia (low sperm counts), where multiple semen collections and pooling may be desirable for use in a single insemination
- Prior to assisted reproductive technologies, such as in vitro fertilization or gamete intrafallopian transfer, to secure a quality semen specimen for the procedure

Long-term cryopreservation is a proven, long-established technique that enables semen specimens to be frozen and stored indefinitely. These are usually kept at an accredited sperm bank but are often prepared through a local or regional facility such as an IVF center. According to the donor's specific wishes, these specimens can later be thawed and used in an attempt to conceive a child through therapeutic insemination or other assisted reproductive techniques.

The purpose of cryopreserving semen is to help assure a chance to father children at some time in the future.

- Some men discover they have diseases or must undergo treatment or surgery which will cause permanent sterilization or genetic damage. As cancer detection techniques and treatment techniques improve, more diseases are being detected at younger ages in men, with better and longer survival rates. Therefore, more men in their child-producing years are now considering this option.
- Some men wish to have a vasectomy, but still desire to keep a possible option open to father children should their circumstances change.
- Some men are engaged in high-risk occupations, including exposure to radiation or dangerous chemicals, and wish to ensure a future chance to father children.

- Some men find circumstances force them to be away from their wives during a period of time in which they had planned to conceive a child. Therapeutic insemination using their cryopreserved semen allows such couples a chance to follow their desired plan.

Prior to the collection of semen, sexual abstinence of at least 2 days but not more than 5 days is recommended to maximize the quality of the sample. The specimen is collected into a sterile container either by masturbation or withdrawal with the use of a special nontoxic condom. Collection may occur at home, provided that it does not take more than one hour to bring the sample to the facility. Otherwise, specimens may be collected at the cryopreservation facility.

Each sample (ejaculate) is mixed with a special media or solution to help provide protection during freezing and thawing. The samples are then placed in special plastic 1- or 2-milliliter vials, which are then sealed, coded, and carefully frozen in liquid nitrogen vapor. Once frozen, the vials are immersed in liquid nitrogen in secure tanks at a temperature of −196°C (−371°F). The liquid nitrogen is independent of any source of power, and is regularly checked and replenished.

THE UPSIDE. This is the maximum preservation of fertility, and the costs for cryopreservation and storage of sperm are relatively low when considering the potential for later reproduction.

THE DOWNSIDE. Some semen/sperm from very healthy donors of proven fertility withstand the freezing and thawing process very poorly. Because sperm is frozen, there is no guarantee that it will either be viable, or capable of initiating a pregnancy. Semen which is cryopreserved is considered property. Very specific instructions should be given as to the final disposition of the specimens.

THE BOTTOM LINE. This is an important adjunct for maximizing or protecting male fertility.

Oocyte Cryopreservation Theory

There are many fewer eggs (oocytes) in the ovary than sperm in the testes. There is no replenishment of the supply of oocytes over time. Access to the egg storehouse is much more difficult, and most oocytes in the ovary are resting in an immature state. These four factors severely limit the possibility of oocyte donation.

Unfortunately attempts at freezing eggs have been largely unsuccessful. Pregnancies after oocyte freezing, thawing, and IVF have been reported, but success rates in several large studies from otherwise successful centers have shown about a 1 percent pregnancy rate. It is not clear what the problem is, but research is under way to unravel the mystery. Theoretically, women who want to prolong their reproductive potential could have ovarian stimulation and follicle aspiration with cryo-preservation of the eggs for later thaw and insemination by the sperm of their choice. Since studies have shown little effect of age on the uterus, this means that pregnancy would be possible at any time.

An exciting procedure, which so far has been shown to work in sheep, is to surgically remove the ovary, or a section of ovary, freeze it, and surgically replace the fragment at some later time. Since the uterus is mostly resistant to the aging process, this means women who want to prolong their reproductive potential could do so. This is a very practical option for women who are facing radiation or possible sterility from radiation or chemotherapy for cancer.

THE UPSIDE. Maximum preservation of fertility.

THE DOWNSIDE. You have to wait until the ethical and legal ramifications are sorted out.

THE BOTTOM LINE. Great hope for future babies!

Part Four

Complementary Approaches to Making a Baby

Chapter 15

Beating the Baby Blues

"There used to be these Stan Freburg TV commercials with an ominous voice from the background warning, 'It's not nice to fool with Mother Nature!'" said Whitney, age 41. *"I have heard that voice frequently over the course of our two-year excursion into the world of high-tech reproduction. Our sex life definitely moved from intimate romance into the on-demand category. As the months came and went, and the clock ticked louder, I pursued a round of testing with my gynecologist to be sure my anatomy checked out. This ranged from blood testing of hormone levels to the hysterosalpingogram. I passed everything.*

"Nonetheless, my disappointment grew. I didn't much want to discuss the issue with anyone other than Nick, as I dreaded constant questions after that. Yes, nature failed us, it was off to the doctor ... again and again and again. I memorized the routine and knew the agony of the wait. I tried hard not to indulge the desire to do a home pregnancy test seven days before it would be valid. To escape my rumination, I headed out of town to visit a friend."

Stress. Just hearing the word can make you cringe. Yet while you may think you know all about stress, trying to get pregnant without success is probably one of the greatest emotional roller coasters you can ever experience. From the constant poking, probing, and prodding that makes you feel so broken and vulnerable; to late-night hormone injections and early-morning blood tests; to sore ovaries, ultrasounds, and even exploratory surgery, the entire focus of your life is toward one goal: making a healthy baby. Yet when the long-awaited pregnancy test comes back negative—month after month after month—your stress levels soar and your self-confidence dwindles. As 33-year-old Adriana said, "I feel as if I'm in constant training for a marathon, yet no matter how hard I try, I keep coming in last."

Ashley's six-year experience with infertility and the subsequent tests and procedures was no less positive. "When you have no control over the outcome of life situations combined with no control over what may happen, it makes for a lethal emotional combination. I constantly felt that if I could just control the outcome of events, I could cope. Or even if I have no control, at least if I know what will happen, I can cope. The entire infertility experience made me feel so fragile and vulnerable."

All Stressed Up and No Place to Go

If you find yourself feeling such symptoms of stress as extreme emotional highs and lows, high anxiety, depression, or isolation, you are not alone. Infertility is an extremely distressing life crisis that is ongoing until your family is completed. The long-term inability to conceive a child can evoke significant feelings of loss. In fact, experts agree that few life experiences rank as high on stress scales as infertility. Coping with the multitude of medical decisions and the uncertainties that infertility brings can create great emotional upheaval, not to mention the strain on your family's finances.

For couples who are trying to conceive, the stress of infertility never ends. Perhaps you have experienced each of the following anxiety-provoking scenarios:

- The first time you and your doctor discussed the term "infertile"
- The first semen sample
- Awaking early to take your temperature to determine ovulation
- The many nights you and your partner had to have sex—no matter how exhausted you felt
- The day your partner was told his sperm count was low or poor quality
- The many home pregnancy tests
- Every period
- The day your period started after IVF; the day it happened again
- The day your doctor said, "The chances are slim"

- The day your doctor said, "Donor eggs"
- The day your doctor said, "Donor sperm"
- Having your first miscarriage
- Having your second miscarriage
- Having a stillborn baby
- A sister-in-law who's pregnant
- A baby shower for your best friend
- Mother's Day
- Your parents' insistence on grandchildren
- Seeing a mother and her newborn

Is there any wonder that experts now believe that all infertile women live with grief, depression, and anxiety—even before treatments such as IVF are started? One infertility patient, Carla, summed up these feelings by saying, "Each time I go to the doctor's office to have blood drawn, it is just one more reminder that I am different and cannot have children. It takes its toll."

Carla's feelings are supported by millions of infertile couples. In a study from the University of North Carolina at Greensboro published in *Obstetrics & Gynecology*, researchers found that all infertile women experience similar levels of grief. This grief is experienced even before treatment and again after treatment fails—no matter what the treatment.

Interestingly, infertility most commonly attacks successful individuals, those that are accustomed to accomplishment. The problem occurs when they work even harder to conceive. While ambition and hard work usually pay off in the business world, unfortunately the reverse is true with infertility. The harder you push to have a baby, the more complex the problem of infertility.

You know the anguish and despair that infertility can bring. The heartbreak of infertility and the feeling of isolation become chronic stress that persists for weeks, months, or even years. This long-term stress can cause interruptions in sleep, erractic mood swings, and feelings of utter hopelessness—all of which can affect your immune system and may even increase your chance of having more health problems. Research from the American Psychological Association reveals that at least four in ten of all adults suffer adverse health effects from stress, and as many as nine in ten of all visits to doctors' offices are for stress-related complaints. Stress has been linked to an increased risk of the following diseases:

- Allergies, asthma, and hay fever
- Backaches
- Cancer
- Heart disease
- High blood pressure
- Migraine headaches
- Stroke
- TMJ (temporomandibular joint) syndrome
- Tension headaches
- Peptic ulcer disease

Not only is chronic stress a leading cause of health problems, it also may negatively affect your chance of conception. Studies from the Department of Physiology at the Medical College of Ohio show that even minimal stress can cause a man's levels of testosterone and sperm count to drop. For women, high levels of stress can affect hormones and menstrual cycles, and can cause irregular ovulation. Studies show that ovulation is delayed in female medical students during exam weeks, and some studies show that high stress levels may cause the fallopian tubes to spasm.

Specific stresses such as jet travel and crossing multiple time zones have been associated with menstrual irregularities and may contribute to infertility. Whether the irregularities result from high altitude, pressurization, or time zone changes is not yet known. A Danish study found excessive noise as a stress factor associated with an increased risk of infertility and delay to conception. Researchers conclude that excessive noise causes vasoconstriction and increased secretion of stress hormones.

When we are exposed to a stressful situation perceived as threatening, our bodies prepare for confrontation. The physical response known as the fight-or-flight response is controlled by our hormones. Though we do not live in the age of fighting wild animals anymore, those wild animals still exist in such forms as traffic jams, long lines, and disputes with our boss or family. If you are undergoing infertility treatment, when you are confronted with a stressful situation such as starting your period after IVF or getting a call from the lab that none of the embryos were fertilized, your body produces adrenaline—and a lot of it. The release of adrenaline is like sending a thousand "red alert" telegrams to different parts of your body at once. These telegrams prepare the body to deal with the stress, whether it is positive or negative.

Increased Cortisol Results in Decreased Immune Function

It is true that the immune system needs a certain amount of cortisol, which is the body's main stress-induced hormone. Yet when cortisol becomes elevated, as it does with chronic stress, and remains so for an extended period, it damages the cells that comprise your immune system. Research has found that while acute stress increases cortisol levels, these do not appear to have long-term effects on reproduction. Nonetheless, the prolonged elevations of cortisol that are seen in chronic stress may lead to inhibition of gonadotropin release. Altered patterns of cortisol secretion also can cause hyperprolactinemia, a condition in which the pituitary gland secretes too much prolactin.

Comprehensive research reveals that women who undergo infertility treatment may have a higher level of stress than women who deal with life-threatening illnesses, even cancer. The amount of stress associated with infertility is equivalent to that connected to the death of a close family member. Perhaps this is because the stress of infertility is chronic and erratic, and there is little chance of gaining control. For example, you may feel great anticipation and excitement as you await the pregnancy test results. When these results come back negative, the excitement and hope you felt turn to despair, anger, and dejection. Now multiply this stressful moment times 12, 24, 36, or more—depending on the number of times you try to get pregnant without success.

Infertility Linked to Depression

Psychological stress can manifest itself in a variety of ways. Among infertile women, depression (technically termed by psychologists and psychiatrists either major depression, in more severe cases, or adjustment disorder with depressed mood, in less severe cases) is a very common response. On average, American women are more than twice as likely to suffer from major depression as American men. Many researchers believe this gender difference is at least in part due to the high rate of depression among infertile women.

Depression is first and foremost a disorder of mood, characterized by profound sadness, discouragement, and hopelessness. When infertility is the cause, the onset tends to be gradual. Perhaps you've experienced how each month without conception weighs heavier than the last. Men and women may complain of a loss of energy, general fatigue, or insomnia, combined with feelings of worthlessness ("My body has failed me!") and guilt ("What have I done to deserve this?"). Seeking treatment for infertility may produce an initial boost in mood ("Maybe this will be the answer!"). Still, this rise often sets you up for even greater disappointment when treatment is unsuccessful. Every new treatment strategy— usually more costly and invasive than the last—produces renewed optimism. Every failed attempt brings you crashing back to earth—and reality. In addition, the hormonal treatments intrinsic to fertility efforts may well exacerbate mood disturbances. Finally, among infertile women who ultimately have to accept the loss of the ability to have their own biological child, depression may turn to grief. Periods of denial, bargaining, and anger will intermingle with depression until, hopefully, a state of acceptance establishes itself.

For those who have experienced the emotional trauma of miscarriage, the risk of depression is substantially higher. In a study published in *The Journal of the American Medical Association* (1977), researchers found that the risk of major depression greatly increases during the month after the loss of the pregnancy. For women who have suffered with depression, the risk of recurrence after pregnancy loss is great.

Each Month the Clock Ticks Louder

Another psychological reaction to infertility, and especially its treatment, is anxiety. After years of frustrating attempts to produce a pregnancy, couples often turn to infertility treatment when a sense of urgency strikes: *Time is running out!* This feeling of racing against the clock is frequently reinforced by specialists, who see age 35 as ancient in gynecological years. You may become obsessed with pregnancy, viewing the world as a minefield of reminders of childlessness. Complaints of general nervousness and irritability, excessive worry, and sleep problems are common. Anxiety may also take the form of specific phobias (such as fear of injections), or realistic concern about the financial burden of infertility treatment. In some situations, you may find yourself angry at your seemingly ineffectual medical consultants as well as at the world in general.

Infertility Can Lead to Bumpy Relationships

Often overlooked is the impact of infertility and infertility treatment on your partner and your relationship. When men are declared infertile, it may be less traumatic than for females, but many men clearly experience significant loss as well. Regardless of where the finger of infertility blame is pointing, both you and your partner experience comparable frustration and stress. You have had to engage in an undue amount of discussion and decision-making, often fraught with conflict. Your sexual relationship has probably suffered when sex has to be perfectly timed—when sex turns from recreation to procreation. Your partner may be more acutely affected by this new mandate to perform on demand. Sperm samples have to be produced on demand, under less than ideal circumstances. Your partner is often a bystander to a complex process, observing pain and discomfort and not knowing how to help. Satisfactory relationships may unravel under the pressures of infertility.

Many women fear that they are infertile as a consequence of past behavior or decisions that they have made. Perhaps an elective abortion resulting in scar tissue or a sexually transmitted disease that has left adhesions is the reason for their infertility. Many women feel they are somehow to blame for their infertility. Or they may see infertility as punishment from God. While it's important to remember that all choices have consequences, most of the causes of infertility involving sperm quality, heredity, anatomy, and hormonal functions are beyond your control. You have enough to deal with today; don't live with unnecessary guilt!

Cope with Stress-Less Strategies

So how can you best cope with the stress of infertility? No one coping strategy is right for everyone. For example, you might benefit from learning more about infertility and its impact. Or you may feel more relief through distraction and distancing yourself from the infertility crisis as much as possible. Understanding that even severe emotional reactions to infertility are both typical and in some sense normal can be helpful. Simple, commonsense strategies of benefit include the following:

- Don't blame yourself.
- Don't blame your partner.
- Realize that this time is stressful, and give yourself permission to avoid baby-focused events.
- Remember the traits and interests that resulted in choosing your partner and expand on these.
- Be hopeful, but understand the reality of each new treatment.
- Get involved in other interests with your partner for diversion.
- Take time off from treatment to gain back perspective.
- To feel more in control, play a key role in making decisions about treatment instead of depending on others.
- Learn about the reproductive process. There can be comfort in knowledge.

Each of the following seven Stress-Less Strategies plays an important role in stopping the ravages of stress that go hand in hand with infertility. As you read each strategy, try to evaluate your life and see how you can implement the suggestions in your daily lifestyle. Then, by using the alternative mind/body relaxation tips in Chapters 16 and 17, you will be well on your way to regaining some control of your stress level in the midst of uncertainty.

Strategy 1. Evaluate Your Stress Level

Evaluate your lifestyle and work habits to see if you are experiencing undue anxiety. Doctors know that the stress of living with infertility can put anyone into overload, resulting in overwhelming feelings of nervousness and anxiety (see the list below). But this increased stress can add to problems of anger, distractibility, and irritability and can even lead to further physical changes that hinder conception.

Signs and Symptoms of Stress

Stress symptoms vary greatly from one person to the next, but besides feeling pressured or overwhelmed, other symptoms include:

- Physical complaints—stomachaches, headaches, diarrhea
- Problems getting along with others
- Changes in behavior at home—outbursts, unexplained anger, crying for no reason
- Regression—behavior that is not age-appropriate
- Sleep patterns—nightmares, too little or too much sleep
- A change in your personality—a withdrawn person requiring a lot of attention or an extrovert becoming withdrawn
- Impatience
- Substance abuse—an increased use of alcohol or drugs

Assess your level of stress using the checklist below. If you are experiencing one or more of these symptoms, chances are good that your level of stress is excessive. If your stress level is at an all-time high, use the mind-body tools in Chapter 17 to unwind. Relaxation techniques—for example, music therapy or deep abdominal breathing—allow your body to heal and elicit the relaxation response, a physiological state characterized by a feeling of warmth and quiet mental alertness. This is the opposite of the fight-or-flight response. Once you learn how to use the mind-body therapies, blood flow to the brain increases and brain waves shift from an alert beta rhythm to a relaxed alpha rhythm.

ASSESSING YOUR LEVEL OF STRESS
____ Physical symptoms such as headache, digestive problems
____ Feeling overwhelmed day after day
____ Anxious upon awakening
____ Impatient for no apparent reason
____ Unable to sleep soundly
____ Difficulty in concentrating on projects at home or work

___ Loss of interest or enjoyment in life
___ Easy to anger or frequently irritable
___ Changes in appetite (eating more or less food)

Stressors with Infertility

Physical stressors (reproductive problems)

Social stressors (seeing friends with babies)

Work stressors (having to take time off work for treatments; inability to concentrate)

Family stressors (feelings of guilt, shame, or grief for being infertile)

Financial stressors (the high cost of treatment not covered by insurance)

Strategy 2. Recognize the Signs of Depression

Living with infertility can cause feelings of depression. While some normal individuals may have one or more of the symptoms of depression at one time or another—hopelessness, tearfulness, and loss of a sense of self-worth—symptoms of depression on a daily basis for at least two weeks constitute a real problem.

Check out the common signs of depression:

- Disturbances in sleep patterns
- Loss of interest in usual activities
- Weight loss or gain (more than 5 percent of body weight)
- Fatigue
- Impaired thinking
- Thoughts of dying or suicide
- Depressed thoughts or irritability
- Mood swings
- Staying at home all the time
- Avoidance of friends
- Difficulty concentrating

- Difficulty getting out of bed
- Feelings of worthlessness or excessive or inappropriate guilt
- Either agitation or a general slowing of intentional bodily activity

If you exhibit any of these signs, talk with your doctor about treatment. Often depression is temporary. Nonetheless, it can stem from a biochemical imbalance or can be a symptom of an underlying ailment. Frequently professional help is needed to maintain, control, and cure depression. There are many excellent prescription drugs and many medical protocols that can help greatly.

Strategy 3: Keep a Daily Journal

Writing in a journal each day can allow you to discover inner feelings and enhance the awareness of who you really are. So often with infertility—or any chronic disease, for that matter—women disguise or are unaware of intense feelings of resentment, anger, and loss. Journaling can open the pathways to discover these destructive inner feelings and deepest concerns.

Strategy 4. Get Healing Sleep

Almost all couples undergoing infertility treatments tell of having difficulty sleeping—waking up frequently during the night, feeling tired during the day, feeling unrefreshed by sleep. Many require more rest periods during the day. Whether as a result of anxiety or hormonal fluctuations, sleep problems are common.

Baby Booster

Keep your journal by your nightstand and let it assist you in tracking your BBT each day. This will give you one more accurate accounting of when ovulation occurs.

You may experience feeling awake or in a shallow state of sleep throughout the night. The problem with this is that during the delta, or deep level, sleep, your body does its repair and replenishment. If deep sleep is reduced over a long period of time, your body may not be able to repair and replenish itself as well.

ASSESSING PROBLEMS WITH SLEEP

___ Many arousals during a night's sleep

___ Awakening in the middle of the night

___ Difficulty in getting to sleep

___ Reduction in total sleep time

___ Long awakenings (10 minutes or more) during sleep

How can you relax and achieve restful sleep? Check out the following:

- Sleep only as much as needed to feel refreshed and healthy the following day, not more. Always awaken at the same time, even if you go to bed late.
- Eat less sugar, which can cause sudden raises in blood sugar. This may then cause you to wake up in the middle of the night when your blood sugar drops.
- Avoid salty foods. Following a low-sodium diet helps some insomniacs sleep sounder.
- A steady daily amount of exercise probably deepens sleep, but do not exercise right before bedtime. Studies show that regular exercise helps you to sleep sounder.
- Make sure your bedroom is sound-attenuated. Wear earplugs if noises bother you while you are sleeping. Some people find that white noise from a machine that produces a humming sound or from turning the radio to a station that has gone off the air helps.
- Eat foods for a calming effect. Foods that are high in carbohydrates, such as breads, cereal, pasta, or sherbet, raise the level of serotonin, a mood-elevating brain chemical, in the brain. When serotonin levels rise, we feel calmer and sleep sounder. Warm milk also has a calming effect for some people, especially when you add a few graham crackers or half a bagel (carbohydrates).
- Hunger may disturb sleep; a light snack may help sleep. Also eat

foods rich in B vitamins—fish, whole grains, peanuts, bananas, and sunflower seeds. These help to counteract the effects of stress.

- Take a hot bath well before bedtime. Sleep usually follows the cooling phase of your body's temperature cycle. After your bath, keep the temperature in your bedroom cool to see if you can influence this phase.
- Spend time outdoors each day, especially during the morning hours, to keep your body's rhythms in harmony. Researchers have found that exposure to daylight and darkness regulates the body's secretion of melatonin.
- Have peace of mind. Anxieties and worries can interfere with healthful sleep. Before you go to sleep, use prayer or meditation to let go of worries about impending tests, or the uncertainty of infertility.

Strategy 5. Widen Your Social Network

Having intimate relationships with family and friends helps us feel cared for, helps maintain optimism, and aids in stress management. All these benefits lead to enhanced immunity, which is vital to keep your reproductive system functioning at its peak. In fact, it is well documented that people who are happily married and/or have large networks of friends not only have a life expectancy greater than those who do not, but they also have fewer incidences of just about all types of disease.

In the midst of infertility stress, close relationships allow you to safely get your burdens off your chest. One study revealed that women who have a confidential relationship with another adult are less likely to be depressed than those women who do not have such a relationship.

While you are out seeking friends, keep in mind that it is the variety of social contacts a person has that helps in protecting the immune system. According to a study from Carnegie Mellon University in Pittsburgh, when 276 health volunteers, ages 18 to 55, were exposed to cold viruses, those who had fewer links to family, friends, and community were more likely to become ill. This study has been reinforced by other similar research such as studies done at Dartmouth-Hitchcock Medical Center in New Hampshire, where scientists report that heart patients are fourteen times as likely to survive surgery if they are socially active and if they find comfort in their religious faith. Another groundbreaking study reported in *The Journal of the American Medical Association* (1997) revealed that people involved in a variety of activities such as work, church, family, soccer, and barbershop quartets get fewer colds than those exposed to the same number of people who have only a few things to occupy them. Researchers speculate that being happy and involved keeps our immune systems strong.

As you seek to de-stress by increasing your social network, make sure you have support in the following areas from friends, coworkers, and family members:

- **Emotional support.** Someone you trust with your most intimate thoughts and fears regarding infertility.
- **Social support.** Someone you enjoy being with, who helps you cope with disappointments, and who celebrates your joys.
- **Informational support.** Someone you can ask for advice on major decisions regarding infertility tests and treatments.
- **Practical support.** Someone who will help you out in a pinch (neighbors or coworkers) when you need to see the doctor.

If infertility has you too overwhelmed to make new friends, try the following ways to increase social contacts:

- Volunteer to help with a political campaign or benevolent organization in your town.
- Join a religious group.
- Start a dinner club with your partner and invite two couples to join you.
- Participate in an interest group such as a community chorus or book club.
- Reignite family relationships and friendships through regular letter-writing or e-mails.
- Use Internet chat rooms to speak with people who are going through the same thing.

Two groups, RESOLVE and INCIID (see the Appendix), may offer you great support. RESOLVE is a national nonprofit support group established to help people cope with infertility. INCIID (pronounced "inside") is a nonprofit consumer advocacy organization educating infertile couples about the latest methods to diagnose, treat, and prevent infertility and pregnancy loss.

Strategy 6. Seek Professional Support

One study from Massachusetts reported in *The Journal of the American Society for Reproductive Medicine* (1998) has shown that psychological intervention in the case of infertile couples has improved their pregnancy rate. The study consisted of 112 women who had been trying to conceive for one to two years. Of these women, 46 were placed in a cognitive-behavior group (a 76 percent pregnancy rate), 41 were placed in a support group (a 68.3 percent pregnancy rate), and 25 were placed in the routine care group (a 28 percent pregnancy rate). The researchers concluded that stress does negatively affect pregnancy rates in infertile couples. However, group therapy seems to improve the infertile couples' chance of pregnancy.

Aware of the psychological consequences of infertility treatment, reproductive endocrinologists often employ a psychologist or clinical social worker to provide psychological assistance to patients. Individual psychotherapy can serve as the social support that so many infertile women do not have. Family and friends frequently respond in less than optimal ways: they may have grown tired of the infertility theme and pulled back, they often offer unsolicited advice ("Have you tried . . . ?"), and they frequently fail to recognize the severity of the impact of infertility.

Therapists who specialize in infertility have the advantage of familiarity not only with the crisis but also with its treatment. Therapists might also employ specific behavioral medicine techniques such as relaxation training, biofeedback, and cognitive-behavior therapy. These interventions serve to relieve adverse reactions as well as to help couples cope with upcoming medical procedures. In addition, therapists can work with couples on relationship issues.

Some therapists also offer support groups to relieve the sense of isolation, or psychoeducational groups (for example, stress management, relaxation) to teach coping skills. Group modalities can be especially therapeutic for women experiencing infertility; members of a support group know

---

Doctor's Rx

While the Internet can be extremely helpful in disseminating information from medical sites or in providing support via online chat groups,
it can also be detrimental to your health. Be sure to take the information or ideas you receive as opinions until you discuss them with your
doctor.

---

what helps and what doesn't. They are familiar with the treatment alter-
natives and therefore can be of help in decision-making. For women with
no support groups in their geographic area, virtual group therapy is available on the Internet (see the Appendix for a list of Internet sites).

There are several options for professional help:

INDIVIDUAL COUNSELING. This is a one-on-one session with
a therapist in which your personal problem areas are addressed.
These sessions may include specific help with alleviating depression,
anxiety, or even relationship difficulties that may go hand in hand with
infertility.

MARRIAGE COUNSELING. Obviously infertility affects both of you.
Therefore, it is often helpful for both husband and wife to understand
and accept the problem, as well as the possible impact this may have on
your relationship. This counseling may open the door to better communication as you openly discuss the problem and possible solutions.

GROUP COUNSELING. No one understands you better than
another person with the same problem. Group sessions led by trained
therapists in the field of infertility allow for the sharing of feelings, as well
as for the development of effective coping strategies. The exchange of
ideas at group sessions is often the most productive way to revamp your
thought processes and get over stumbling blocks as others in the group
share experiences, as well as what has worked for their situations.

SUPPORT GROUPS. In a support group, you can share your feelings
with others suffering from infertility and receive comfort and encouragement from each other. The latest treatments available can be discussed
and members can give suggestions for coping while affirming the positive

experiences of each other. The realization that "someone else knows what I am going through" is helpful as people share their struggles. Being able to confide in someone will have a positive effect on your physical well-being.

Keep in mind that while support groups can offer great comfort, they are not meant to be professional therapy groups. Those who would benefit from standard psychological or psychiatric intervention should seek professional treatment.

Stay in a Network

Perhaps most important is to stay in a strong network of people who know the latest information on infertility. Jessica's story is just one example of how others can guide you to find the right doctor with answers for your infertility problem.

"Hit the alarm. Take your temperature. Chart it on the calendar. Then face the day teaching adorable preschoolers knowing that you cannot have children. My life wasn't much fun." That's how Jessica described her typical day.

"Since I was a teenager, I longed to have a family. I mean, that's all I ever wanted in life. So when my doctor said the odds were against me because of PCOS, I wanted to run away. I became very introverted and quit seeing my friends. I even lost interest in my teaching for several months and gained thirty pounds until my husband jarred me into reality. He insisted that I go to counseling to talk about my emotions and the sense of loss I was feeling."

Jessica found great comfort in talking with a therapist who had also been diagnosed as infertile yet was now the mother of twin boys. The therapist referred Jessica to a clinic in a neighboring state that was known for successfully treating women with PCOS and helping them get pregnant. Eighteen months later, Jessica also delivered twins—a girl and a boy.

Finding support from others who have been through all the tests and procedures is crucial in moving from infertility to making a baby, and this is one part of your life that only you can control.

Chapter 16

Ancient Therapies to New Age Trends

*"After trying to conceive for six years, I had given up on having a baby,"
said Diane, age 42. "Because of a host of problems, I was even considering a hysterectomy. Then I visited a Chinese acupuncturist for my
chronic lower back pain. This man spoke little English but had such a
kind, healing demeanor. While I was there for a totally unrelated issue,
he felt my liver and talked about the enormous amount of heat it was
producing. 'You want baby,' he uttered in broken English. I tried to inter-
rupt him and explain that I came to see him for my back pain. Still, he
would not stop saying, 'You want baby.'*

*"The next month, I missed my period. In a few weeks, my doctor
confirmed the unbelievable—I was pregnant."*

While each couple's response to the stress of infertility is different,
many believe that alternative or complementary therapies may
help. *Alternative medicine* is an umbrella term for treatments that fall outside standard medical practice. Using alternative therapies may help you
to reduce stress and regain control of your life. This control is essential
for wellness. Instead of prescribing an expensive drug as a cure, alternative practitioners focus on holistic medicine and lifestyle balance—ideas
that must be explained and taught by the practitioner.

From nonwestern medicine to massage therapy, complementary or
alternative medicine is a billion-dollar business in the world today. In the
past three decades, this type of doctoring has skyrocketed in popularity.
Studies show that four of every ten Americans use some form of alternative treatment. Some, like tai chi and acupuncture, are steeped in
ancient Asian traditions; others, like light therapy or mindfully visual-

izing a cool mountain scene, are strictly New Age; all have proponents from every walk of life who vouch for their healing powers.

First a Word of Caution

A common mistake made by many when they use alternative medicine therapies is to stop traditional medical treatment altogether. This mistake can often lead to life-threatening setbacks and may even hinder your chances of getting pregnant. As a rule of thumb, just because something is natural does not mean that it is always safe. While some alternative treatments for stress reduction such as deep muscle massage or hydrotherapy may be perfectly safe, some natural supplements and herbs are highly toxic and can raise blood pressure, cause liver damage, and even lead to death. Because alternative medicine is often not regulated by the government, most people do not know this until they ingest the product and become ill. For example, hemlock, a poisonous plant, is very natural—but it is also deadly!

In a new study from Loma Linda University, scientists suggest that some popular herbs commonly taken by millions of people—Saint-John's-wort, echinacea, and ginkgo—could block conception. The study mentions genetic damage to sperm, raising questions of whether these abnormalities could cause problems for the resulting babies. Some herbal products contain hormones that mimic estrogen and could possibly interfere with your fertility.

Doctor's Rx

At the Office of Alternative Medicine (OAM) at the National Institutes of Health (NIH), the budget for studying alternative medicine has grown from $2 million in 1993 to $20 million today. If you want more information on the safety of any alternative treatment, check with the OAM's public information clearinghouse (888-644-6226) for the results of all OAM studies conducted.

If you want to try the alternative therapies explained in Chapters 16 and 17 to reduce the anxiety of infertility, be sure to continue your regular medical treatment. This is important to staying well and increasing your chances of conception. Also get your physician's approval before starting any unproven alternative therapy.

Ayurvedic Medicine

Ayurveda is a holistic Indian healing science that focuses on preventive health care using natural therapies. According to Ayurvedic belief, health is the state of balance, and disease is the state of imbalance. The body's functions are composed of combinations of five elements: air, fire, space, water, and earth. There are three other physiological forces called doshas (Vata, Pitta, and Kapha) in which the five elements are manifest. Ayurvedic practitioners believe that we are made of a combination of doshas that give us a particular metabolic type, yet we have one dosha that dominates. For example, Vata people are thin and energetic, while Pittas are hot tempered and Kaphas are slow and solid.

To make a diagnosis, an Ayurvedic practitioner may feel the pulse in your wrist to determine the imbalance in your body. Then using such therapies as meditation, detoxification, breathing, herbal and mineral preparations, exercise, and dietary advice based on your particular body type, the practitioner will guide you back to balance or wellness.

THE UPSIDE: TEACHES A HEALTHY LIFESTYLE. Because Ayurveda focuses on lifestyle changes, many healthy practices are incorporated in your daily routine. Some conditions which may respond to Ayurvedic medicine include:

- Allergies
- Anxiety
- Depression
- Digestive disorders
- Headaches
- High blood pressure
- Insomnia
- Respiratory problems
- Stress

Baby Buster

While Ayurveda can provide healing benefits when combined with conventional treatments, avoid taking any herbs without consulting with your physician.

THE DOWNSIDE: NOT SCIENTIFICALLY SUBSTANTIATED. Whether or not Ayurvedic methods can help you make a baby is not scientifically proven. However, reducing stress and anxiety and curing insomnia may help to boost immune function, leading to an increased chance of conception.

THE BOTTOM LINE. If you wish to undergo Ayurvedic treatment, you may find it difficult to locate a qualified practitioner in the United States, as there are no schools and no licensing is required. Also, this type of treatment is not covered by insurance unless the services are provided by a licensed medical doctor.

Transcendental Meditation

Transcendental meditation (TM) is a technique in which you sit comfortably with your eyes closed and mentally repeat a Sanskrit word or sound (mantra) for 15 to 20 minutes, twice a day. This meditation is alleged to help you think more clearly, recover from stress, and appreciate life more fully. While there are no studies on the use of TM to boost fertility, it may help lower the anxiety you feel during testing or treatment and keep your blood pressure normal. Research reported in the journal *Hypertension* (1996) concluded that TM was found to surpass other forms of relaxation therapies at lowering blood pressure. In this study, 111 African-American men and women, ages 55 to 85, were asked to practice TM daily. The blood pressure reductions they experienced were similar to those commonly achieved with antihypertensive medicines. In long-term drug studies, such reductions have been associated with about 35 percent fewer strokes and heart attacks.

Yoga

Yoga is a classical Indian practice that is built on the foundation of ethics (yama) and personal discipline (niyama). It is used to relieve stress, achieve mind/body connectedness, and heal pain.

Because yoga is a type of mind/body therapy, the postures or movements are structured to stretch the mind and body beyond their normal limits, then make them act in unison again. Using deep breathing, concentration techniques, and body poses, you learn to calm your mind and increase your flexibility and strength. Pranayama, which is the conscious focus on and control of breath to heal disease, is an important part of yoga.

Yoga postures can relieve mild aches and pains, menstrual cramps, and lower back pain. They can also increase flexibility and coordination, reduce stress, and promote deep relaxation. Breath exercises done with different yoga positions can increase blood circulation.

Besides providing relaxation, yoga can help improve breathing, ease constipation, and improve skin tone. Relaxation, flexibility, and muscle strength are important outcomes of yoga, making it a good exercise to keep you in shape for pregnancy and delivery.

To experience optimum results, yoga should be practiced daily in the form of meditation and postures. Learning yoga can cost as little as the money to purchase a how-to book or instructional video, or you can join a yoga class at your local gym or YMCA.

Baby Booster

Some proponents of yoga believe that it can help boost reproductive function as you increase blood flow through the abdomen. This is not proven one way or the other, but it may be a healthy stress reducer with a potentially added benefit.

Chinese Medicine

Chinese medicine seeks to diagnose disturbances of vital energy, called qi, in health and disease. Health is said to exist when qi (vital energy) and blood flow smoothly through all parts of the body. External factors can disrupt qi, including climate, diet, emotions, and lifestyle factors. The Chinese doctor interprets any symptoms as an imbalance within the entire system of the body and uses holistic therapies such as acupuncture, acupressure, shiatsu, and herbs to balance the body.

Traditional Chinese medicine practitioners believe that infertility occurs because of an imbalance between the yin and the yang. To treat this imbalance, daily doses of herbal teas are ingested, and your basal body temperature (BBT) is charted over a period of three to six months. Although not grounded by scientific research, many claim this has brought about conception.

Acupressure

Acupressure is a well-known ancient Chinese form of physical therapy. It works by stimulating your body's main trigger points to release energy or unblock qi. Today, acupressure exists mainly in Asian countries such as India, China, Japan, and Korea and is used to relieve everyday aches, pains, and stress, as well as specific conditions like sinus pressure, leg cramps, headaches, temporomandibular joint disorder (TMJ), and carpal tunnel syndrome.

Acupuncture

According to advocates of acupuncture, natural energy or qi travels along fourteen pathways or meridians in the body to keep your body nourished. These meridians are connected to specific organs and bodily functions. When qi is blocked or thrown off balance, illness or symptoms result.

The practitioner sticks very thin stainless-steel needles into your skin at any of the 800 designated points on the body. The acupuncturist places the instruments along these meridian lines and may also turn the needles, or use heat, pressure, friction, suction, or electromagnetic impulses to stimulate these points. When one portion of the body is stimulated, an effect is obtained in the same or another portion of the body.

It is believed that acupuncture causes the body to release endorphins—your body's natural pain relievers—which explains the pain relief felt when the pinpricks occur. Acupuncture may also trigger the release of certain hormones including serotonin, a chemical in the brain that makes you feel calm and serene.

Qigong

Tagged as the "mother of Chinese self-healing," qigong (pronounced *chee-gong*) is said to be one of the most powerful healing traditions ever developed in human history. This technique includes acupuncture, massage, and herbal medicines. Of these, qigong is the one that can be most easily initiated by oneself.

The Chinese believe that the primary mechanism triggered by the practice of qigong is a spontaneous balancing and enhancing of the natural healing resources in the human system. Because it involves specific physical postures that dissolve tension, the practice of qigong triggers a wide array of physiological mechanisms with profound healing benefits, including:

- The delivery of oxygen to the tissues
- The elimination of waste products as well as the transportation of immune cells through the lymph system
- Shifts in the chemistry of the brain and the nervous system

There are at least a thousand varieties of qigong, yet all focus on getting qi or energy moving smoothly through the body. When qi is obstructed, you will have fatigue and illness.

Proponents of qigong claim that this discipline increases energy, decreases fatigue, and alleviates pain. Some believe that it can help to heal back pain, carpal tunnel syndrome, circulatory problems, depression, high blood pressure, insomnia, menopause, neuralgia, chronic pain, and TMJ syndrome.

Experts conclude that qi has to be cultivated daily, so the rudimentary exercises should be done each morning to build qi. You may have to pay a practitioner to teach you qigong, but once you understand the positions, you can do this at any time at no cost. Some people feel results instantaneously, while for others it may take days or weeks before a difference in mood, energy, and wellness is noticed.

Shiatsu

This type of therapy also draws on the Chinese notion of qi or energy flowing along meridians throughout the body. Each session focuses on relieving pain and helping the body rid itself of any toxins before they develop into illness.

With shiatsu, a practitioner applies firm, rhythmic pressure for three to ten seconds on specific points. This pressure is given to wake up the meridians or healing channels of the body. The pressure may help to stimulate the body's endorphins to produce a tranquilizing effect, or it may help by loosening up muscles and improving blood circulation. Shiatsu is said to help ease or eliminate back pain, sciatica, digestive problems, headaches, insomnia, leg and menstrual cramps, respiratory problems, and stress.

Tai Chi

Tai chi is an ancient Chinese defensive martial art similar to shadowboxing. With tai chi, you follow a series of slow, graceful movements that mimic the movements you do in daily life. Tai chi requires you to move forward, backward, and from side to side in a carefully coordinated manner—flowing together in continuous harmony as though your body were doing one continuous movement.

Tai chi is based on the theory that continuous practice will help to train the body to respond quickly in a crisis. Since the movements emphasize complete relaxation and passive concentration, they can be compared with "meditation in motion," which is said to be healing to the nervous system. The gentle, graceful movements, along with deep-breathing patterns, help lower blood pressure and heart rate.

Tai chi speeds healing, improves circulation, boosts immune function, and decreases stress. The exercise emphasizes deep abdominal breathing that could help to maintain better lung function. Even though tai chi is considered a low-impact exercise, it does increase the heart rate during exercise and helps to improve overall cardiovascular function.

THE UPSIDE: APPROVED BY NIH FOR SOME AILMENTS. The National Institutes of Health (NIH) confirms that acupuncture works with such ailments as nausea during pregnancy, nausea from chemotherapy, and dental problems. In scientific studies, tai chi has been found to increase flexibility and agility.

THE DOWNSIDE: NO CONCLUSIVE STUDIES FOR INFERTILITY. There are no conclusive studies on other therapeutic values for traditional Chinese medicine, including the use of this modality for infertility treatment. Although some studies report that acupuncture and some herbs may have medicinal value, most Chinese therapies need to be studied in the United States using the highest research criteria.

THE BOTTOM LINE. If you want to try acupuncture to alleviate stress or insomnia, be sure to go to a licensed practitioner who uses only disposable needles, and get your medical doctor's approval. While acupuncture has very few contraindications, certain disorders such as easy bleeding or local infection may stop you from receiving treatments. At this time there are about 15,500 certified and licensed practitioners who specialize in acupuncture, and more than 3,000 of these are conventional medical doctors. You can write or call the American Academy of Medical Acupuncture (AAMA) for names of certified and licensed practitioners. (Write to 5820 Wilshire Blvd., Suite 500, Los Angeles, CA 90036, or call 213-937-5514.) Acupuncture is covered by some medical insurers.

To learn tai chi or qigong, purchase a book or video on these ancient disciplines, or enjoy doing this with others at a local health spa or YMCA.

Naturopathic Medicine

Naturopathy is based on the belief that diseases are a violation of nature's laws. Naturopathic doctors (N.D.) claim to remove the underlying causes of disease while also stimulating the body's natural healing processes. They state that diseases are the body's way of defending itself and that cures result from increasing the patient's vital force by ridding the body of waste products and toxins.

Naturopaths use a variety of therapies to balance the physical, mental, and spiritual roots of an illness. Using a combination of nutrition, botanical medicine, homeopathy, acupuncture, Chinese medicine, hydrotherapy, and naturopathic manipulative therapy, along with scientific medical diagnostic science and standards of care, the N.D. will help you rev up your immune system and, hopefully, end the illness.

THE UPSIDE: STRENGTHENS THE MIND-BODY CONNECTION. Naturopathic doctors believe that the natural approach to healing strengthens healthy body functions so that complications associated with illnesses may be prevented. The N.D. also handles psychological medicine, believing that mental attitudes and emotional states may influence, or even cause, physical illness.

THE DOWNSIDE: NO MEDICATIONS ARE USED. Many naturopathic practitioners believe that all diseases—strokes, myocardial infarctions, cancers—are manifestations of the body's attempt to heal itself and that all a physician needs to do is to assist this process. Consequently, there have been many documented cases in which people under the care of naturopaths were told, as they worsened, that they were actually getting better.

THE BOTTOM LINE. The naturopathic therapies are intended to be incorporated into your lifestyle. You would see a naturopathic practitioner as needed for instruction or healing. While you may trust a naturopathic doctor for a stress-related ailment that can be treated naturally, be cautious when you are hit with the big stuff and need strong medications or surgery to get well. Eleven states license N.D.s at this time, and some insurance companies are now covering naturopathic services.

Baby Buster

An N.D. cannot prescribe pharmaceuticals, which are necessary for many infections and illnesses. These practitioners have various levels of training and may be practicing with a mail-order diploma.

Hydrotherapy

One popular therapy naturopathic doctors use is hydrotherapy—the use of water in all forms, from ice to steam, to promote healing. You may have used hydrotherapy in ice packs for a sprained ankle, a hot compress for sinus pain, or a cold compress to reduce a fever. Other forms include sitz baths, spas, douches, whirlpools, colonic enemas, and steam.

Some common forms of hydrotherapy—ice and moist heat—are right at your fingertips. The next time you get an injury, immediately apply the R.I.C.E. theory—rest, ice, compression, and elevation. Moist heat—a warm shower, a moist heating pad, a whirlpool spa, or even running warm water over the injury, sore muscle, or aching arthritic joint—can greatly alleviate pain and inflammation.

THE UPSIDE: STIMULATES THE BODY'S HEALING FORCE. Hydrotherapy acts to stimulate the body's own healing force. Cold compresses reduce swelling by constricting blood vessels to control minor internal bleeding. Moist heating pads, whirlpools, or even a warm shower can reduce the soreness of aching muscles. Even the simple act of running cool water over a wound can help rid it of dangerous bacteria and aid in healing.

THE DOWNSIDE: STEAM BATHS AND COLONICS ARE DANGEROUS. You have felt the healing benefit of moist heat on a sore muscle, but watch out for some forms of hydrotherapy such as colonics, as they deplete important electrolytes from the body. Steam baths are also dangerous for pregnant women, young children, the elderly, those with heart problems, and diabetics.

THE BOTTOM LINE. As with all alternative treatments, be discerning. Ask for scientific proof before agreeing to use water-based remedies that are not substantiated by research. Some therapies are downright dangerous, such as sweating to release toxins from the body. On the other hand, keep that moist heating pad or ice pack around for sprains, muscle soreness, or aching joints—it really will work!

Bodyworks

Bodyworks is the umbrella term that describes the hands-on technique of massage, touch, and movement used to align the spine, muscles, and joints to promote the flow of energy.

With more than eighty different varieties, massage is one of the most popular forms of alternative medicine. Although the therapist focuses on different muscles or trigger points on the body, the goal is to affect the body as a whole. Massage acts as a mind-body form of stress release and increases flexibility and mobility.

Several popular massage techniques include:

• *General Swedish* is the foundation for all other types of massage, with particular attention paid to the back and chest. The therapist uses a system of long strokes, kneading, and friction techniques on the more superficial layers of the muscles. This is combined with active and passive movements of the joints. The therapist will apply pressure and rub the muscles in the same direction as the blood flows to the heart. Swedish massage is said to help flush the tissue of lactic and uric acids and other metabolic wastes, as well as to improve circulation without increasing the load on the heart. Oil is used to help reduce friction on the body.

• *Tapotement* involves a percussion-type movement that includes short, quick strikes made with the hands or fingertips.

• *Trigger point* is a massage and pain-relief technique that alleviates muscle spasms and cramping. The therapist will locate active and latent trigger points and mild to moderate pressure is applied for a short time (7 to 10 seconds). The muscles are then gently stretched to help the relaxation process.

• *Vibration* is a type of massage in which the therapist uses the heel of her right hand for vibration. The left hand is placed on top of the right for light compression.

THE UPSIDE: MASSAGE PROMOTES RELAXATION. This alternative therapy promotes relaxation, especially with the musculoskeletal system, enhances the circulation of blood and lymph, and relieves muscle tension. Massage helps to relieve chronic headaches, TMJ, and sports injuries, and can alleviate symptoms of muscle spasms, lower back pain, and other common chronic pain. If you are trying to avoid pain relievers, massage may be helpful as a nondrug form of relief.

Studies released from the University of Miami School of Medicine's Touch Research Center found that the benefits of massage include heightened alertness, relief from depression and anxiety, an increase in the number of natural killer cells in the immune system, lower levels of the stress hormone cortisol, and reduced difficulty in getting to sleep.

THE DOWNSIDE: CAN BE DANGEROUS FOR THOSE WITH HYPERTENSION. If you have high blood pressure, ask your doctor before getting a massage. Some studies show that it may cause a brief increase in blood pressure. Also, if you have heart disease or circulatory problems, check with your doctor.

THE BOTTOM LINE. Check the credentials of the massage therapist you use to make sure she is certified and licensed (L.M.T.) by a state or local government. Better still, try to find someone who is nationally certified in therapeutic massage and bodywork (NCTMB), which means they have passed a national certification exam. You medical doctor may refer you to a professional who is qualified. You also can contact the American Massage Therapist Association for a copy of the membership directory. Write to them at AMTA, 820 Davis Street, Suite 100, Evanston, IL 60201-4444, or call at 708-864-0123. Some insurance companies cover massage as a form of alternative treatment.

Zone Therapy

Zone therapy or reflexology is a healing art based upon the theory that there are reflex areas, or specific points, in the feet and hands that correspond to all the glands and organs in the body. The term *reflex* refers to the fact that these points are responsive to stimulus.

Practitioners believe that nerve pathways exist throughout the body. When any of these pathways are blocked, the body experiences discomfort. Reflexology will help to revive your energy flow and bring your body back into homeostasis, or a state of balance. The theory behind zone therapy states that there are ten zones throughout the body—five zones on the right side, five on the left. Reflexes travel through the zones similar to the electrical wiring in your home. These zones are used in determining various locations of reflexes within the hands and feet. All the body parts within any one zone are connected by the nerve pathways and are mirrored in the corresponding reflex zone on the hands and feet.

THE UPSIDE: RELAXES THE BODY. There are different theories regarding the uses of reflexology. Some claim that it releases pain-blocking endorphins into the bloodstream. Others say that it relaxes the body and improves circulation. Although not scientifically proven, people have experienced relief from allergies, headaches, sinus problems, asthma, backaches, carpal tunnel syndrome, constipation, kidney stones, menstrual problems, prostate problems, and arthritis.

THE DOWNSIDE: NO SCIENTIFIC SUBSTANTIATION. Although reflexology is said to stimulate healing to different zones in the body, this is not scientifically proven.

THE BOTTOM LINE. A good foot rub might give you a soothing stress-free benefit, but stay in touch with your conventional medical doctor for serious problems.

REFLEX POINT	CORRESPONDING BODY ZONE
Metatarsal (balls of the feet)	Chest, lung, and shoulder area
Toes	Head and neck
Upper arch	Diaphragm and upper abdominal organs
Lower arch	Pelvic and lower abdominal organs
Heel	Pelvic and sciatic nerve
Outer foot	Arm, shoulder, hip, leg, knee, and lower back
Inner foot	Spine
Ankle area	Reproductive organs and pelvic region

Chapter 17

Chilling Out with Mental Aerobics

"I married for the first time at age thirty-seven, and within two years I miscarried twice," said Heather, age 41. "I had waited so long and was desperate to have a baby. Just before I was to undergo fertility testing, my period was late. I did a home pregnancy test, but it came back negative. A week later, feeling nauseous and light-headed, I knew either I was pregnant or very ill. This time my ob-gyn did a pregnancy test. The nurse said she'd give me a call later that morning, so I planted myself by the telephone. Morning turned to afternoon, and there was no call. Each time the phone would ring I knew it was the nurse saying I wasn't pregnant. By 4:00 P.M., my hands were shaking, my face was flushed, and my heart was racing.

"My doctor finally called later that evening and apologized for taking so long. When she confirmed that I was pregnant, I felt as if I were an inflated balloon and someone had popped me with a pin. Within seconds, my heart rate returned to normal and my anxiety diminished. Later that week when I met with my doctor she explained to me the mind-body connection. I realized that my brain knows only what I tell it, and if I tell it something horrible might happen, it will react accordingly.

"During the entire pregnancy, I focused on healing, positive thoughts, and the result was a gorgeous baby boy."

An increasing number of physicians, psychiatrists, and psychologists are acknowledging that the way we think, feel, act, and react can be a powerful determinant of our physical and mental health. The scientific field that explores this mind-body interplay, psychoneuroimmunology

(PNI), is a comparably new discipline and centers on the connection between the mind and the immune system.

While most studies are not yet conclusive on the benefit of mind-body therapies to enhance fertility, one recent study at the Mind/Body Institute at Beth Israel Medical Center suggests that stress reduction techniques such as guided imagery and deep relaxation may increase conception rates among women who have sought the help of fertility specialists. In this study, researchers stated that depression interferes with all sorts of hormones that may adversely affect ovulation and the implantation of embryos. After attending a stress management program for ten weeks, within six months of completion, 44 percent of the 174 infertile women who were severely depressed had achieved conception and 38 percent had given birth. The women were taught relaxation responses as well as various stress management strategies during the program.

Whether mind-body modalities will increase the incidence of conception is not known. Nonetheless, there are many couples who believe in complementary therapies to help ease the stress and anxiety that result from infertility. Especially when the anxiety of undergoing tests and procedures causes stress hormones to skyrocket, you can use mind-body therapies to block the fight-or-flight response before it occurs.

The main strategy in dealing with stress is to identify and remove or reduce its source. Identification of the source may be relatively easy, but elimination is a challenge, especially when the source is a chronic disease such as infertility. Knowing you have little control over your stressor (infertility), you must find ways to practice "safe stress." For example, an acute or prolonged tense state may cause your heart rate and blood pressure to increase; other possible effects are a dry mouth, enlarged pupils, sweaty palms, and fast, shallow chest breathing. However, slow, deep abdominal breathing helps break the tension cycle, which enables bodily functions to return to normal. Allowing yourself to take ten slow deep breaths at tense times, as well as throughout the day, will help you to stay loose and relaxed.

Some people report experiencing benefits from mind-body tools within minutes of doing them. For example, deep abdominal breathing actually alters your psychological state, diminishing the intensity of a stressful moment. Think about how your respiration quickens when you are fearful. Then consider how taking a deep, slow breath calms you immediately. Likewise, music therapy can lower your heart rate.

The following mind-body therapies can be done alone or with your partner. If you need help in learning these therapies, talk with a licensed mental health counselor. Once you get used to doing these, lean on them regularly to decrease the negative impact of stress on your immune system.

Aromatherapy

Aromatherapy is an ancient art that uses highly concentrated oils, usually distilled from herbs, flowers, fruits, roots, grasses, leaves, and seeds, to affect our sense of smell and thus our sense of well-being. Each different aroma (or essential oil) is said to have a specific healing power, whether to reduce stress and anxiety, increase productivity, or serve as an aphrodisiac. An essential oil is an extract or essence that has been distilled, usually by steam, from the seed, leaves, stem, flower, bark, root, or other parts of a plant. Essential oils are often diluted in a carrier oil such as sweet almond, grapeseed, olive, or canola oil before being used with massage.

It is said that certain fragrances spark immediate reactions in our bodies and can possibly be beneficial in helping us to relax from days filled with stress and anxiety. For example, the smell of lemon or jasmine is said to increase the beta activity in the front of the brain associated with greater alertness. Lavender and chamomile are said to increase the alpha wave activity in the back of the brain, leading to relaxation.

Although scientists are not totally sure how aromas affect your moods, researchers do know that when you inhale aromatic molecules, they connect to receptors and build electrical impulses that move up the olfactory nerves to the brain. The optimum target is the limbic system, where your emotions and memory are processed.

In a study at the Smell and Taste Research Foundation in Chicago, researchers fitted male medical students' penises with gauges that detected erection and then exposed them to dozens of fragrances. The one that got a rise was the smell of hot cinnamon buns! Still, other aromas can also add sensuality to sex, including jasmine and rose. If relaxation is a problem, then use lavender, chamomile, sandalwood, orange blossom, or spiced apples—all said to aid in reducing anxiety.

If you have allergies, aromatherapy may trigger an allergic reaction. If you are allergy-free, then try various aromas to reduce stress and the stress response.

ESSENTIAL OILS THAT RELIEVE STRESS

ESSENTIAL OIL	EFFECT ON THE BODY
Lavender and chamomile	Relieve insomnia
Frankincense and marjoram	Soothe raw nerves
Lavender, vanilla, and chamomile	Reduce stress
Basil, geranium, and orange oil	Elevate mood

Autogenics

Autogenics is a method of "cuing" yourself to calm down and relax. It's easy to perform and can be done anywhere. Because the brain needs only a few reminders to calm down, autogenics teaches you to concentrate on raising the temperature of your hands and feet. Proponents claim that autogenics will give your heart a break from pumping so hard, open blood vessels, reduce breathing rate and pulse, and lower blood pressure.

With autogenics, you sit quietly and put your left hand in your lap, palm up. Lay your right palm on top of it, and clasp your fingers together. Concentrating on the feeling in your hands, "mindfully" work to raise the temperature of your hands for ten minutes, then do the same with your feet. Counselors claim that if this is done correctly, you will feel the heat rise in your hands and feet, signaling that your body is relaxing.

Deep Abdominal Breathing

Perhaps you know all too well how breathing can measure and alter your psychological state, making a stressful moment more stressful or diminish in intensity. Yet did you know that breathing is the only involuntary activity of the body that we can consciously control? The problem arises when you breathe from your chest, taking shallow, rapid breaths. This type of breathing only hinders relaxation. Taking slow, deep abdominal breaths not only oxygenates the brain but helps end the stress cycle and enables your heart rate and blood pressure to return to normal.

Your brain makes its own morphine-like pain relievers, called endorphins and enkephalins, that are associated with a happy, positive feeling. These hormones can help relay "stop-stress" messages. During deep abdominal breathing, you will add oxygen to the blood and cause your body to release endorphins while decreasing the release of stress hormones.

Use the following steps to learn deep abdominal breathing. Then remember how this is done when you have to undergo an uncomfortable test or treatment for infertility.

1. Lie on your back in a quiet room with no distractions.
2. Place your hands on your abdomen and take in a slow, deliberate deep breath through your nostrils. If your hands are rising and your abdomen is expanding, then you are breathing correctly. If your hands do not rise, yet you see your chest rising, you are breathing incorrectly.
3. Inhale to a count of five, pause for three seconds, then exhale to a count of five. Start with ten repetitions of this exercise, then increase to twenty-five, twice daily.

Faith

Even many scientists agree that the human body has a powerful sacramental dimension to it. Those who acknowledge this with a strong sense of higher purpose—a body-soul connectedness—are the ones who are more likely to stay with programs that lead to optimal health. This does not mean that faith or a belief in God or a higher power should ever replace medicine. However, faith in something greater than yourself offers a type of curative power, helping you to disconnect from unhealthy worries and replace these with soothing belief. Many recent studies have found that people who are active in religious organizations and attend group functions regularly are also healthier, with lower blood pressure, less depression, and greater longevity.

At the National Institute for Healthcare Research, such experts as research psychiatrist David Larson, M.D., have compiled scientific studies supporting the positive link between faith and good health. One study concludes that people who attend church regularly have fewer stress-related health problems than those who do not.

Laughter Therapy

Can a laugh a day help you get pregnant? That's not scientifically proven. Yet, according to many researchers, laughter is crucial for healthy immune function. Laughter increases the activity of body cells that attack tumor cells and viruses. It helps to relieve anxiety, decreases stress-producing hormones, and increases immune system activity—definitely a bonus when tests are negative and you are faced with disappointment. In fact, many doctors are now prescribing humor therapy for chronically ill patients. Laughter may even have an aerobic benefit. Dr. William F. Fry, a psychiatrist at the Stanford University School of Medicine, has studied the aerobic, physical, and emotional benefits that laughter can give and found that one hundred laughs are equivalent to ten minutes spent rowing.

How does laughter strengthen the immune system? Some studies have shown that people who laugh hard produce more immunoglobulin A, which strengthens your ability to fight infection. Your heart rate increases, the oxygen to the brain is boosted, and your blood flow improves. When you relax afterwards, your body calms down.

Meditation

Remember when transcendental meditation was thought to be a cult? Today meditation is recognized as a viable way to lower blood pressure, alleviate insomnia, and reduce chronic pain. This stress releaser seeks to integrate the mind, body, and spirit through intentionally focusing on the silent repetition of a focus word ("love"), sound ("om"), phrase ("peace heals"), or prayer ("thank you"). As thoughts intrude, you will continue to mindfully chant while facilitating the relaxation response.

This technique can guide you beyond the negative thoughts and agitations of the mind and allow you to become "unstuck" from your fear and other disturbing emotions. Mindfulness is a traditional Buddhist approach to meditation and allows your mind to be full of whatever you are doing at that moment, whether you are dancing, gardening, writing, or listening to music. An intense focus is the key to mindfulness, as well as the ability to keep negative thoughts from intruding on the moment.

Some people who meditate only occasionally have reactions such as increased anxiety or fear during the session. Researchers believe that these feelings may be responses to the sensation of being totally relaxed and uninhibited.

Music Therapy

Music therapy is an effective nondrug approach to help reduce fear, anxiety, stress, or grief. Music therapy is effectively used for treating neurological, mental, or behavioral disorders such as developmental and learning disabilities, Alzheimer's disease and other aging-related problems, brain injuries, and acute and chronic pain.

Music may also have therapeutic value during surgery, as doctors report performing better when they could select the music played in the operating room. Composer and researcher Steven Halpern says that certain musical forms can transport the listener's brain into the alpha wave, a state of relaxation much like meditation.

At Saint Agnes Hospital in Baltimore, patients in critical care units listen to classical music. Researchers claim that listening to half an hour of classical music produces the same effect as 10 milligrams of Valium.

Baby Booster

If you have an impending infertility test or treatment coming up, let music relax your body, mind, and spirit. Take your headset and favorite CD or tape with you to your doctor's office, and focus on the soothing melody instead of dwelling on your anxiety.

Progressive Muscle Relaxation

Also known as deep muscle relaxation, progressive muscle relaxation involves concentrating on different muscle groups as you contract, then relax, all of the major muscle groups in the body. You will begin with the head, then go down the body to the neck, arms, chest, back, stomach, pelvis, legs, and feet. To do this exercise, lie on your back on the floor or bed. Close your eyes, then focus on one set of muscles at a time, tensing to the count of 10 and releasing to the count of 10. Along with progressive muscle relaxation, use deep abdominal breathing, inhaling while tensing the muscles and exhaling while relaxing them. Add a classical CD playing in the background, light an aromatic candle, and turn the lights down low to get an added de-stressing benefit.

The Relaxation Response

Dr. Herbert Benson of the Harvard Medical School was one of the first medical researchers to study the interplay between the mind and body. According to Benson's studies, the relaxation response brings about the opposite of the fight-or-flight reaction, helping to decrease cortisol secretion so optimal immune function can be restored. Benson realized that inducing the relaxation response at will can reduce physical strain and emotional, negative thoughts—and increase your ability to self-manage stress.

The relaxation response slows down the sympathetic nervous system, leading to:

- A decreased heart rate
- Lower blood pressure
- Less sweat production
- Lowered oxygen consumption
- Lowered production of catecholamines (dopamine and norepinephrine, brain chemicals associated with the stress response)
- Lowered production of cortisol (stress hormone)

Achieving relaxation is important in reducing the emotional stress of dealing with infertility. With the relaxation response, you will develop an inner quiet and peacefulness, a calming of negative thoughts and wor-ries, and a focus on something other than your problems.

Relaxation can reduce negative thoughts and increase your ability to manage your daily problems. Use the following steps to learn the relax-ation response. Then practice this several times each day until it becomes second nature to you.

1. Set aside a period of about 20 minutes that you can devote to relaxation practice.
2. Remove outside distractions that can disrupt your concentration: turn off the radio, the television, even the ringer on the tele-phone, if need be.
3. Lie flat on a bed or floor, or recline comfortably so that your whole body is supported, relieving as much tension or tightness in your muscles as you can. You can use a pillow or cushion under your head if this helps.
4. During the 20-minute period, remain as still as possible; try to focus on the immediate moment, and eliminate any outside thoughts competing for your attention.
5. As you go through these steps, in your own way try to imagine that every muscle in your body is now becoming loose, relaxed, and free of any excess tension. Picture all of the muscles in your body beginning to unwind; imagine them going limp.
6. Concentrate on making your breathing even. As you exhale, pic-ture your muscles becoming even more relaxed, as if you somehow breathe the tension away. At the end of 20 minutes, take a few moments to focus on the feelings and sensations you have been able to achieve. Notice whether areas that felt tight and tense at first now feel more loose and relaxed, and whether any areas of tension remain.

Visualization

Visualization or guided imagery is a stress-release activity that you can do wherever you are, any time of the day or night—even while you are waiting at the doctor's office for test results or a painful procedure. This mind-body technique involves mentally seeing pictures of relaxing situations, such as a sunset on the beach, a mountain waterfall, or a brilliant sunrise. One researcher suggests that experiencing an event through imagination is equivalent to actually having the experience. Perhaps imagery could increase the chance of conception!

Using the following steps, you can allow your imagination to take over as you focus on your senses to create a desired state of relaxation in your mind.

1. Find a place where you can be comfortable and allow about 15 minutes for this exercise. Take several deep breaths while sitting or lying down, and close your eyes.
2. Imagine a relaxing place—somewhere you have been before, so you can see it in your mind. This might be sitting on the seashore at sunset or sunrise, being in a mountain cabin next to a babbling brook, or floating on a raft in the lake on a sunny day.
3. Continue to breathe slowly and keep this image in your mind. As you explore your mental picture of your relaxing spot, imagine all the stress, worries, and tension leaving your body. Feel the temperature of your special place. See the colors surrounding you. What sounds do you hear? Smell the freshness of the air. Touch the gentleness of the moment. Take in all the sensory details of your relaxing place and continue to de-stress.
4. After about 15 minutes, slowly open your eyes and acclimate yourself to the surroundings in the room. Stretch your arms and legs; gently move your head from side to side and feel the tension release. Carry the calm feeling you now have with you through the day.

If you have trouble imagining scenes and images to de-stress, listen to sounds of nature or waves to trigger thoughts of natural settings. Relaxation tapes and CDs can be purchased in any bookstore or music store.

Art Therapy

Art therapy is based on human developmental and psychological theories. Using a broad spectrum of creative and artistic methods, the art therapist will help you identify, then change emotional conflicts and behavioral problems, as well as increase your self-awareness and develop self-esteem. Call your local mental health association for a list of qualified therapists, or enjoy using creative and artistic methods on your own to express your inner feelings.

Dance Therapy

Dance or movement therapy came from the modern dance era in the 1940s. Using movement, positions, and various postures, the dance therapist helps you to get in touch with your innermost feelings. Once these feelings are brought out and identified, you can move forward in a healthy manner. This form of mind-body treatment is often used with adults who have buried painful memories or those who are too depressed to talk about inner conflicts and resulting emotions.

Drama Therapy

Drama therapy uses theater methods to help you reduce symptoms, integrate the mind and body, or move toward personal growth. Using such techniques as role play, theater games, mime, puppetry, and improvisation, among many, you can enjoy creative expression and actually deactivate stress aging.

Biofeedback

This relaxation technique teaches you to read and control such body functions as skin temperature, heart rate, and brain waves. The main idea of biofeedback is that you may not be able to control what goes on around you, but you can learn to alter the way that you respond to it.

With biofeedback, sensors are placed over specific muscle sites and you are connected to a machine that informs you and your therapist when you are physically relaxing your body. The therapist will read the tension in your muscles, heart rate, breathing, sweat, or body temperature.

The ultimate goal of biofeedback is to use this new skill outside the therapist's office when you are facing the real lions and tigers of life. If learned successfully, biofeedback can help you control your heart rate, blood pressure, breathing patterns, and muscle tension when you are not hooked up to the machine.

While biofeedback is not always easy, the skills acquired might be well worth the effort. For many people, biofeedback provides relatively fast, effective, long-lasting relief from the physical symptoms of stress.

Hypnotherapy

Hypnosis is a temporary condition of altered attention, whereby your brain shuts out external events. This mind-body technique allows you to concentrate deeply and fully on a single idea while also including such factors as role playing, imagination, motivation, and the power of suggestion. It also requires that you truly desire to change a type of behavior.

Studies show that only about 15 percent of the population is thought to be highly hypnotizable, while 25 percent are thought to be not hypnotizable at all.

Doctor's Rx

Because hypnosis is endorsed by the American Psychiatric Association and the American Psychological Association, seek a qualified clinical psychologist or psychiatrist to see if hypnosis would be helpful and safe for you.

Light Therapy

Light therapy involves using natural or artificial light to cause physiological changes in the human body. Broad-spectrum light is used to give people the effect of having a few extra hours of daylight each day. Using specially made light boxes, people are exposed to bright light and subsequently produce serotonin, a neurotransmitter in the brain that is associated with a calming, anxiety-reducing reaction. Because of this rise in serotonin, scientists believe that light therapy may ease depression. At night, when it is dark, the brain produces less serotonin and more melatonin, a hormone naturally produced in the brain that helps us sleep deeply.

Most recently, doctors are using bright light therapy to relieve the symptoms associated with seasonal affective disorder (SAD), a psychological problem that occurs with the change of seasons and less exposure to daylight. Those who have SAD feel depressed and fatigued, and may crave carbohydrates, as these carbohydrates boost levels of serotonin in the body. Light therapy is also thought to be helpful for alleviating PMS, migraines, high blood pressure, stress, and insomnia.

In some studies using light therapy, women with PMS reported less depression, less moodiness, better sleep, and better concentration. Researchers have shown that serotonin levels drop just before ovulation in women, and this drop correlates with the onset of PMS symptoms. Serotonin levels also rebound with the onset of menstruation or when PMS symptoms decrease. Recent research suggests that PMS occurs in women with low base levels of serotonin; when serotonin levels drop further at ovulation, these levels fall low enough in PMS sufferers for symptoms to appear. Using phototherapy, women with PMS can keep their serotonin/melatonin levels high enough to prevent their PMS.

The intensity of light is a vital factor in determining your physiological response. Two standard intensities are suggested for use: 2,500 lux for an average of 2 hours per day or 10,000 for an average of 30 minutes per day. Many insurance companies have reimbursed the purchase price of light fixtures for the treatment of seasonal affective disorder (SAD), PMS, sleep disorders, and problems adapting to shift work.

You may experience improvement with just 30 minutes of bright light exposure, while some people may need up to two hours daily.

•   •   •

Again, if an alternative treatment is proven harmless and won't delay your continuing medical evaluation and treatment, then try it. First talk to your doctor and make sure the therapy will benefit you. This will allow you to take advantage of the safest alternative or mind-body treatments and avoid those that may cause more harm than relief.

Part Five

Insurance and Legal Issues

Chapter 18

Who's Paying the Bill?

"I recently represented a woman who had a laparoscopy with an inci-
dental chromotubation because of complaints of pelvic pain," said Britt-
nye, 34, an attorney. "The insurance carrier denied the claim, stating it
was for the treatment of infertility. Because we took the claim through
the grievance process, eventually the insurance company decided to pay
the benefits. We established that the laparoscopy was done not for
infertility, but for pelvic pain.

"More important, the contract excluded only 'treatment' of infer-
tility. Since the procedure was diagnostic, the insurance company deter-
mined that it was required to make the payment. Thus, it is very
important that you determine what is excluded and ultimately the
reason the insurance company is denying the claim."

Not only does infertility cause great stress and emotional pain, but
there's another enormous hurdle to overcome. The treatment is
unbelievably expensive, and someone has to foot the bill.

"My insurance company should pay. After all, this is a real health
problem," you might say. Before you are convinced that the test, medication, or treatment will be covered by your health insurance company,
there are some obstacles you need to consider. According to Foster Hig-
gins, a benefits consulting firm, only about 25 percent of traditional
insurance plans and 37 percent of HMOs offer coverage for infertility
treatment, and these still may not pay the full cost of infertility treatment, or may cover only diagnosis and not treatment.

Insurance companies usually provide benefits for infertility if the
charges are related to diagnostic testing, prescription drugs, or surgery.

Historically, insurance coverage for infertility has been arbitrary and inconsistent, with most insurers calling it elective or experimental. Nonetheless, if you read your insurance policy yet do not see infertility coverage, don't throw in the towel just yet. Check out the following guidelines designed to help you to overcome any legal and financial restrictions.

Insurance Coverage and Infertility Treatments

Many insurance companies do not provide health insurance coverage for infertility treatment or provide only very limited insurance coverage. Insurance reimbursement falls into a gray area and is open to interpretation. If your claims for infertility treatment have been denied, *you* are your best advocate for coverage. No one is as concerned about insurance coverage for infertility as you are, so consider the following questions, and don't stop until you get the answers you need to help fund having a baby.

Does Your State Mandate Coverage?

Do you live in a state that mandates infertility insurance coverage? As of this writing, the thirteen states that mandate coverage for infertility to some extent or under certain conditions include:

- Arkansas
- California
- Connecticut
- Hawaii
- Illinois
- Maryland
- Massachusetts
- Montana
- New York
- Ohio
- Rhode Island

- Texas
- West Virginia

Although these states require some coverage in infertility care, the laws differ significantly. For example, only six states (Arkansas, Hawaii, Illinois, Maryland, Massachusetts, and Rhode Island) require insurance companies to cover in vitro fertilization and other high-tech conception treatments. While Massachusetts mandates the coverage of infertility treatments, California only requires the insurance company to offer the coverage to employers. Arkansas exempts HMOs from its law, and employers who are self-insured, which includes many, do not have to follow the state's mandates. A summary of these statutes can be found at the American Society for Reproductive Medicine's website at www.asrm.org/patient/insur.html.

Is Your Company Policy an ERISA Plan?

If your insurance is provided through your employer, you need to determine whether it is an ERISA (Employees Retirement Income Security Act) plan. ERISA is a federal law regulating employer benefits that applies to self-funded employer insurance plans. You can determine this by looking in your plan booklet or by asking your employer. If you have an ERISA plan, it preempts state law, meaning that even if you live in one of the states listed above, the law is not applicable to you because your health insurance is governed by ERISA.

Is the Company in Compliance with State Laws?

If the state mandate is applicable to you, then you need to decide whether the insurance company is in compliance with the law. In Massachusetts, this would be simple enough—i.e., if the policy does not include infertility diagnosis and treatment, then it is violating the law. In California, you would need to determine whether the coverage was in fact offered to your employer.

Should You Appeal Law Violations?

If the law has been violated, then you need to write an appeal to your insurance company, explaining the law to them and saying that you believe they are violating the state mandate. You would then request that they pay for your medical care and correct the violation.

Understanding Your Insurance Contract

Now that you know what you're up against as far as the state you live in mandating infertility coverage, get to know your own insurance plan. Carefully read your summary plan description, as well as your entire insurance contract. Most people obtain their health insurance through their employer, who provides a "summary" of the health insurance plan. Although this is helpful to some extent, you must read the actual contract, as it controls your health insurance. If a procedure is not listed in the exclusions section, it is reasonable to surmise that it is covered.

Request the Contract in Writing

The benefits booklet your employer hands you is not a legal document and is nonbinding in court. You want to see the actual contract, a notarized legal document with dates and signatures. If you do not have a copy of the contract between your employer and the insurance company, ask your employer for a copy. If ERISA is applicable to your situation, your employer or the plan administrator is required to provide you with a copy.

When you request a copy of your insurance contract, do so in writing. If your employer fails to provide the information that is requested within thirty days, he may be held personally liable to you (the participant or beneficiary) in the amount of up to $100.00 per day from the date of such failure or refusal to provide the information. Keep a copy of the letter sent to your employer requesting this contract.

Make a Copy of the Contract

Once you receive the contract, ask for a copy to be made, and keep this for future reference. The reason you need a copy is that employers can request changes in insurance policies at any time, sign the new contract, and put this into effect at that date for all employees.

Check for Infertility Exclusion

Insurance contracts are construed against the insurance company. Thus, if they are going to deny you benefits, *it must be clearly stated in the contract*. Read your contract to determine if there is a specific exclusion for infertility. If there is no exclusion, you should have coverage. If there is an exclusion, carefully read what it excludes. Does it exclude treatments only, or does it also exclude diagnosis? You may find that certain aspects of treatment may be covered while others are not. Or the insurance company may pay for diagnostic but not treatment procedures. Generally speaking, if the contract does not have an exclusion for infertility, the insurance company must pay benefits.

Appealing the Denial of a Claim

If you have read your contract and believe you should have coverage (and your insurance company has denied a claim, or stated you do not have coverage when preauthorization is requested), be persistent. Write your insurance company and ask for identification of the specific reasons for the denial and under what provision of the contract your claim is being denied. Approximately 80 percent of all costs to diagnose and treat infertility are eventually paid by insurance companies—if you stay on top of what is lawfully covered.

Identify the Reasons for a Denial

In the past, insurance companies that do not have exclusions have denied claims for one of the following three reasons:

1. Infertility is not an illness.
2. Treatment of infertility is not medically necessary.
3. Treatment of infertility is experimental.

These are invalid reasons to deny your claim. Infertility is an illness. *Medically necessary* is usually defined by insurance policies as medically required and medically appropriate for diagnosis and treatment of an illness or injury under professionally recognized standards of health care. (Again, read your policy and determine how *medically necessary* is defined.) Treatments such as GIFT, IVF, and ZIFT/PROST have been off the American Medical Association's experimental list since the late 1980s.

Review the Policy for Inconsistencies

If the insurance company gives you another reason, you should review your policy carefully and determine if the reason given is consistent with the insurance contract. The language in many insurance policies is difficult to understand and unclear. This makes it hard to decide what infertility treatments or procedures are covered.

Get Substantiation in Writing from Your Doctor

Once the insurance company has identified the reasons for the denial of the claim, you can then present evidence that their reasoning is incorrect. This may include a letter from your doctor explaining the reasons for a particular procedure. You should also write a letter to the insurance company explaining why you believe its denial was inappropriate. You should attempt to make all contacts with the insurance company through written communication. If you should need to contact them by telephone, take extensive notes, which should include the date and time you called, the name of the person you spoke with, and what was said.

Violation of Discrimination Laws

Even if the exclusion is valid under the insurance contract, it may nevertheless be invalid under federal discrimination laws. These laws are currently being tested in some courts throughout the country as to how they should be applied to persons with infertility. The law is not settled and the result may be different from jurisdiction to jurisdiction.

Infertility Is a Disability

The Americans with Disabilities Act (ADA), which was passed in 1991, provides that it is unlawful to discriminate against persons with disabilities. To be disabled under the ADA, a person must have a physiological disorder that affects a major life activity. The definition of a disability includes any physiological disorder or condition of the reproductive system. The United States Supreme Court has ruled that reproduction is a major life activity under the ADA. *Thus infertility is a disability.* It is unlawful under the ADA to treat persons with disabilities differently from other employees in the terms or conditions of employment, including fringe benefits.

The ADA defines a disability as a "physical or mental impairment that substantially limits one or more of the major life activities of such individual." Thus, to be protected under the ADA, a person must establish that he or she has a physical or mental impairment that affects a major life activity.

A physical or mental impairment has been defined in the Code of Federal Regulations to mean:

> Any physiological disorder, or condition, cosmetic disfigurement, or anatomical loss affecting one or more of the following body systems: Neurological, musculoskeletal, special sense organs, respiratory (including speech organs), cardiovascular, reproductive, digestive, genital-urinary, hemic and lymphatic, skin, and endocrine; or . . .

The Code of Federal Regulations also defines major life activities to include walking, seeing, breathing, and caring for oneself, among others.

Reproduction is not included in the list of major life activities in the regulations. However, the regulations do state the list is not exclusive but is given by way of example. Thus, there are major life activities that are not listed.

Since the enactment of the ADA there have been many cases where persons with infertility or HIV have sought protection under the ADA. The major issue in these cases was whether reproduction is a major life activity under the ADA. There was a split in the decisions. The majority of the federal district courts have ruled that reproduction is a major life activity.

Under the ADA your employer, and, if relevant, your insurance carrier, cannot discriminate against you based on your disability—infertility. They must treat you the same as other people. They cannot deny you leave to seek medical treatment if they provide leave for other persons. They cannot fire you for seeking medical treatment or because of your infertility if they would not do the same to others.

Seeking Safe Harbor

Of course the big question is, how does this affect my health insurance, which excludes or limits infertility treatments? Under the ADA an additional provision known as the safe harbor affects insurance. Basically what this provision states is that the ADA is not intended to affect how insurance companies do business or how your employer sets up its health insurance coverage unless it is a "subterfuge" under the ADA. The courts are still not in agreement as to what this provision of the ADA means.

Check the EEOC Guidelines

Although the ADA has a specific section that protects some insurance plans, the Equal Employment Opportunity Commission (EEOC) has issued guidelines in interpreting this provision that are very favorable to persons whose health insurance excludes infertility. The guidelines state that in order to have the protections of the insurance provision for a disability-based distinction, the insurer must establish that it is financially impossible to include the coverage. Studies have clearly shown that the costs to cover infertility are minimal. Various studies have revealed the costs to be in the range of $0.34 to $2.00 per family plan per month.

Limitations in Court

Unfortunately, the insurance provision of the ADA remains unsettled in the courts. Some courts have followed the EEOC's interpretation but have limited its application. Other courts have held that this provision means that when insurance is involved, the employer must discriminate in a non–fringe benefit aspect of employment. This means that the person is not hired or fired because of the cost implications for insurance coverage.

Is It Sex Discrimination?

Title VII of the Civil Rights Act provides that sex discrimination includes discrimination based on pregnancy, childbirth, or related medical conditions. It has been held that infertility is a medical condition related to pregnancy. Therefore, an employer cannot treat you any differently from its other employees as far as providing insurance benefits, time off from work, or other factors related to infertility testing and treatment. There is no provision relating to insurance under the Pregnancy Disability Act. Thus, the costs of providing the coverage are irrelevant; the law simply prohibits discrimination in the terms or conditions of employment, including fringe benefits.

You must keep in mind that to recover money under these laws you will most likely have to take legal action against your employer. This prospect frightens most people in that they are afraid their employer will retaliate by terminating their employment. This is a legitimate fear, but it is illegal to retaliate against any person who has made a claim of discrimination. Even so, there is little that can be done to stop the retaliation. The only remedy for such retaliation is to bring an additional claim for the retaliation and ask for reinstatement or money damages.

It may be possible to bring an action directly against the insurance carrier under the ADA. However, there are only a few court cases that interpret how the law is to be applied to insurance policies. Again, the courts are in disagreement.

Taking Time Off from Work

The provisions of the ADA and the PDA also protect you when you need to take time off work for treatments. Your employer must treat you the same as all other employees when making decisions as to utilization of sick leave or vacation leave or other provisions for time off from work for medical reasons.

Lean on the Family Medical Leave Act

In addition, under the Family Medical Leave Act, or FMLA, any employer that has 50 or more employees must give you time off from work for medical treatment. There are certain limitations on this requirement, and it has not been conclusively determined whether infertility would be a covered condition. However, there is a good probability that it would be included under the language of the statute.

The Family Leave Act:

- Covers only certain employers
- Affects only those employees eligible for the protections of the law
- Involves entitlement to leave
- Maintains health benefits during leave
- Restores an employee's job after leave
- Sets requirements for notice and certification of the need for leave
- Protects employees who request or take leave
- Includes certain employer record-keeping requirements

The law contains provisions on employer coverage; employee eligibility for the law's benefits; entitlement to leave, maintenance of health benefits during leave, and job restoration after leave; notice and certification of the need for FMLA leave; and protection for employees who request or take FMLA leave. The law also requires employers to keep certain records.

Who's Covered by the FMLA?

The FMLA applies to:

- All agencies, including state, local, and federal employers, local education agencies (schools)
- Private-sector employers who employed 50 or more employees in 20 or more workweeks in the current or preceding calendar year
- All who are engaged in commerce or in any industry or activity affecting commerce—including joint employers and successors of covered employers

Who's Eligible for Benefits?

To be eligible for FMLA benefits, an employee must:

- Work for a covered employer
- Have worked for the employer for a total of 12 months
- Have worked at least 1,250 hours over the previous 12 months
- Work at a location in the United States or in any territory or possession of the United States where at least 50 employees are employed by the employer within 75 miles

Involve Your Doctor

If your employer is reluctant to give you time off from work to obtain your treatments, then you should specifically tell your employer (assuming that there are more than 50 employees) that you are requesting time off as dictated by the Family Medical Leave Act, and ask your supervisor what you need to do to obtain such leave. Generally, you will be given a form to complete that will require a statement from your doctor that it is necessary for you to miss work.

Involve an Attorney

While this chapter summarizes some of the legal protections you may have under various federal laws, you may still have protection under your state law. If you have any concerns, contact an attorney. Most attorneys will provide a free initial consultation. Try to locate an attorney that specializes in the area of employment and/or insurance law.

No Easy Answers

There are no easy answers about payment for infertility treatment. Many insurers still feel that covering payments for infertility tests and treatment is expensive and unnecessary. Conversely, these same companies pay for impotence treatments, such as penile implants, that involve surgery and can cost in excess of $15,000 to $20,000. Compared to the cost of high-tech conception, this cost is outrageous, not to mention questionable as a priority.

A current resource for seeing if your state has an infertility insurance law or if a specific test or treatment should be covered is *The Infertility Insurance Advisor: An Insurance Counseling Program for Infertile Couples*, which is available for a fee from RESOLVE, an infertility patient advocacy and information organization.

If your reproductive body clock is running out of time, you might consider moving to a state where fertility tests and treatment are already available. Still, be cautious! If you work for a large company (usually, one that employs over 500 employees), this company is probably considered self-insured and does not have to comply with the fertility statutes of that state.

Because the courts are still in a state of flux as to whether an employer or insurance carrier may exclude or limit treatments for infertility, the only way of getting the answer regarding payment for infertility treatments is to pursue litigation and attempt to get a case before the United States Supreme Court.

Part Six

Choosing a Practitioner and Clinic

Chapter 19

Guidelines for
Choosing a Specialist

"I read everything I could on the Internet about infertility," said Ursula, age 34. "The site alt.infertility said we needed an RE. I eventually decoded this to mean a reproductive endocrinologist. Everybody on alt.infertility had one. In fact, the Internet buzz said one of the best (not to mention cheapest) was in a neighboring town.

"Dr. Barnes is a polar bear of a man. He smacks of the rumpled Ivy League professor he had been before moving back home to start his own practice. By the time of our first appointment, he had devoured our medical records and personal histories. He summarized our situation while examining my carefully compiled (some might say obsessive) ovulation charts; at last, someone who could not only decipher them but could also appreciate the data!

"Dr. Barnes's style was a combination of therapist, detective, and scientist. Clearly, he was sensitive to the issue of blame, noting that we probably both contributed to our fertility problem, but trying hard not to point the finger."

Your doctor plays the first, most significant role as you get answers to your infertility problem. Not only does he or she serve as the one who can accurately run tests, diagnose, and prescribe proper treatment for your problem, this health care professional may become a close, dependable friend to talk to when concerns turn into ongoing worries and anxieties. The combination of managed care constraints and infertility problem specifics can make it hard to find the right specialist.

The only physician many people see is a general practitioner, more commonly called a primary care physician. These doctors are concerned with the overall health and well-being of the patient. The primary care physician is familiar with all aspects of general medicine and should be a good diagnostician. This doctor often sees many members of the same family (family medicine) and often provides cradle-to-grave care. Women often see their general practitioner for annual exams, Pap tests, and even obstetric care, if available.

Many women rely on their gynecologist or ob-gyn. In addition to providing treatment for female medical conditions, many of these doctors offer infertility treatment as part of a comprehensive ob-gyn practice. An ob-gyn may provide ultrasounds, semen analysis, clomiphene therapy, intrauterine inseminations, or surgery to treat infertility. Most gynecologists work closely with reproductive endocrinologists when a referral is needed.

If there are extensive problems contributing to infertility, or if six months or so of clomiphene or other therapy has been unsuccessful, you may want to consider an infertility specialist known as a reproductive endocrinologist (RE). This physician is an ob-gyn who has additional training in the subspecialty area of reproductive endocrinology. An RE should be board certified in reproductive medicine.

Situations in which an RE may be considered:

- Unable to conceive, yet have tried to conceive for more than two years without birth control
- Age 35 or older
- 6 months on clomiphene with no success of conception
- Irregular menstrual periods
- Irregular or no ovulation
- Need treatment for reproductive diseases such as endometriosis
- Need treatment or microsurgery for tubal damage
- Had three or more pregnancy losses
- Have a history of PID
- Partner has male-factor infertility

Infertility Specialists

All doctors with "M.D." after their names have completed four years of medical school. The medical student then goes on to do an internship, either in a specified field or a so-called rotating internship, which exposes him or her to many areas of medicine. If a doctor decides to specialize in a specific field such as ob-gyn, he or she must complete a residency program in this area. In general, infertility training in medical school internship and residency is limited to a few weeks at best. Little emphasis is placed on the intricate endocrinology and physiology that can contribute to female and male infertility. Rarely is time devoted to understanding ways to help couples deal with the emotional component of infertility.

To become board certified in obstetrics and gynecology the doctor must graduate from college and medical school and complete a four-year residency training in ob-gyn. In addition, he or she must pass a written examination in ob-gyn, complete a two-year practice experience, and then pass an oral examination in ob-gyn.

If the doctor decides to become board certified in reproductive endocrinology, he or she must successfully complete requirements for board certification in ob-gyn and in addition attend a two- to three-year fellowship in reproductive endocrinology, pass a written examination on the topic, finish a two-year practice experience in reproductive endocrinology, and then pass a three-hour oral examination in reproductive endocrinology. Some doctors have completed all but the oral examination and are still in their practice experience in reproductive endocrinology. These doctors are board eligible in reproductive endocrinology.

There are about 500 board-certified reproductive endocrinologists in the United States. Another 800-plus doctors are board eligible. It should also be noted that some doctors can also "learn by doing" and are considered to have expertise in infertility.

Urologists with a subspecialty called andrology are the most highly qualified physicians to deal with all aspects of male-factor infertility. These doctors have completed a two-year fellowship and have passed an examination to become a board-certified andrologist.

Used with permission from RESOLVE

Consider Age, Gender, and Credentials

Undergoing the invasive infertility tests and high-tech procedures requires a tremendous commitment of emotional energy and money, not to mention time. While many basic infertility tests and treatments can be done by your gynecologist, if you are having no results with treatment or feel that your doctor is not current with the latest assisted reproductive methods, you may want to check out your other options.

When choosing an RE and fertility clinic, you need to evaluate many factors, including the services available, the convenience of the clinic, and the staff's "personality"—the rapport they have with each other and with the patients. Some women are fortunate enough to get referrals from friends who have undergone infertility procedures. Others depend on referrals from their primary care physicians or ob-gyns. In this age of managed care, the reality is that you need to check the list of doctors who will accept your insurance provider. Nevertheless, none of these methods is foolproof in finding a qualified RE with whom you can feel comfortable to share your innermost feelings and concerns.

Perhaps one of the most important steps to take when selecting an RE is to know yourself, including your personal likes and dislikes. Do you feel more comfortable with a man or a woman? Should your physician be older than you, the same age, or younger? Do you have a preference as to educational background? These questions are important to consider when making your appointment.

Ask the following questions as you go through the process of choosing a specialist.

- *Where did the doctor go to medical school?* Your local medical society can provide this information. Or check out *The Directory of Medical Specialists*, published by Who's Who, which gives basic information on about 400,000 practicing physicians. This is available at most public libraries. Other sources include the AMA's doctor finder, which is an online service. Or check your health plan. The plan administrator may be able to update you on the doctor's qualifications.
- *Is the doctor board certified in reproductive endocrinology?* This means that the doctor has passed a standard exam and has completed other requirements issued by the governing board. Many fertility specialists are

not board certified or even board eligible. Check the American Board of Medical Specialties website on the Internet, or call 800-776-2378 to see if the doctor is board certified.

- *Is the doctor a member of the Society of Reproductive Endocrinologists?* What other professional organizations does he belong to? All REs should be members of the American College of Obstetricians and Gynecologists. Many are members of RESOLVE, a national support organization that provides education and information for infertile couples.

- *How long has the doctor been involved in assisted reproductive technology?* Experience is vital with such invasive procedures as ART. You also need to have an RE who is up-to-date on the latest developments in the field. The American Society for Reproductive Medicine (ASRM) recommends that each physician supervise a minimum of twenty follicular recruitment cycles for a year. Clinics should also have access to a reproductive surgeon, who specializes in correcting obstructions, endometriosis, and other abnormalities of the reproductive system, and a reproductive immunologist, who specializes in immunological barriers to achieving pregnancy. A reproductive urologist, an M.D. with further residence in treating urinary tract and male reproductive disorders and two years of surgical training, should be available in case male-factor infertility is the problem.

- *Is the doctor involved in any academic pursuits, such as teaching, writing, or research?* This doctor may be more up-to-date in the latest developments in the field of reproductive endocrinology. If the clinic is associated with a teaching medical center, you may benefit from cutting-edge breakthroughs in tests and treatments.

- *Where does the RE have hospital privileges, and where are these hospitals located?* Some doctors may not admit patients to certain hospitals, and this is an important consideration. Your state's licensing board can let you know if any disciplinary action has been taken against the doctor.

- *Does the clinic provide a copy of the past year's statistics?* Check to see how many egg retrievals have been performed. How many patients undergo embryo transfers per month, and how many result in pregnancy and live births? What is the program's miscarriage rate? Make sure the success rates are broken down by the ages of the women involved.

- *If this is a group practice, will you be able to choose your personal doctor?* Often the RE who does the many tests and evaluates your situation is not the one who is on call when an emergency occurs. Find this out ahead of time and make sure you are in agreement with the practice policy.

• *Does the doctor accept your particular health insurance, or is the doctor a member of the medical panel associated with your HMO?* Find out what procedures are covered under your policy (see Chapter 18). Be sure to get in writing the cost of the services, including any medications you may need. If a cycle is canceled because of poor ovulation response, what is your financial responsibility?

• *What services are offered at the clinic?* Some programs are equipped to handle sperm/egg donors and cryopreservation of embryos. Others may offer combined IVF/GIFT (in vitro fertilization/gamete intrafallopian transfer), ICSI (intracytoplasmic sperm injection), ZIFT (zygote intrafallopian transfer), PROST (pronuclear stage transfer), and TET (tubal embryo transfer).

• *Does the clinic follow specific regulations?* Ask if it meets the American Society for Reproductive Medicine's (ASRM) guidelines. Federal legislation passed in 1988 by the Clinical Laboratory Improvement Amendment (CLIA) requires all laboratories to be accredited. Is the IVF lab accredited by the Commission on Laboratory Accreditation (COLA), the College of American Pathologists (CAP), and the ASRM? Is the program a member of the Society for Assisted Reproductive Technology (SART), a society affiliated with the ASRM?

• *Are the office hours convenient with your work schedule?* Ask for information about emergency availability and charges. Also see if the lab and ultrasound offices are opened during evening hours, weekends, and holidays. Clinics should be available seven days a week for women in treatment cycles. A doctor at the clinic must be on call 24 hours a day.

• *Is the support staff amenable?* The support staff will help you with prescriptions, necessary lab work, x-rays, and appointments with hospitals or other professional services. Even the receptionist's responses might set the tone for the practice and help you decide if this is the right office. Be sure to get their names and introduce yourself so they will know you when you need to call. Find out if the nurses have a time that you can call with pertinent questions about your case.

Plan a Consultation

Plan an initial consultation with the doctor during which you can get to know each other. This will include a detailed interview and physical examination. Make sure the RE has copies of your medical records, including any past tests or procedures. Having your partner join you is important, for infertility is a family problem. Keep in mind that patient-physician communication is important to receive the highest quality of care and also comfort needed during anxious moments.

At the end of this initial interview, ask questions as to the preferred methods of treatment.

- Does the physician appear to relate well to you?
- Do you feel at ease, or is the doctor strictly business?
- Are your questions answered?

Especially with a stressful illness such as infertility, your physician needs to be accessible. When you are taking fertility medications, having a procedure, or believe there is a problem with a pregnancy, popularity is not important, but availability is. Make sure your RE is not only an excellent doctor but one who is available and attentive to your personal needs.

Assessing a Fertility Clinic

As you assess the fertility clinic using annual statistics, remember that a clinic's success rate will change from year to year, depending on the number of cycles that it carries out. The larger the number of cycles that a clinic carries out, the less its rates should vary. Yet the smaller the number of cycles, the greater the margin of error and the more variability in success rates from year to year. For example, if the clinic performed only three ART cycles and all were successful in presenting live births, the success rate would be 100 percent. If none were successful, the rate would be zero! Clinics that accept a higher percentage of women who have had many previous unsuccessful ART cycles will usually have lower success rates than clinics that do not.

Success rates of any clinic will be affected by:

- The quality of eggs (largely related to the woman's age)
- The quality of sperm (including its motility and ability to penetrate the egg)
- The skill and competence of the treatment team
- The general health of the woman
- Genetic factors

The Fertility Clinic Success Rate and Certification Act of 1992 directs the selection of a secretary of health and human services to develop a model program for the certification of embryo laboratories. This act also mandates that ART programs must provide their success rates to the Centers for Disease Control (CDC) for annual review and publication. This law is slated to get clinics to report the success rates that reflect real numbers of actual pregnancies in relation to completed ART cycles.

The Centers for Disease Control and RESOLVE, an infertility organization, have compiled a list arranged by state that provides a full assessment of fertility clinics. These vital statistics provide success rates (also called the take-home baby rate) and evaluate clinic quality. To see this report, go to www.cdc.gov/nccdphp/drh/arts/index.htm on the Internet, or call 888-299-1585 to order a copy.

When Is a Second Opinion Necessary?

With the increased demands of our health care system, doctors can make mistakes. Medical errors can result when the doctor does not ask for enough tests to make an evaluation, or when the doctor requests more tests than necessary. Either way can lead to a misdiagnosis, the wrong medication, or unnecessary expense. Clearly, the only way to reduce the chances that this will happen to you is to be assertive and knowledgeable as you take responsibility for your health.

If you feel your doctor is not communicating openly with you or if you feel that testing or treatments are not thorough, you have every right to seek another opinion. Remember, it's your body, and you must do all you can to protect your fertility and future family. Be sure to check with your health plan before you get a second opinion. Usually this expense is not covered.

Get it in Writing

Once you've chosen an RE, ask for a written treatment plan; this will ensure that you and your partner don't progress too slowly or too aggressively through your fertility treatment. According to RESOLVE, this written plan should recommend a stepped-care approach to treating infertility as well as a rationale for initiating each new treatment or test. This plan should include time or cycle limits for each treatment modality before the couple is moved on to the next level of therapy.

Be the Captain of Your Ship

Whatever treatment you decide upon, remember, it is your body. You have the right to become an informed, educated, and active participant in your own wellness. You have the right to ask your doctor questions, to get a second opinion, to change physicians, and to refuse a procedure if you feel it is not in your best interest. Working in partnership with conventional and complementary practitioners, you can choose the safest and most effective treatments that will work with your body's own healing power.

No Matter What
the Odds, Have Hope

No matter what, have hope. It doesn't take much. Just a glance. A maybe. A word from a friend that she is finally pregnant after years of trying. A new medication. A promising procedure. A nod from your doctor that things look positive.

I know it's hard to stay optimistic when it seems as if all the doors are closing on your chances of getting pregnant. But hope will keep you going when pregnancy tests continue to show negative results. Try to disconnect unhealthy worries and replace these with the belief that things will work out in the near future.

Create your own network of friends and acquaintances who are in the same situation as you. Read fertility success stories on the Internet. Talk with other patients in your RE's office. Most important, have faith that if just one infertile couple can overcome the odds to make a baby, so can you.

Lorri was told by her doctor that she should consider adoption. Yet her true story shows how keeping alive the faith or hope that you can get pregnant—even when the statistics are against you—can often be the key to making a baby:

"Jack and I married when we were both 25, but we put off having children for a few years. He was searching for the right career while I was experiencing great opportunities at my job. We bought a house, then decided it was the right time to start our family. So we tried and tried and tried.

"Finally, as I was approaching my thirtieth birthday, we decided to get some real help. I wasn't thrilled with my gynecologist, and I visited three other doctors before I found one with whom I was comfortable. We had the usual tests. I'll never forget the evaluation visit when all the results were in. My doctor's first question was whether we were interested in adoption. The news wasn't great. Both my husband and I had fertility obstacles that were not going to be resolved naturally.

"I was put on Clomid and Synthroid (for hypothyroidism) and was given the guidelines for artificial insemination. We left the office stunned and embarrassed. We didn't know anyone who had had trouble getting pregnant, we didn't know how to face the questions our families would inevitably ask, and we sure didn't know where we were going to find the money to pay for the procedures.

"We did the inseminations for six months. I remember driving to the doctor at eight on a Saturday morning, a vial of semen tucked in my bra to keep it warm, looking at the three other couples huddled in the cold office waiting their turn. Infertility usually strains marriages, but there's nothing that brings two people together more than trying to have intercourse right after artificial insemination. I experienced bleeding and cramping every time, so you can imagine how sexy I was feeling afterward. But we did what we were supposed to. Then, nothing.

"Every month my period would arrive, and every month I said this would be the last month we would try. I couldn't take the disappointment. Though I wouldn't tell anyone, for those two weeks between ovulation and menstruation, I spent almost every minute thinking I was pregnant. I was so hopeful that I calculated the due date, planned a nursery, and even picked out names for this phantom baby who would never be. It broke my heart.

"We took a break, then tried another six-month cycle. Nothing for the first five attempts. Then two weeks after the last insemination, my period was late. I waited 24 hours, then bought the pregnancy test. I carried the results to work with me that morning to show to a friend to make sure I was seeing the plus sign. She cried, I cried, Jack bought the baby a teddy bear. Rachel was born nine months later. And now Rachel has a little brother, also through artificial insemination. I can't help but feel we've somehow cheated nature . . . twice."

Tavia's story is yet one more miracle. "After trying for months to get pregnant, we finally did it. We were so thrilled the day the pregnancy test came back positive. Then our lives took a dismal turn. In my second month, I awoke with excruciating pain and nausea. I immediately called my ob-gyn. He said it sounded like a possible tubal pregnancy and to get to the hospital just in case.

"After a series of tests, which confirmed the diagnosis, then emergency surgery, my doctor came to me during recovery. I'll never forget the grim look on his face as he explained that the pregnancy was in my tube, and that in the process of removing it, he'd been forced to cut out the tube—it was distended from the pregnancy. My other tube wasn't functional, so the doctor explained that Jeff and I were now technically infertile. He suggested we talk to one of the other doctors in his office about a procedure called in vitro fertilization (IVF). The terms he was throwing around were foreign at best.

"The road was very rocky for a while—test after test, insurance appeals to gain coverage for high-tech infertility procedures, making appointments for lab work while trying to manage a home and a full-time career. We had orientation in January 1998 for the IVF program. A woman at work heard what we were going through and told me she and her husband had gone through IVF with the same doctors and their program was actually one of the best in the nation. I had hope.

"To prepare for the IVF, we began our medications in March 1998. The nurse taught me how to give myself injections and taught Jeff how to give them to me as well. (Before this whole experience, Jeff got queasy if someone even suggested needles. Now he's a pro at giving injections.) I spent most of March at the doctor's office, having blood drawn and getting ultrasounds. Everything was progressing nicely. At one ultrasound to check the number of eggs I was producing, the ultrasonographer said, 'Holy cow, woman! There's an army of eggs here! I think we're ready for harvesting.' With that, we set up the appointment for the harvesting and transfer. We took the last of the injections and waited for Friday.

"The doctor's office, usually a bevy of activity, was oddly quiet and serene that Friday afternoon. After my doctor explained the entire procedure of harvesting and preparing the eggs, Jeff and I sat in our room, waiting and praying that all would go well.

"The doctor told us he was able to harvest sixteen eggs and they'd be able to tell us the next day how many had been fertilized. The next day, a nurse called us to say that fifteen had been fertilized. She emphasized that everything went very well and we should be pleased with our progress so far. When we went back on Sunday for the embryo transfer, my doctor explained that twelve of the fifteen fertilized eggs were viable embryos. Three had not fertilized well. We chose to implant three of the embryos, though the doctor's recommendation was to transfer two. He thought we were good candidates for multiple gestation and he thought triplets would be a little risky.

"As Jeff and I entered the sterile room, an embryologist wheeled in an incubator with a small petri dish in it. She had the dish set up under a microscope so we could see the embryos before the transfer. It was our future family and so surreal.

"The IVF worked. I was pregnant. Because of a myriad of problems throughout the pregnancy, including blood clots and preeclampsia, my doctor decided to induce labor the day after Thanksgiving. After I went through thirty-four hours of labor and finally a C-section, our gorgeous daughter was born. She is the light of our lives, our angel. And you know what? I'd repeat the whole procedure in a heartbeat—for such a wonderful result."

Keeping in mind that despite the odds couples with fertility problems still get pregnant can sustain you in the most anxious moments. Millions of women like Lorri and Tavia conceive even when the doctors give no hope—so can you.

When life gets tough, remember that:

- Hope keeps on keeping on when you want to give up.
- Hope is strong because it believes in the future.
- Hope copes.
- Hope breeds courage and confidence.
- Hope is optimistic.
- Hope helps you remember what you do have—not what you don't have.
- Hope keeps you focused on your strengths instead of your weaknesses.
- Hope moves forward when you have setbacks.
- Hope gives you reason to laugh even in tough times.

As you take advantage of the wealth of information in this book and follow the baby-making tips and lifestyle suggestions, you will be well on your way to getting pregnant. The success stories show that no matter what your infertility situation is, there are answers. No matter what the test results are today, you have to hold on to the hope for tomorrow that your goal of making a baby will be realized.

And the greatest of these . . . is hope.

Appendix

Acronyms and Abbreviations

ACTH = adrenocorticotropic hormone

AFP = alpha-fetoprotein

AH, AZH = assisted hatching

AI = artificial insemination

AID = artificial insemination (donor)

AIH = artificial insemination (husband)

ANA = anti-nuclear antibodies

APA = anti-phospholipid antibodies

ART = assisted reproductive technology

ASA = anti-sperm antibody

ASRM = American Society for Reproductive Medicine

BBT = basal body temperature

βHCG = beta human chorionic gonadotropin

CASA = computer-assisted semen analysis

CCCT, CCT = clomiphene citrate challenge test (Clomid challenge test)

CVS = chorionic villae sampling

Cx = cervix

D&C = dilation & curettage

DE = donor eggs

DES = diethylstilbestrol

DHEAS = dihydroepiandrosterone sulfate

DI = donor insemination

DNA = deoxyribonucleic acid

DOST = direct oocyte-sperm transfer
E2 = estradiol
ENDO = endometriosis
EPT = early pregnancy test
ET = embryo transfer
ETA = embryo toxicity assay
FET = frozen embryo transfer
FSH = follicle-stimulating hormone
GIFT = gamete intrafallopian transfer
GnRH = gonadotropin-releasing hormone
GTT = glucose tolerance test
hCG = human chorionic gonadotropin
HEPA = hamster egg penetration assay
HIV = human immunodeficiency virus
HMG = human menopausal gonadotropin
HPT = home pregnancy test
HRT = hormone replacement therapy
HSG = hysterosalpingogram
IBT = immunobead binding test
ICSI = intracytoplasmic sperm injection
IOR = immature oocyte retrieval
IR = insulin resistant
IU = International units
IUI = intrauterine insemination
IVF = in vitro fertilization
IVIg = intravenous immunoglobulin
LAP = laparoscopy/laparotomy
LH = luteinizing hormone
LIT = leukocyte immunization therapy
LPD = luteal phase defect
MESA = microsurgical epididymal sperm aspiration
MRI = magnetic resonance imaging
OHSS = ovarian hyperstimulation syndrome
OPK = ovulation predictor kit
PCOS = polycystic ovarian syndrome (PCOD)
PCT = postcoital test
PESA = percutaneous epididymal sperm aspiration
PID = pelvic inflammatory disease

PMS = premenstrual syndrome
PN = pronuclear (stage of development)
POF = premature ovarian failure
RPL = recurrent pregnancy loss
SA = semen analysis
SART = Society of Assisted Reproductive Technology
SPA = sperm penetration assay
STD = sexually transmitted disease
TESA = testicular sperm aspiration
TESE = testicular sperm extraction
TET = tubal embryo transfer
TSH = thyroid-stimulating hormone
U/S = ultrasound
UTI = urinary tract infection
ZIFT = zygote intrafallopian transfer

Internet Sites

http://fertilethoughts.net
http://www.resolve.org   RESOLVE
http://www.ihr.com/infertility/index.html   Infertility Resources
http://www.reutershealth.com/   Reuters Health Information
http://jazz.san.uc.edu/~pranikjd/infertil.html   GYN Web Library
http://www.ihr.com/infertility/drugs.html   Infertility Drugs
http://womenshealth.miningco.com   Women's Health—Mining
   Company
http://www.homepage.holowww.com/lf.htm   Fertility Weekly (weekly
   digest on fertility and human reproduction)
http://www.womens-health.com/inf_ctr/index.html   Women's
   Health Interactive—Infertility Center
http://www.noah.cuny.edu/pregnancy/fertility.html   Ask Noah About
   Pregnancy—Fertility and Infertility
http://www.asrm.org/   The American Society for Reproductive
   Medicine
http://www.vgme.com/jarl.htm   The Journal of Assisted Reproductive Law

http://search.intelihealth.com   Johns Hopkins Health Information

http://www.goaskalice.columbia.edu/Cat7.html   Go Ask Alice! Sexual
Health at Columbia University

http://www.merck.com   The Merck Manual

http://www.inciid.org   INCIID (International Council on Infertility
Information Dissemination)

http://www.inciid.org/links.html#Barriers   Infertility and Pregnancy
Loss INCIID Links and Online Resources

http://www.betterhealth.com/BetterHealth   iVillage Better Health

http://search.onhealth.com   OnHealth

http://pregnancy.tqn.com/msubmiscarriage.htm   Miscarriage links

http://www.fertilethoughts.com   Ask Fertile Thoughts

http://www.asrm.abstracts.org   American Society for Reproductive
Medicine (ASRM)

http://www.ncbi.nlm.nih.gov/PubMed   Medline (copies of journal
articles)

http://www.ama-assn.org   Journal of the American Medical Association

http://www.acupuncturecenter.com   New York Center for Acupuncture and Alternative Medicine

http://www.pinelandpress.com/toc.html   Fertility Plus

http://www.fertilitext.org   Fertilitex

http://medlineplus.nlm.nih.gov/medlineplus/serachdatabases.html
Medline Plus (National Library of Medicine)

http://www.healthfinder.gov/   A gateway consumer health and human services consumer website

http://www.hon.ch/   Health on the Net Foundation

http://www.stairway.bc.ca/tickle/adopt.html   Infertility and adoption
resources available on the net

http://webcom.com/~tapestry/welcome.html   Adoption and infertility books available

http://www.surrogacy.com   The American Surrogacy Center

http://www.pcosa.org   Polycystic ovarian syndrome support organization

Newsletters

RESOLVE National Newsletter
Phone: 617-623-1156

A 16-page quarterly newsletter free with RESOLVE membership.

INCIID National Newsletter
Phone: 520-554-9548

A quarterly newsletter free with INCIID membership.

Donors' Offspring
P.O. Box 37
Sarcoxie, MO 64862

A quarterly newsletter that covers issues concerning donor insemination.

Support Groups and Organizations

American Society for Reproductive Medicine
1209 Montgomery Highway
Birmingham, AL 35216
205-978-5000

Professional society of reproductive endocrinologists and ob/gyns involved in infertility treatment.

RESOLVE
1310 Broadway
Somerville, MA, 02144
Business office: 617-623-1156
Helpline: 617-623-0744

RESOLVE's mission is to provide timely, compassionate support and information to people who are experiencing infertility and to increase awareness of infertility issues through advocacy and public education.

INCIID
P.O. Box 91363
Tucson, AZ 85752
520-554-9548

The mission of the International Council on Infertility Information Dissemination (INCIID, pronounced "inside") is to promote the exchange of information between fertility experts and those who suffer from infertility and pregnancy loss.

Glossary

abortion Pregnancy loss by any cause before 20 weeks of gestation.

    spontaneous Pregnancy loss during the first 20 weeks of gestation.

    habitual Three or more miscarriages.

    incomplete Abortion after which some tissue remains inside the uterus. A D&C must be performed to remove the tissue and prevent complications.

    missed The fetus dies in the uterus, but there is no bleeding or cramping. A D&C will be needed to remove the fetal remains and prevent complications.

    therapeutic A procedure used to terminate a pregnancy before the fetus can survive on its own.

    threatened Spotting or bleeding that occurs early in the pregnancy. May progress to spontaneous abortion.

ACTH A hormone produced by the pituitary gland to stimulate the adrenal glands. Excessive levels may lead to fertility problems.

adhesion Scar tissue in the abdominal cavity, fallopian tubes, or inside the uterus, which can interfere with the pickup or transport of the egg and implantation of the embryo in the uterus.

adrenal androgens Male hormones produced by the adrenal gland which in excess may lead to fertility problems in men and women. Elevated levels of androgens are associated with PCOS.

amenorrhea Cessation of the menstrual periods for 6 months or more at a time. *Primary amenorrhea* is when a woman has never menstruated. *Secondary amenorrhea* is when a woman has menstruated at one time but has not had a period for 6 months or more.

American Society of Reproductive Medicine (ASRM)   A large organization serving as a platform for education, innovation, and advocacy in fertility and reproductive medicine issues.

amniocentesis   A sampling of a small quantity of the fluid that surrounds the fetus. It permits the detection of certain abnormalities.

andrologist   A physician-scientist (M.D. or Ph.D.) who performs laboratory evaluations of male fertility.

anovulation   Absence of ovulation, yet a menstrual period may still occur.

antibodies   Chemicals made by the body to fight or attack foreign substances entering the body. Normally they prevent infection; however, when they attack the sperm or fetus, they cause infertility. Sperm antibodies may be made by either the man or the woman.

artificial insemination (AI)   A high-tech method of placing sperm into the vagina, uterus, or fallopian tubes through artificial means instead of by intercourse.

Asherman's syndrome   A condition usually caused by uterine inflammation whereby the uterine walls adhere to one another.

aspiration   The removal of fluid and/or cells by suction through a needle.

assay   Test.

assisted hatching   A microscopic procedure that chemically or mechanically dissolves the protein halo around the embryo surface to facilitate implantation.

assisted reproductive technologies (ART)   A group of procedures including IUI, IVF, GIFT, and ZIFT; these employ manipulation of the egg and/or sperm to establish a pregnancy.

asthenozoospermia   Low sperm motility.

azoospermia   Semen containing no sperm, either because the testes cannot make sperm or because of blockage in the reproductive tract.

basal body temperature (BBT)   The body temperature at rest. It is taken orally each morning immediately upon awakening and recorded on a calendar chart. The readings are studied to help identify the time of ovulation.

beta hCG test   A blood test used to detect very early pregnancies and to evaluate embryonic development.

bicornuate uterus   A congenital malformation of the uterus in which the uterus is Y-shaped rather than heart-shaped.

blighted ovum (egg)   A fertilized egg that fails to survive after implantation in the uterus.

bromocriptine (Parlodel) An oral medication used to reduce prolactin levels and reduce the size of a pituitary tumor when one is present.

canceled cycle Discontinuation of the cycle due to one of the following: poor response, no oocyte recovery, or failed fertilization.

candidiasis A yeast infection that has a burning and a "curdy" discharge.

CBC (complete blood count) A routine preoperative blood test that gives information regarding infection and anemia.

cervical factor Infertility due to previous surgery or structural abnormality of the cervix. Also applied when there are factors associated with the cervix that inhibit sperm function.

cervical mucus Mucus produced by the cervix that permits or inhibits the passage of sperm to the uterus and fallopian tubes depending on time in the menstrual cycle. It increases in volume, elasticity, and clarity before ovulation.

cervical smear A sample of the cervical mucus examined microscopically to assess the presence of estrogen and white blood cells, indicating possible infection (Pap smear).

cervical stenosis A narrowing of the cervical canal from a congenital defect or from complications of surgical procedures.

cervix The lower section of the uterus that protrudes into the vagina and serves as a reservoir for sperm. The cervix remains closed during pregnancy and dilates during labor and delivery to allow the baby to be born.

cervix, incompetent A weakened cervix that opens prematurely during pregnancy and can cause the loss of the fetus. A *cervical cerclage* is a procedure in which a stitch or two is put around the cervix to prevent its opening until removed when the pregnancy is to term.

chemical pregnancy A positive pregnancy test, but with levels of pregnancy hormone too low for the ultrasound documentation of a pregnancy.

chocolate cyst A cyst in the ovary that is filled with old blood and tissue from endometriosis; endometrioma. This occurs when endometriosis invades an ovary, causing the ovary to swell.

chromosome The structures in a cell that carry the genetic material (genes); the genetic messengers of inheritance (DNA). The human has 46 chromosomes, 23 coming from the egg and 23 coming from the sperm.

cilia Tiny hairlike projections lining the inside surface of the fallopian tubes. The waving action of these hairs sweeps the egg toward the uterus and the sperm toward the egg.

clinical pregnancy A pregnancy in which the beating fetal heart has been identified by ultrasound.

clomiphene citrate An oral fertility drug that stimulates ovulation through the release of gonadotropins from the pituitary gland.

controlled ovarian hyperstimulation The use of fertility drugs to stimulate multiple follicle growth.

corpus luteum A portion of the ovary that forms from the follicle after ovulation. It produces progesterone during the second half of the cycle, which is necessary to prepare the uterine lining for implantation.

cryopreservation Controlled freezing and storage.

Cushing's syndrome A condition characterized by an overproduction of adrenal gland hormone cortisol.

cycle This refers to the period of time when infertility treatment is initiated and continues until treatment is discontinued or completed—usually one month.

cyst A fluid-filled structure. May be normal or abnormal depending on circumstances.

D&C (dilation and curettage) A procedure used to dilate the cervical canal and scrape out the lining and contents of the uterus.

Danazol (danocrine) A medication used to treat endometriosis. Suppression of LH and FSH production by the pituitary causes a state of amenorrhea, during which the endometrial implants are reduced. Many women experience oily skin, acne, weight gain, abnormal hair growth, deepening of the voice, and muscle cramps with this medication.

DES (diethylstilbestrol) A medication prescribed to women during the 1950s and 1960s to prevent miscarriage. Male and female fetuses exposed in utero to this drug developed numerous deformities, including blockage of the vas deferens, uterine abnormalities, cervical deformities, miscarriages, and unexplained infertility. DES is no longer prescribed for miscarriage.

DHEAS (dehydroepiandrosterone sulfate) An androgen produced primarily by the adrenal gland. A high level suggests too much adrenal androgen output and may be associated with polycystic ovaries.

donor insemination The introduction of sperm from a volunteer donor into a women's vagina, cervix, or uterine cavity in order to achieve a pregnancy.

donor embryo transfer The transfer of a fertilized egg from a volunteer (may be paid or unpaid) donor to an otherwise infertile recipient.

ectopic pregnancy A pregnancy in which the fertilized egg implants outside the uterine cavity (usually in the fallopian tube, the ovary, or the abdominal cavity).

egg retrieval A procedure used to obtain eggs from ovarian follicles for use in in vitro fertilization. The procedure may be performed during laparoscopy or by using a long needle fitted to an ultrasound transducer.

ejaculate The semen and sperm expelled during ejaculation.

embryo The early stages of fetal growth from conception through the eighth week of pregnancy.

embryo transfer Placing an egg fertilized in the laboratory into a woman's uterus or fallopian tube.

endocrinology The study of hormones, their function, the organs that produce them, and how they are produced.

endometrial biopsy The extraction of a small piece of tissue from the endometrium (lining of the uterus) for microscopic examination.

endometriosis The presence of endometrial tissue in abnormal locations such as the fallopian tubes, ovaries, and peritoneal cavity, which often causes painful menstruation and infertility.

endometrium The inner lining of the uterus, which grows and sheds in response to estrogen and progesterone stimulation.

endorphins The body's natural narcotics manufactured in the brain to reduce sensitivity to pain and stress.

epididymis A tubular structure attached to the male's testis that serves as a reservoir where sperm mature and are stored.

estradiol The principal hormone produced by the growing ovarian follicle.

estrogen A female sex hormone.

fallopian tube Either of a pair of tubes that transfer sperm, pick up eggs, serve as a site of fertilization, and nurture the embryo on its path to the uterus.

fertility specialist A physician specializing in the practice of fertility. The American Board of Obstetrics and Gynecology certifies a subspecialty for ob-gyns who receive extra training in endocrinology (the study of hormones) and infertility. Those who acquire certification are reproductive endocrinologists (REs).

fertilization The union of a sperm with an oocyte.

fetus A term used to refer to a baby during the period of gestation between 8 weeks and term.

fibroid (myoma) A benign tumor of the uterine muscle and connective tissue.

fimbria The finger-like extensions from the end of the uterine tube that aid in gathering the oocyte at ovulation.

follicle A small cyst in the ovary which nurtures and eventually ruptures to release ovulation.

follicle-stimulating hormone (FSH) A hormone produced by the pituitary gland that causes the ovarian follicles to grow.

follicular fluid The fluid inside the follicle that cushions and nourishes the ovum. When released during ovulation, the fluid stimulates the fimbria to grasp the ovary and coax the egg into the fallopian tube.

follicular phase The first part of the menstrual cycle, when ovarian follicular development occurs.

galactorrhea A clear or milky discharge from the breasts, possibly associated with elevated prolactin.

gamete A reproductive cell (sperm in men; the egg in women).

gamete intrafallopian transfer (GIFT) A technique that may be used instead of in vitro fertilization for women with patent (clear and open) tubes. After egg retrieval, the eggs are mixed with the husband's sperm and then injected through the fimbria into the woman's fallopian tubes for in vivo fertilization.

gestation The period of the pregnancy from conception to birth, usually considered to be 40 weeks in humans from the last menstrual period.

gonad The gland that makes reproductive cells and sex hormones: the testicles, which make sperm and testosterone, and the ovaries, which make eggs (ova) and estrogen.

gonadotropin A hormone that stimulates the ovary or testis.

gonadotropin-releasing hormone (GnRH) The hormone controlling the production and release of gonadotropins. Secreted by the hypothalamus every ninety minutes or so, this hormone enables the pituitary to secrete LH and FSH, which stimulate the gonads to produce estrogen and testosterone. *See* FSH *and* LH.

hamster test   A test of the ability of human sperm to penetrate a hamster egg stripped of the zona pellucida (outer membrane). Also called sperm penetration assay (SPA).

hirsutism   The overabundance of sexual body hair, such as a mustache or pubic hair growing upward toward the navel, found in women with excess androgens.

HIV   A retrovirus that causes acquired immune deficiency syndrome (AIDS). It is transmitted by the exchange of bodily fluids or blood transfusions.

hormonal assay   A chemical substance produced in the body by an organ or cells of an organ that has a specific regulatory effect on the activity of another organ.

hostile mucus   Cervical mucus that impedes the natural progress of sperm through the cervical canal.

host uterus (surrogate gestational mother)   A couple's embryo is transferred to another woman. She carries the pregnancy to term and returns the baby to the genetic parents immediately after birth.

human chorionic gonadotropin (hCG)   The hormone produced in early pregnancy that keeps the corpus luteum producing progesterone. Also used via injection to trigger ovulation after some fertility treatments, and used in men to stimulate testosterone production.

human menopausal gonadotropin (HMG)   A purified extract of LH and FSH, hormones secreted from the pituitary gland that stimulate the ovary. It is a commercial preparation used by injection to facilitate development of multiple follicles.

hydrocele   A swelling in the scrotum that contains fluid.

hyperprolactinemia   A condition in which the pituitary gland secretes too much prolactin. Prolactin can suppress LH and FSH production, reduce male sex drive, and directly suppress ovarian function.

hyperstimulation (ovarian hyperstimulation syndrome—OHSS)   A potentially life-threatening side effect of fertility drugs. Ovaries become markedly enlarged. In severe cases, fluid may collect in the lungs or abdominal cavity. The most serious complication can be blood clots. Symptoms include rapid weight gain and abdominal pain. Cycles stimulated with these drugs must be carefully monitored with ultrasound scans. OHSS may be prevented by withholding the hCG injection when ultrasound monitoring indicates that too many follicles have matured.

hyperthyroidism Overproduction of thyroid hormone by the thyroid gland.

hypoestrogenic Having lower than normal levels of estrogen.

hypothalamus A part of the brain, the hormonal regulation center, located adjacent to and above the pituitary gland. In both men and women this tissue secretes GnRH every ninety minutes or so. The pulsatile GnRH enables the pituitary gland to secrete LH and FSH.

hypothyroidism A condition in which the thyroid gland produces an insufficient amount of thyroid hormone. The resulting lowered metabolism causes lethargy and weight gain. Men will suffer from a lowered sex drive and elevated prolactin (see hyperprolactinemia), and women will suffer from elevated prolactin and estrogen, both of which will interfere with fertility.

hysterectomy The removal of the uterus, which can be total (including the removal of the cervix) or partial (just the upper uterus).

hysterosalpingogram (HSG) An x-ray procedure in which a special dye is injected into the uterus to illustrate the inner contour of the uterus and degree of openness (patency) of the fallopian tubes.

hysteroscope A telescopic device, much like the laparoscope, that enables examination of the uterine cavity.

idiopathic infertility Unexplained infertility.

immature sperm A sperm that has not matured and gained the ability to swim. In the presence of illness or infection, such sperm may appear in the semen in large numbers.

implantation The embedding of the fertilized egg into the lining of the uterus.

impotence (erectile dysfunction) The inability of the man to have an erection and to ejaculate.

in vitro fertilization (IVF) Literally means "in glass." A method of assisted reproduction that involves surgically removing an egg from the ovary and combining it with prepared sperm in the laboratory to permit fertilization.

infertility The inability to conceive after a year of unprotected intercourse or the inability to carry a pregnancy to term.

insemination Transfer of semen or sperm for the purpose of establishing a pregnancy.

intracytoplasmic sperm injection (ICSI) The placement of a single sperm into an oocyte (egg) using a small glass needle to penetrate the outer coatings of the egg.

intrauterine insemination (IUI)   A relatively low-tech ART that deposits washed sperm directly into the uterus through the cervix.

karyotyping   A test performed to analyze chromosomes for the presence of genetic defects.

Klinefelter's syndrome   A genetic abnormality characterized by having one Y (male) and an extra X chromosome; it may cause a fertility problem.

laparoscope   A small, lighted telescope that can be inserted into a hole in the abdominal wall for viewing the pelvic cavity, ovaries, fallopian tubes, and uterus. (This procedure is called laparoscopy.)

laparotomy   Major abdominal surgery in which reproductive organ abnormalities can be corrected (for example, tubal repairs and the removal of adhesions) and fertility restored.

Leydig cell   The testicular cell that produces the male hormone testosterone. The Leydig cell is stimulated by LH from the pituitary gland.

LH (luteinizing hormone)   A hormone secreted by the anterior pituitary that causes the mature egg to be released by the ovary (ovulation). In the male, LH stimulates testosterone production.

LH surge   A spontaneous release of large amounts of luteinizing hormone (LH). This normally results in the release of a mature egg (ovulation).

luteal phase   The final part of the menstrual cycle that occurs after ovulation and ends either with embryo implantation or menstruation.

luteal phase defect (or deficiency) (LPD)   A condition that occurs when the uterine lining does not develop adequately because of inadequate progesterone stimulation; or because of the inability of the uterine lining to respond to progesterone stimulation. LPD may prevent embryonic implantation or cause an early abortion.

male-factor infertility   The term used to describe the condition when the couple's infertility is attributed to the male partner.

menorrhagia   Heavy or prolonged menstrual flow.

menses   The cyclic (monthly) flow of blood (menstruation) signifying ovulation, but failure to achieve pregnancy. The onset of bleeding is considered cycle day 1.

metrorrhagia   Bleeding from the uterus that is not associated with menstruation.

micromanipulation A process manually performed with the help of a microscope.

miscarriage Spontaneous loss of an embryo or fetus from the womb (*see* abortion).

mittelschmerz The abdominal discomfort felt at the time of ovulation.

myomectomy The surgical removal of fibroid tumors from the wall of the uterus.

oligomenorrhea Infrequent menstrual periods.

oligospermia Abnormally low sperm numbers.

oocyte (ovum, gamete) The female gamete or egg.

oocyte retrieval A surgical procedure to collect the eggs contained with the ovarian follicles.

ovarian cyst A fluid-filled sac of the ovary. An ovarian cyst may be found in conjunction with ovulation disorders, tumors of the ovary, and endometriosis. *See also* chocolate cyst.

ovarian failure The failure of the ovary to respond to FSH stimulation from the pituitary because of damage to or malformation of the ovary. Diagnosed by elevated FSH in the blood.

ovary The female sex gland with both a reproductive function (releasing oocytes) and a hormonal function (production of estrogen and progesterone).

ovulation The release of a mature egg from the surface of the ovary.

ovulation induction The use of female hormone therapy to stimulate oocyte development and release.

ovulatory phase When discharge of a mature egg occurs, usually around midcycle.

ovum (ova, egg) A mature oocyte.

Pap test A screening test named after Dr. George Papanicolaou to determine the presence of cervical cancer. It is done by gently touching a cotton swab on the cervix and then wiping the swab on a slide, which is treated and examined under a microscope.

patent Open.

pelvic inflammatory disease (PID) An infection of the pelvic organs that causes severe illness, high fever, and extreme pain. PID may lead to tubal blockage and pelvic adhesions.

pituitary gland The gland stimulated by the hypothalamus that controls all hormonal functions.

placenta The embryonic tissue that invades the uterine wall and provides a mechanism for exchanging the baby's waste products for the mother's nutrients and oxygen. The baby is connected to the placenta by the umbilical cord.

polycystic ovarian syndrome (PCOS, or Stein-Leventhal syndrome) A condition found in women who don't ovulate, usually characterized by obesity, excessive production of androgens (male sex hormones), irregular periods, and the presence of cysts in the ovaries.

postcoital test (PCT) A microscopic examination of the cervical mucus best performed twelve or more hours after intercourse to determine compatibility between the woman's mucus and the man's semen; a test used to detect sperm-mucus interaction problems, the presence of sperm antibodies, and the quality of the cervical mucus.

premature ovarian failure A condition where the ovary runs out of follicles before age 40.

progesterone A hormone produced by the corpus luteum of the ovary after ovulation has occurred; it prepares the uterus for a possible pregnancy.

prolactin A hormone that stimulates the production of milk in breastfeeding women. Excessive prolactin levels when one is not breastfeeding may result in infertility.

pronuclear stage tubal transfer (PROST) (ZIFT) A procedure whereby oocytes are aspirated, allowed to fertilize in vitro, and the conceptus transferred before cell division.

prostaglandins Hormone-like substances found in men and women. It is hypothesized that prostaglandins secreted by active young endometrial implants may interfere with the reproductive organs by causing muscular contractions or spasms. Also, prostaglandins not washed from sperm can cause severe cramping during IUI procedures.

prostate gland A gland in the male reproductive system that produces a portion of the semen, including a chemical that liquefies the coagulated semen 20 minutes to an hour after entering the vagina.

retrograde ejaculation A male fertility problem where sperm are ejaculated into the bladder instead of out the opening of the penis due to a failure in the sphincter muscle at the base of the bladder.

salpingectomy Surgical removal of the fallopian tube.

scrotum The bag of skin and thin muscle surrounding the man's testicles.

secondary infertility   The inability of a couple to achieve a pregnancy after having been pregnant.

secondary sex characteristics   The physical qualities that distinguish man and woman, such as beard, functional breasts, and deep voice. Formed under the stimulation of the sex hormones (testosterone or estrogen), these characteristics also identify those people who have gone through puberty (sexual maturity).

semen   The fluid portion of the ejaculate consisting of secretions from the seminal vesicles, prostate gland, and several other glands in the male reproductive tract. The semen provides nourishment and protection for the sperm and a medium through which the sperm can travel to the woman's vagina. Semen may also refer to the entire ejaculate, including the sperm.

semen analysis   A laboratory test used to assess semen quality: sperm quantity, concentration, morphology (form), and motility. In addition, it measures semen (fluid) volume and whether or not white blood cells are present, indicating an infection.

semen viscosity   The liquid flow or consistency of the semen.

septate uterus   A uterus divided into right and left halves by a wall of tissue (septum). Women with a septate uterus have an increased chance of early pregnancy loss.

sonogram (ultrasound)   Use of high-frequency sound waves for creating an image of internal body parts. Used to detect and count follicle growth (and disappearance) in many fertility treatments. Also used to detect and monitor pregnancy.

sperm penetration assay (SPA)   A test where sperm are incubated with nonviable hamster eggs to determine the capacity of the sperm to fertilize (*see* hamster test).

sperm   The male reproductive cell.

sperm motility   The ability of sperm to swim. Poor motility means the sperm have a difficult time swimming toward their goal—the egg.

sperm morphology   A semen analysis factor that indicates the number or percentage of sperm in the sample that appear to have been formed normally. Abnormal morphology includes sperm with kinked, doubled, or coiled tails. The higher the percentage of misshapen sperm, the less likely fertilization can take place.

sperm maturation   A process during which the sperm grow and gain their ability to swim. Sperm take about 90 days to reach maturity.

sperm penetration   The ability of the sperm to penetrate the egg so it can deposit the genetic material during fertilization.

sperm bank   A place where sperm are kept frozen in liquid nitrogen for later use in artificial insemination.

sperm wash   A technique for separating sperm from seminal fluid.

sterility   An irreversible condition that prevents conception.

stillbirth   The death of a fetus before the twentieth week of gestation and birth.

superovulation   Stimulation of multiple follicle growth with fertility drugs; also known as controlled ovarian hyperstimulation (COH).

surrogate mother   A woman carries a pregnancy for another woman; may be a traditional surrogate, inseminated, and genetically related to the child, or gestational, carrying an embryo conceived by IVF for an infertile couple and not genetically related to the child.

testicles   The two male sexual glands (testes) and associated structures.

testicular/epididymal sperm aspiration (TESA)   The removal of sperm directly from the testis or the epididymis, using a needle for aspiration.

testosterone   The male hormone responsible for the formation of secondary sex characteristics and for supporting the sex drive. Testosterone is also necessary for spermatogenesis.

TET (tubal embryo transfer)   A process in which a fertilized and divided egg is transferred to the fallopian tubes.

Turner's syndrome   The most common chromosomal defect contributing to female fertility problems. The ovaries fail to form and appear as slender threads of atrophic ovarian tissue, referred to as streak ovaries. Karyotyping will reveal that this woman has only one female (X) chromosome instead of two.

ultrasound (sonogram)   High frequency sound waves that can be used painlessly, safely, and without radiation to view the internal portions of the body.

unicornate uterus   An abnormality in which the uterus is one-sided and smaller than usual.

ureaplasma (mycoplasma)   A genus of bacteria that may cause an infection; this may result in the formation of sperm antibodies and an inflammation of the uterine lining, either of which may interfere with implantation of the embryo.

urethra   The tube that allows urine to pass between the bladder and the outside of the body. In the man, this tube also carries semen from the area of the prostate to the outside.

urologist A physician specializing in the genitourinary tract.

uterine tube (fallopian) The anatomic and physiologic connection between the uterus and the ovary. It serves to transport the egg and sperm, as the site of fertilization and support, and to transport the conceptus en route to the uterus.

uterus (womb) The reproductive organ that houses, protects, and nourishes the developing embryo and fetus.

vaginal ultrasound Visualization of soft tissue by projecting sound waves through a probe inserted into the vagina. A baseline ultrasound shows the ovaries in their normal state. A follicular ultrasound shows egg follicle maturation. A pregnancy ultrasound shows if a pregnancy is intrauterine or tubal and measures growth.

vaginitis Yeast, bacterial vaginosis, or trichomonas infections of the vagina.

varicocele A varicose vein around the ductus deferens and the testes that may cause male infertility.

vasectomy The accidental or elective surgical separation of the vasa deferentia; a procedure used for birth control.

venereal diseases Any infection that can be sexually transmitted, such as chlamydia, gonorrhea, ureaplasma, and syphilis. Many of these diseases will interfere with fertility and some will cause severe illness. *See also* pelvic inflammatory disease.

zygote A fertilized egg that has not yet divided.

zygote intrafallopian transfer (ZIFT) An ART that transfers a zygote, or fertilized egg, into a fallopian tube one day after its fertilization.

References

A Committee Opinion: Intravenous Immunoglobulin (IVIG) and Recurrent Pregnancy Loss. *American Society for Reproductive Medicine: A Practice Committee Report*, October 1998.

Akira, S., et al. Gasless laparoscopic ovarian cystectomy during pregnancy: comparison with laparotomy. *American Journal of Obstetrics and Gynecology* 180:554–57, March 1999.

Allen, S.E., et al. Prevalence of hyperandrogenemia among nonhirsute oligo-ovulatory women. *Fertility and Sterility* 67:567–72, March 1997.

American Dietetic Association 1997 Nutrition Trends Survey, American Dietetic Association, September 1997.

Arcaini, L., J.P. Balmaceda, L.N. Weckstein, et al. Reproductive performance in women aged 40 and over: analysis of different infertility treatments. Read before the 46th annual meeting of the American Fertility Society, October 15–18, 1990, Washington, D.C.

Asch, R.H., T. Ord, S. Stone, et al. Assisted reproductive techniques in women over 40 years of age: IVF, GIFT, ZIFT, egg donation: is there a best alternative? Read before the 39th annual meeting of the Pacific Coast Fertility Society, April 10–14, 1991, Scottsdale, Arizona.

Ballagh, S., et al. Is curettage needed for uncomplicated incomplete spontaneous abortion? *American Journal of Obstetrics and Gynecology* 179: 1279–1282, November 1998.

Bartels, C.L., and S.J. Miller. Herbal and related remedies. *Nutrition in Clinical Practice* 12(2):5–19, 1998.

Beisel, W. History of nutritional immunology: introduction and overview. *Journal of Nutrition.* 122:591–596, 1992.

Benson, Herbert, and Marg Stark. Reason to believe. *Natural Health.* May–June 1996, 74.

Bjorkman, D.J. The effect of aspirin and nonsteroidal anti-inflammatory drugs on prostaglandins. *American Journal of Medicine* 105(b): 8S–12S, July 1998.

Bonjour, J.P., et al. Nutritional aspects of hip fractures. *Bone* 18(3 Suppl):139S–144S, March 1996.

Bowman, M.A., and J.G. Spangler. Osteoporosis in women. *Primary Care* 24(1):27–36, 1997.

Bussen, S., et al. Endocrine abnormalities during the follicular phase in women with recurrent spontaneous abortion. *Human Reproduction* 14:18–20, January 1999.

Caan, B., et al. Caffeine consumption does not impair fertility. *American Journal of Public Health* 88:270–74, March 1998.

Callahan, Maureen, M.S., R.D. Antioxidants and fewer health problems. *Bottom Line Personal.* January 15, 1996, 8.

Camara, E.G., and T.C. Danao. The brain and the immune system. *Psychosomatics* 30(2):140–48, 1989.

Center, J., et al. Mortality after all major types of osteoporotic fracture in men and women: an observational study. *The Lancet* 353:878–882, March 13, 1999.

Chandra, R.K. Nutrition and the immune system: an introduction. *American Journal of Clinical Nutrition* 66(2):460S–63S, 1997.

Chew, B.P. Antioxidant vitamins affect food animal immunity and health. *Journal of Nutrition* 125(6 Suppl):1804s–1808s, June 1995.

Clamlan, H.N. The biology of the immune response. *Journal of the American Medical Association.* 268(20):2790–2801, 1992.

Cohen, S., and T.B. Herbert. Health psychology: psychological factors and physical disease from the perspective of human psychoneuroimmunology. *Annual Review of Psychology* 47:113–42, 1996.

Cohen, S., D.A. Tyrrell, and A.P. Smith. Psychological stress and susceptibility to the common cold. *New England Journal of Medicine* 325: 606–12, 1991.

Dulitzki, M., et al. Effect of very advanced maternal age on pregnancy outcome and rate of cesarean delivery. *Obstetrics and Gynecology* 92:935–944.

Esplin, M., et al. Thyroid autoantibodies are not associated with recurrent pregnancy loss. *American Journal of Obstetrics and Gynecology* 179:1583–86, December 1998.

Fahey, M.T., L. Irwig, and P. Macaskill. Meta-analysis of Pap test accuracy. *American Journal of Epidemiology*. 141:680–89, 1995.

Fenster, L., et al. Effects of psychological stress on human semen quality. *Journal of Andrology* 18:194–202, March/April 1997.

Ferris, D.G., T.C. Wright, Jr., M.S. Litaker, et al. Triage of women with ASCUS and LSIL Pap smear reports: management by repeat Pap smear, HPV DNA testing, or colposcopy? *Journal of Family Practice*. 46:125–34, 1998.

Fruzzetti, F., et al. Treatment of hirsutism: comparisons between different antiandrogens with central and peripheral effects. *Fertility and Sterility* 71:445–51, March 1999.

Gentile, G. Is there any evidence for post-tubal sterilization syndrome? *Fertility and Sterility* 69:179–86, February 1998.

Glatstein, I.Z., B.L. Harlow, and M.D. Hornstein. *Fertility and Sterility*. 70:2:263–69, August 1998.

Grodstein, F., R. Levine, L. Troy, et al. Three-year follow-up of participants in a commercial weight loss program. Can you keep it off? *Archives of Internal Medicine* 156(12):1302–1306, 1996.

Hafen, Brent O., Ph.D., et al. *Health Effects of Attitudes, Emotions, and Relationships*. Utah: EMS Associates, 1992.

Hall, Nicholas, Ph.D., ed. *Mind-Body Interactions and Disease and Psychoneuroimmunological Aspects of Health and Disease*. Orlando: Health Dateline Press, 1996.

Hata, T., et al. Assessment of embryonic anatomy at 6–8 weeks of gestation by intrauterine and transvaginal sonography. *Human Reproduction* 12:1873–76, September 1997.

Hewitson, L., et al. Unique checkpoints during the first cell cycle of fertilization after intracytoplasmic sperm injection in rhesus monkeys. *Nature Medicine* 5:431–33, April 1999.

Hickman, T., et al. Timing of estrogen replacement therapy following hysterectomy with oophorectomy. *Obstetrics and Gynecology* 5:673–77, May 1998.

Hirsch, Cheryl. Insidious allergies caused by immune system's overreaction. *Health News and Review*, Winter 1995; 9 (2).

Hoffman-Goetz, L. Influence of physical activity and exercise on innate immunity. *Nutrition Reviews* 56(1):S126–S130, 1998.

House, J.S., et al. Social relationships and health. *Science* 241:540, 1988.

Ilich, J.Z. Primary prevention of osteoporosis: pediatric approach to disease of the elderly. *Woman's Health Issues* 6(4):194–203, July–August 1996.

Imani, R., et al. Predictors of patients remaining anovulatory during clomiphene citrate induction of ovulation in normogonadotropic oligomenorrheic infertility. *Journal of Clinical Endocrinology and Metabolism* 83:2361–65, July 1998.

Johnson, M. Genetic risks of intracytoplasmic sperm injection in the treatment of male infertility: recommendations for genetic counseling and screening. *Fertility and Sterility* 70:397–411, September 1998.

Kalden, J.R., et al. Immunological treatment of autoimmune diseases. *Advances in Immunology*. 69:333–417, 1998.

Kendler, K.S. Social support: a genetic-epidemiologic analysis. *American Journal of Psychiatry* 154:1398–1404, October 1997.

Kraemer, W.J., and L.P. Koziris. Muscle strength training: techniques and considerations. *Physical Therapy Practice* 2(1):54–68, 1992.

Levin, J.S. Religion and health: is there an association, is it valid, and is it causal? *Social Science Medicine* 38:1475–82, 1994.

Lipscomb, G., et al. Management of separation pain after single-dose methotrexate therapy for ectopic pregnancy. *Obstetrics and Gynecology* 93:590–93, April 1999.

Lundberg, S., et al. Radionucleotide hysterosalpingography is not predictive in the diagnosis of infertility. *Fertility and Sterility* 69:216–20, February 1998.

McGrady, A., P. Conran, D. Dickey, et al. The effects of biofeedback-assisted relaxation on cell-mediated immunity, cortisol, and white blood cell count in healthy adult subjects. *Journal of Behavioral Medicine* 15(4): 343–54, 1992.

McLaughlin, T., et al. Differences in insulin resistance do not predict weight loss in response to hypocaloric diets in healthy, obese, nondiabetic women. *Journal of Clinical Endocrinology and Medicine* 84: 578–81, February 1999.

Meldrum, D.R., F. Hamilton, B. Mann, et al. Oocyte donation (OD) increases the proportion of embryos implanting and reverses the age-related decline of fertility. Read before the 38th annual meeting of the Pacific Coast Fertility Society, April 25–29, 1990, Scottsdale, Arizona.

MMWR, Centers for Disease Control. Use of folic acid–containing supplements among women of childbearing age—United States, 1997. *Journal of the American Medical Association* 18:1430, May 1998.

Modica, Peter. The ancient art of acupuncture gets FDA approval. May 24, 1996. Medical Tribune News Service.

Moss, R.B., H.B. Moss, and R. Peterson. Microstress, mood, and natural killer-cell activity. *Psychosomatics* 30(3):279–83, 1989.

Muzii, L. Postoperative adhesion prevention with low dose aspirin: effect through the selective inhibition of thromboxane production. *Human Reproduction* 13:1486–89, June 1998.

Nahum, G. Uterine anomalies: how common are they, and what is their distribution among subtypes? *The Journal of Reproductive Medicine* 10:877–87, October 1998.

Nehlsen-Cannarella, S.L., D.C. Nieman, et al. The effects of moderate exercise training on immune response. *Medicine and Science in Sports and Exercise* 23(1):64–70, 1991.

Nestler, J.E., et al. Ovulatory and metabolic effects of d-chiro-inositol in the polycystic ovary syndrome. *New England Journal of Medicine* 340:1314–20, April 1999.

Nielsen, H.B., N.H. Secher, N.J. Christensen, et al. Lymphocytes and NK cell activity during repeated bouts of maximal exercise. *American Journal of Physiology* 40:R222–27, 1996.

Oei, S., et al. Effectiveness of the post-coital test: randomized controlled trial. *British Medical Journal* 317:502–505, August 1998.

Padilla, S.L., and J.E. Garcia. Effect of maternal age and number of in vitro fertilization procedures on pregnancy outcome. *Fertility and Sterility* 52:270, 1990.

Paulson, P., et al. Successful pregnancy in a 63-year-old woman. *Fertility and Sterility* 67:949–51, May 1997.

Pedersen, B.K., and H. Brunnsgaard. How physical exercise influences the establishment of infections. *Sports Medicine* 19:393–400, 1995.

Piette, C., J. de Mouzon, A. Bachclet, et al. In-vitro fertilization: influence of women's age on pregnancy rates. *Human Reproduction* 5:56, 1990.

Quesenberry, C., Jr., et al. Obesity, health services use, and health care costs among members of a health maintenance organization. *Archives of Internal Medicine* 158:466–72, March 1998.

Reilly, David, et al. Is evidence for homeopathy reproducible? *The Lancet.* December 10, 1994 v344, n8937 p1601(6).

Sauer, M.V., R.J. Paulson, and R.A. Lobo. A preliminary report on oocyte donation extending reproductive potential to women over 40. *New England Journal of Medicine* 323:1157, 1990.

Schulz, P. J.P. Walker, L. Peyrin, et al. Lower sex hormones in men during anticipatory stress. *Neuroreport* 7(18):3101–4. 1996.

Schwartz, P., and M.J. Mayaux. Female fecundity as a function of age. *New England Journal of Medicine* 306:404,

Shimizu, Y., et al. Spontaneous conception after the birth of infants conceived through in vitro fertilization. *Fertility and Sterility* 71:35–39, January 1999.

Shushan, A., et al. How long does laparoscopic surgery really take? Lessons learned from 1,000 operative laparoscopies. *Human Reproduction* 14:101–105, January 1999.

Singh, N.A., et al. A randomized controlled trial of the effect of exercise on sleep. *Sleep* 20(2):95–101, 1997.

Sohn, S., et al. Administration of progesterone before oocyte retrieval negatively affects the implantation rate. *Fertility and Sterility* 71:11–14, January 1999.

Surrey, E., et al. Add-back therapy and gonadotropin releasing hormone agonists in the treatment of patients with endometriosis: can a consensus be reached? *Fertility and Sterility* 71:420–24, March 1999.

Taylor, A., et al. Impact of binge eating on metabolic and leptin dynamics in normal young women. *Journal of Clinical Endocrinology and Metabolism* 84:428–34, February 1999.

Tietze, C. Reproductive span and rate of reproduction among Hutterite women. *Fertility and Sterility* 8:89, 1957.

Tonor, J.P., C.B. Philpot, G.S. Jones, et al. Basal follicle-stimulating hormone level is a better predictor of in vitro fertilization performance than age. *Fertility and Sterility* 55:784, 1991.

Tulandi, T., et al. Reproductive outcome after treatment of mild endometriosis with laparoscopic excision and electrocoagulation. *Fertility and Sterility* 69:229–31, February 1998.

Uchino, B.N., et al. The relationship between social support and physiological processes: a review with emphasis on underlying mechanisms and implications for health. *Psychological Bulletin* 119(3):488–531, 1996.

Valdimarsdottir, H.B., and A.A. Stone. Psychosocial factors and secretory immunoglobulin A. *Critical Review Oral Biology Medicine* 8(4):461–74, 1997.

Wang, H., et al. Total antioxidant capacity of fruits. *Journal of Agricultural and Food Chemistry* 44(3):701–705, 1996.

Wang, P., et al. Ovarian tumors that complicate pregnancy. *Journal of Reproductive Medicine* 44:279–87, March 1999.

Warburton, D., and F.C. Fraser. Spontaneous abortion risks in man: data from reproductive histories collected in a medical genetics unit. *Human Genetics* 16:1, 1964.

Warren, M., et al. Functional hypothalamic amenorrhea: hypoleptinemia and disordered eating. *Journal of Clinical Endocrinology and Metabolism* 84:873–77, March 1999.

Witz, C., et al. Whole explants of peritoneum and endometrium: a novel model of the early endometriosis lesion. *Fertility and Sterility* 71:56–60, January 1999.

Index

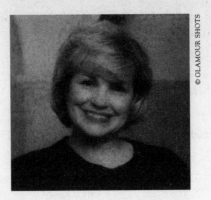

DEBRA FULGHUM BRUCE is an expert health writer who has published more than 2,500 magazine articles and authored or coauthored many books, including *The Super Aspirin Cure for Arthritis* and *The Snoring Cure*. She lives in Atlanta, Georgia.

Medical editor SAM THATCHER, M.D., Ph.D., is a reproductive endocrinologist and director at the Center for Applied Reproductive Science in Johnson City, Tennessee. He received his training in reproductive medicine at Yale and Edinburgh Universities. He is a noted educator and patient advocate with numerous clinical and scientific publications.